ENCYCLOPEDIA OF MEDICINE IN THE BIBLE AND THE TALMUD

ENCYCLOPEDIA OF MEDICINE IN THE BIBLE AND THE TALMUD

FRED ROSNER

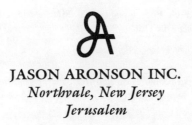

JASON ARONSON INC.
Northvale, New Jersey
Jerusalem

This book was set in 10 pt. Galliard by Alpha Graphics of Pittsfield, NH. and printed and bound by Book-mart Press, Inc. of North Bergen, NJ.

Library of Congress Cataloging-in-Publication Data
Rosner, Fred.
    Encyclopedia of medicine in the Bible and the Talmud / Fred
Rosner.
       p. cm.
    Includes bibliographical references and index.
    ISBN 0-7657-6102-5
    1. Medicine in the Bible Encyclopedias. 2. Medicine in rabbinical
literature Encyclopedias. I. Title.
R135.5.R663 2000   99-20306
610'.89'924—dc21   CIP

Printed in the United States of America on acid-free paper. For information and catalog write to Jason Aronson Inc., 230 Livingston Street, Northvale, NJ 07647-1726, or visit our website: www.aronson.com

To my wonderful grandchildren:

עטרת זקנים בני בנים (משלי יז:ו)

The crown of elders is grandchildren
(Proverbs 17:6)

CONTENTS

Contents

Contents

Contents

Contents

Contents

Contents

Contents

Contents

PREFACE

In 1978, I published an English translation of Julius Preuss's classic book *Biblical and Talmudic Medicine* (New York: Hebrew Publishing Company). A second printing was issued in 1983. Due to the book's popularity, it was reprinted in 1993 (Northvale, NJ: Jason Aronson).

In 1977, I published an original work entitled *Medicine in the Bible and the Talmud* (New York: Ktav and Yeshiva University Press) containing in-depth analyses of biblical and talmudic sources relating to a variety of specific diseases, body organs, ethics and prayers for the Jewish physician, and other general subjects of interest. An augmented second edition of this book was published in 1995.

Jewish medicine and Jewish medical history seem to interest and fascinate more and more people, Jews and non-Jews alike. To respond to this new or renewed interest in medical topics in classical Jewish sources, I recently published a *Medical Encyclopedia of Moses Maimonides* (Jason Aronson, 1998). The present *Encyclopedia of Medicine in the Bible and the Talmud* provides the interested reader with a starting point on several hundred medical and medically related topics. Each section provides the key biblical and talmudic citations relating to that topic with occasional analyses of some of these citations. The reader is encouraged to consult the original sources for the content of the citations and for more detail. Some sections provide bibliographical material for further reading. A work such as this *Encyclopedia* is obviously fraught with the possibility of errors in omission and commission, for which I take full responsibility.

I am indebted to my mentor, teacher, colleague, and advisor Lord Immanuel Jakobovits, whose written works and oral presentations have been an inspiration to me for several decades, for writing the Foreword. I am grateful to Rabbi Dr. Edward Reichman for his introductory chapter and bibliography, which will assist readers who wish to read further about some of the topics briefly presented in this *Encyclopedia*. Mr. Louis (Luzer) Gross reviewed the manuscript and offered helpful suggestions. I am thankful to Christine Trudel for the typing of large segments of this work. I express my gratitude to my wife Saranne and my children Mitchel and Lydia, Miriam and Motty, Aviva and Michael, and Shalom and Tamar for their patience, support, and encouragement during my writing of this *Encyclopedia* as well as my other books on Jewish medical ethics and the medical writings of Moses Maimonides. Finally, I offer my admiration to Mr. Arthur Kurzweil and his expert staff of dedicated professionals for the high standards they maintain in publishing books of enduring value in attractive and valuable formats.

Fred Rosner, M.D.
New York City

FOREWORD

As the most prolific contemporary writer on Judaism and medicine, Fred Rosner hardly requires any introduction. He has contributed a veritable library of books and articles on the subject, and his name has become virtually synonymous with it.

His own previous magnum opus—the translation from German into English of Julius Preuss's *Biblical and Talmudic Medicine* (Hebrew Publishing Company, 1978)—testifies to the extraordinary proclivity for medicine among Jews.

In the Middle Ages, the majority of the best-known Jewish thinkers, philosophers, poets, and grammarians were physicians by occupation—men like Maimonides, the Ibn Ezras, the Tibbons, Immanuel of Rome, and many others.

One needs only to look at the extraordinarily high number of Jews among Nobel prizewinners for medicine and physiology in the present century (at thirty, about twenty times as high as the corresponding number among Gentiles) to realise that this is an age-old phenomenon that still persists.

Lately the subject has been greatly enriched by the addition of an entirely new rubric: Jewish medical ethics. Though deeply embedded in all earlier biblical and rabbinic literature, as a distinct discipline Jewish medical ethics has been featured only over the past forty years or so, especially in response to the growing demand for ethical guidelines consonant with classic Jewish teachings. This volume, too, reproduces a fair amount of material on this now-flourishing department of Jewish medicine.

The phenomenal expansion of medical research and technology has brought numerous new ethical problems to the fore. Apart from its intrinsic historical worth, this volume will also contribute much useful guidance to the growing band of professionals and laymen who seek to guide their moral attitudes by classic Jewish teachings.

May the work succeed in strengthening and enlarging their ranks as a valuable contribution of the application of timeless Jewish teachings to timely new challenges.

Lord Immanuel Jakobovits

BIBLICAL AND TALMUDIC MEDICINE: A BIBLIOGRAPHICAL ESSAY

RABBI EDWARD REICHMAN, M.D.

As you pick up this book and begin to leaf through its pages, you are sharing a centuries-old fascination of the study of medicine in the Bible and Talmud with quite an eclectic group of people. Since the first systematic treatises on medicine in the Bible were published in the seventeenth century, a great number of people—Jews and non-Jews, physicians, scientists, historians, clergy, and laymen—have contributed, in varying degrees, to this field.

Dr. Rosner's contributions to the fields of Jewish medical history and ethics are legion. Aside from his many original articles on biblical and talmudic medicine, his translation of Julius Preuss's classic work *Biblisch-Talmudische Medizin* (see below), first published in 1978, opened the world of biblical and talmudic medicine to the English-speaking public. My own interest in the field was sparked, in large part, by reading Rosner's translation, as well as his original works.

The current volume represents another significant effort intended to generate interest and inform the lay reader about the Jewish history of medicine. The encyclopedia format, while allowing for the breadth of entries, must by definition sacrifice detail, and consequently often leaves the reader thirsting for more. My objective in this brief essay is twofold: to place this work into its proper historical and literary context by mentioning the works in the field that precede it; and, secondly, to provide direction for those wishing to use the current volume as a starting point for further research.

Studies of the eighteenth century were devoted primarily to the medicine in the Bible, one of the earliest of these works being that of the prominent seventeenth-century physician Thomas Bartholin.[1] Dealing with topics such as Jacob's limp, Moses' withering hand, leprosy, and King Asa's arthritis, Bartholin applied the then-

1

current understanding of medicine as a means of textual interpretation. For example, in claiming that Jacob suffered from a dislocation of the hip, he marshals support from the works of Celsus and Galen.

The earliest work on biblical medicine written by a Jewish physician is that of Benjamin Mussaphia.[2] This 173-page work, published in 1640, lists all the verses from the Bible that relate, in the broadest sense, to medicine. Each of the roughly 650 verses cited is followed by a brief explanation.

The earliest treatise to include talmudic medicine was that of Wolff Gintzburger, whose dissertation on talmudic medicine completed in 1743 fulfilled his requirement for graduation from the medical school of the University of Gottingen.[3] Gintzburger attempted to place the medicine of the Talmud into an historical context, stating that a small portion of the Talmud precedes the time of Galen, while the remainder is either coeval or of a later date. That is why, he claims, much of the Talmud agrees with the Galenic tradition.

Gintzburger was apparently a religious student who encountered conflict between his religious obligations and his medical training, as evidenced by a question he posed to one of the leading rabbinic figures in Germany of his time, Rabbi Jacob Emden. The query, published in Rabbi Emden's collected responsa, regards the permissibility of performing dog dissec-tion on the Sabbath. Rabbi Emden's response, addressing both human and animal dissection, serves as a basis for modern discussions on autopsy and anatomical dissection in Jewish law.[4]

Gintzburger concludes his dissertation with the following comment:

Here I will stop. I could further diverge in this enormous field, entered by few, and collect scattered opinions by using a less unsystematic method, also compare them more precisely with the medicine of a more recent kind. But as this would require more work, reading, and contemplation, I rest for now with this first outline of Talmudic medicine.[5]

The nineteenth century saw more extensive contributions to the field of biblical and talmudic medicine. Eliakim Carmoly's *Histoire des Medicins Juifs Anciens et Modernes*, published in 1844, is one such work. However, despite its breadth and chronological precedence to the works of Wunderbar and Ebstein (see below), it is of little consequence in the history of the study of biblical and talmudic medicine, as Carmoly's theories are considered by many to be baseless and fantastical.[6]

The Dutch medical historian Abraham Hartog Israels contributed a volume on talmudic gynecology in 1845. However, R. J. Wunderbar's *Biblisch-Talmudische Medizin*, completed in 1860, is the first systematic and comprehensive modern treatise of biblical and talmudic medicine. I. M. Rabino-wicz followed Gintzburger in composing a treatise restricted to talmudic medicine. Published in Paris in 1880, *La Medicine du Thalmud* is organized according to the tractates of the Talmud, with the tractate of *Chullin* occupying a disproportionately large part. Rabinowicz later included a section on talmudic medicine in his introduction to the Talmud.[7] Wilhelm Ebstein also produced an important two-volume work: *Die Medizin im Alten Testament* (Stuttgart, 1901), devoted to biblical medicine; and *Die Medizin im Neuen Testament und im Talmud* (1903), devoted to talmudic medicine.

Despite the aforementioned ventures into the world of biblical and talmudic medicine, it is Julius Preuss who truly accomplished what Gintzburger only contemplated doing. His *Biblisch-Talmudische Medizin*, first published in 1911, remains the definitive reference work in this field. Arranged topically, it covers all organ systems and diseases mentioned in the Bible and Talmud with accompanying medical and historical commentary. Although others had endeavored to cover the entire field of biblical-talmudic medicine before him, Preuss considered his work to be a first for two reasons: it is the first composed by a physician, and the first derived from the study of the original sources.[8] Wunderbar was a layman, and Ebstein relied on translations to compile his work. All work subse-quent to this magnum opus can only be considered supplemental in nature.

Despite the comprehensiveness of Preuss's work, there have been a number of noteworthy contributions since. Dr. Judah Loeb Katznelson, a Russian-Jewish physician, poet, and novelist, wrote extensively on biblical and talmudic medicine.[9] After completing his medical training, Katznelson opted to write a dissertation and take special exams in order to practice academic hospital-based medicine. The topic of his dissertation in Russian was normal and abnormal anatomy in ancient Hebrew literature in relation to ancient Greco-Roman medicine. This was followed by the publication of a small volume in Hebrew on talmudic anatomy in 1886 entitled *Remach Eivarim*, wherein Katznelson posits a creative physiological explanation to account for the rabbinic description and enumeration of 248 limbs in the body. This anatomical essay, in a revised form, was later incorporated into his magnum opus, *HaTalmud VeChokhmat haRefuah*, which was written in Hebrew and published posthumously in 1928 by his family. This work contains essays on hemophilia as described in the Talmud; the dermatological conditions of the Bible, including *zara'at*, from a medical perspective; a dictionary of medical terminology translated into Greek, Russian, and Hebrew; and a commentary on the section of the Talmud that deals with the laws of *kashrut*.

In 1926, Moshe Pearlman published *Midrash haRefuah*, a compilation and brief commentary of all passages relating to medicine and health found in the Babylonian and Jerusalem Talmuds and Midrashim. Pearlman relates that he sent a copy of the third draft of his completed manuscript to Dr. Katznelson, and it was the latter who first informed him that others before had ventured into the field of biblical and talmudic medicine.[10] Aside from sharing his own works with Pearlman, Katznelson informed him of the works of Rabinowicz, Ebstein, and Preuss, none of which Pearlman had seen. In Pearlman's introduction, he says, "Had I known then that others had already done research in this field, I clearly would not have continued this work. However, I did not know . . . that voluminous works had been written by scholars versed in these topics . . . and I thought myself to be the redeemer of this long forgotten discipline."[11] While, admittedly, there is significant overlap with earlier works, *Midrash haRefuah*, published with the notes of Dr. Katznelson, is still a novel and valuable contribution.

In 1936 appeared a novel contribution to the field of biblical medicine by Charles Brim, a New York physician.[12] In his introduction to Brim's book, Victor Robinson best describes the nature of Brim's work:

In method and interpretation it does not follow any predecessor. It follows only the Hebrew text of the Torah and the commentary of Rashi (Rabbi Shlomo Yitzchaki, eleventh-century Biblical commentator). With the original text before him, the author brings to the subject a rare clinical insight, an unusual diagnostic ability. He perceives symptoms hidden from previous investigators, and determines conditions not told in contemporary Gath or published in the streets of modern Ashkelon.

Much of the literature since the 1930s has appeared either in periodicals or as book chapters. Between 1937 and 1943 five volumes of the journal *Medical Leaves* were published. This journal of Jewish medical history contains many articles on biblical and talmudic medicine. Examples include R. Isaacs, "Hematology in the Bible and Talmud";[13] S. R. Kagen, "Talmudic Medicine";[14] D. I. Macht, "The Bible as a Source of Subjects for Scientific Research";[15] and S. Boorstein, "Orthopedic Passages in the Bible and Talmud."[16]

The contributions of Dr. David Macht merit special mention. Born in Moscow in 1882, he emigrated to the United States where he completed his medical training at Johns Hopkins University in 1906. Macht was a prolific writer, publishing three books and over nine hundred original articles in the fields of science and medical/scientific history. Of the roughly one hundred works he wrote on medical history, many are devoted to biblical and talmudic medicine, with special emphasis on the pharmacological and physiological interpretations of biblical and rabbinic passages.[17]

Other medical historians who devoted articles or chapters to biblical or talmudic medicine include M. B. Gordon,[18] B. L. Bordon,[19] and S. R. Kagan.[20]

Another journal devoted largely to Jewish medical history is *Koroth*, first published in April, 1952. For its first twenty years the journal was edited by a triad consisting of Professor J. O. Leibowitz, Dr. S. Muntner, and Dr. David Margalit, all of whom contributed significantly to the field of Jewish medical history. Dr. Margalit devoted some of his efforts to biblical and talmudic medicine,[21] as did Professor Leibowitz, although to a lesser extent.[22] Professor S. Kottek joined the editorial staff of *Koroth* in the 1980s, and after the passing of the founding editors, assumed the editorial mantle, a position he maintains to this day. Professor Kottek has written more extensively on biblical and talmudic medicine than his predecessors and currently contributes a serial column in the *Israel Journal of Medicine and Science* entitled "Gems from the Talmud."[23]

Throughout the years of its publication *Koroth* has included numerous articles relating to biblical and talmudic medicine. Authors with multiple contributions in this field in the pages of *Koroth* include A. Shoshan,

H. Kook, and M. Michael. Volume 8:7–8 (Fall 1982) is devoted entirely to biblical medicine, and a special issue of volume 9 (1988) contains the Proceedings of the Third International Symposium on Medicine in the Bible and Talmud.

For the past thirty years, the contributions to this field can largely be found in the periodical literature of three disciplines: medical history, Judaic studies, and medicine. The topic of artificial respiration in the Bible, which merits an entry in this encyclopedia, is illustrative, as articles on this topic have appeared in all the aforementioned literatures as listed by discipline below:

MEDICAL LITERATURE

F. Rosner, "Artificial Respiration in Biblical Times," *New York State Journal of Medicine* 69:8 (April 15, 1969): 1104–05; Z. Rosen, "Rhinological Aspects of Biblical Resuscitation," *Archives of Otolaryngology* 95:5 (May, 1972): 488–89; Z. Rosen and J. Davidson, "Respiratory Resuscitation in Ancient Hebrew Sources," *Anesthesia and Analgesia* 51:4 (July–August, 1972): 502–05; L. Wislicki, "A Biblical Case of Hypothermia-Resuscitation by Rewarming (Elisha's Method)," *Clio Medica* 9:3 (September, 1974): 213–14; R. B. Howard, ". . . And There Is Nothing New Under the Sun," *Postgraduate Medicine* 65:3 (March,

1979): 25; J. H. Comroe Jr., ". . . In Comes the Good Air," *American Review of Respiratory Diseases* 119:6 (June, 1979): 1025–31.

JUDAIC STUDIES LITERATURE

A. S. Abraham, "Hanshamah Melakhutit bi-Tanakh," *Ha-Ma'ayan* 28:3 (Nisan, 5748): 72–76.

MEDICAL HISTORY LITERATURE

E. Tratner, "Intubation Mentioned in the Talmud and by Jacob ben Asher," *Koroth* 8:7–8 (August, 1983), 333–338; J. A. Paraskos, "Biblical Accounts of Resuscitation," *Journal of the History of Medicine and Allied Sciences* 47:3 (July, 1992): 310–21.

Access to this vast and diverse literature is no longer restricted to the expert of any particular field, nor does it require visitation to obscure libraries. Computer databases now make this material easily accessible to any interested researcher, and the searches can be performed on the internet. A search on Histline, the National Library of Medicine's (NLM) database on medical history, will yield roughly five hundred items relating to biblical and talmudic medicine; a search on NLM's Medline, which includes hundreds of contemporary medical journals in its database, will likewise yield hundreds of entries on these topics. My objective is not to provide a list of these works, which can be easily accessed by the reader, but I should like to point out a few trends that can be found in the literature.

Determining the medical diagnosis of biblical or talmudic personalities still occupies a significant part of the research, and articles of this nature can be found in the literature of varied disciplines. Not dissimilar to Bartholin's essay some three hundred years ago, one author has endeavored to provide modern medical explanation for Jacob's limp.[24] Many others have applied the same diagnostic principles to other personalities.[25]

The identification of biblical diseases, in particular the skin disease *zara'at*, continues to maintain the interest of physicians and historians, with enough material being produced so as to necessitate bibliographical articles restricted exclusively to this topic.[26]

Another common trend is to interpret biblical and talmudic cases as being "the first reported case" of a particular disease. While it is true that the Bible and the Talmud, by virtue of their antiquity, often contain early descriptions of certain diseases, many of these articles involve reinterpretation of passages based on modern understanding of medicine.[27]

These are just three trends found in the literature, but the evolution of the study of biblical and talmudic medicine parallels the evolution of medicine itself. As new discoveries continue to affect our understanding of medicine and human disease, there will always be those who will apply this new knowledge to the interpretation of the medical passages in the Bible and Talmud. One author employs a modern understanding of the transmission of infectious diseases to advance the theory that the requirement to eliminate the storage houses of grain for Passover served in the Middle Ages to effectively prevent the spread of plague amongst the Jewish people by eliminating the rodent vectors.[28] The veracity of this theory notwithstanding, it could not have been advanced until but a few decades ago. What does the future hold for the field of biblical-talmudic medicine? I suspect we will have to follow the developments in medicine in order to find out.

ADDENDUM: BIBLIOGRAPHICAL LITERATURE ON BIBLICAL AND TALMUDIC MEDICINE

The earliest bibliography of ancient medicine was published in the *Dictionare des Sciences Medicales* in Paris, 1819, listing twenty-six items. In 1842, J. L. Choulant included many entries about biblical and talmudic medicine in his classic *Bibliotheca Medico-Historica*.[29] As part of his monumental contribution to Jewish bibliography in general, Moritz Steinschneider published, in 1886, *Schriften uber Medicin in Bibel und Talmud*.[30] Wunderbar and Ebstein both included bibliographies in their works. Preuss wrote an extensive bibliography covering the literature up to his time. However, it was not comprehensive and was apparently completed by Adolph Levinger, who circulated this supplement in stencil form.[31] In 1935, Friedenwald, like Preuss before him, compiled an extensive bibliography of the works that had appeared until his day.[32] S. R. Kagan supplemented and updated Friedenwald's bibliography in 1948.[33] A bibliography of Jewish bibliographies, including those relating to biblical-talmudic medicine, was compiled by S. Shunami.[34] Nahum Rakover's *Bibliography of Jewish Law*, first published in Hebrew in 1975, with second editions in both Hebrew and English published in 1990, contains a section on medical Jewish law (*halakha*), wherein numerous entries are devoted to biblical and talmudic medicine. Finally, the contemporary bibliographical periodical *Current Works in the History of Medicine*, published by the Wellcome Institute of the History of Medicine, contains entries on Bible and Talmud.

Here I will stop. I could further diverge in this enormous field, entered by many. But, alas, I rest for now with this outline of the bibliography of biblical and talmudic medicine.

———

1. J. Willis, trans., *Thomas Bartholin On the Diseases of the Bible: A Medical Miscellany, 1672* (Copenhagen: Danish National Library of Science and Medicine, 1994).
2. See H. Friedenwald, "Bibliography of Ancient Hebrew Medicine," in his *The Jews and Medicine* (Baltimore: Johns Hopkins Press, 1944), p. 112; D. Margalit, "Rav Binyamin Mussaphia," *Koroth* 2:7–8 (1960): 307–318.
3. F. Schiller, "Benjamin Wolff Gintzburger's Dissertation on Talmudic Medicine," *Koroth* 9:7–8 (Fall 1988): 579–600.
4. *She'ilat Yavetz*, n. 41.
5. Schiller, op. cit., p. 600.
6. See S. Muntner, "*Yulius Preuss. Micholel haMechkar biToldot haRefuah halvrit haKedumah,*" *Koroth* 2:9–10 (May, 1961): 410. Carmoly only merits citation by Preuss for purposes of refutation. See F. Rosner, trans., *Julius Preuss' Biblical and Talmudic Medicine* (New York: Hebrew Publishing Company, 1978), pp. 42 and 162.
7. *Mavo haTalmud* (1894).
8. F. Rosner, trans., *Julius Preuss' Biblical and Talmudic Medicine* (New York: Hebrew Publishing Company, 1978), p. 1.
9. See H. A. Savitz, "Judah Loeb Katznelson (1847–1916): Physician to the Soul of His People," in his *Profiles of Erudite Jewish Physicians and Scholars* (Chicago: Spertus College Press, 1973), pp. 56–61.
10. M. Pearlman, *Midrash haRefuah* (Tel Aviv: Devir Publishers, 1926), IX–XI.
11. Ibid.
12. C. J. Brim, *Medicine in the Bible* (New York: Froben Press, 1936).
13. *Medical Leaves* 1 (1937): 76–80.
14. *Medical Leaves* 3:1 (1940): 164–173.
15. *Medical Leaves* 3 (1940): 174–184.
16. *Medical Leaves* 5 (1943): 49–55.
17. David Wilk composed a brief bio-bibliography of Macht's medical historical contributions that was published in *Koroth* 8:7–8 (August 1983): 305–317.
18. "Medicine Among the Ancient Hebrews," *ISIS* 33 (1941): 454–485.
19. "Ancient Hebrew Medicine," in his *Medicine Throughout Antiquity* (Philadelphia: F. A. Davis, 1949), pp. 25–294.
20. "Ancient Jewish Medicine," in his *Jewish Medicine* (Boston: Medico-Historical Press, 1952), pp. 27–63.
21. See bibliography of his works until 1973 in *Koroth* 6:5–6 (November 1973): 367–372.
22. See bibliography of his works in *Koroth* 8:11–12 (Summer 1985): 7–23.
23. See bibliography of his works until 1991 in *Koroth* 9:11–12 (Summer 1991): 755–766.
24. L. J. Hoenig, "Jacob's Limp," *Seminars in Arthritis and Rheumatism* 26:4 (February 1997): 684–688.
25. See, for example, A. de Vries and A. Weinberger, "King Asa's Presumed Gout," *Koroth* 6:9–10 (December 1974): 561–567; A. Shoshan, "The Illness of Rabbi Judah the Patriarch," *Koroth* 7:5–6 (November 1977): 521–524; S. Levin, "Isaac's Blindness: A medical Diagnosis," *Judaism* 38:1 (Winter 1988): 81–83.
26. See, for example, A. D. Rabinowitz and Bezalel Naor, "The Medical Aspects of *Zara'at*: Selected Bibliography," *Orot* 1 (1991): 30–32; G. Milgram, "On *Zara'at*: A Bibliographical Overview," *Koroth* 9:11–12 (Summer 1992): 818–825. Some have applied medicine looking to interpret biblical passages in a new light. See, for example, E. V. Hulce,

"Joshua's Curse and the Abandonment of Ancient Jericho: Schistosomiasis As a Possible Medical Explanation." *Medical History* 15:4 (October 1971): 376–86.

27. S. Leons, "The First Reported Case of Radial Nerve Palsy," *Southern Medical Journal* 86:7 (July 1993): 808–11; M. A. Goldenhersh, "Rapid Whitening of the Hair First Reported in the Talmud: Possible Mechanisms of this Intriguing Phenomenon," *American Journal of Dermatopathology* 14:4 (1992): 367–368; H. Decher, "Brachiocervical Syndrome: First Case Report Over 3,000 Years Ago," *Laryngorhinootologie* 75:4 (April 1996): 255–6; I. Schiff and M. Schiff, "The Biblical Diagnostician and the Anorexic Bride," *Fertility and Sterility* 69:1 (January 1998): 8–10.

28. M. J. Blaser, "Passover and Plague," *Perspectives in Biology and Medicine* 41:2 (Winter 1998): 243–256.

29. See H. Friedenwald, *The Jews and Medicine* (Baltimore: Johns Hopkins Press, 1944), pp. 109–110; S. R. Kagan, "The Bibliography of Ancient Jewish Medicine," *Bulletin of the History of Medicine* 22 (1948): 480–485.

30. In *Wiener Klinische Rundschau* 10 (1896): 433–435 and 452–453.

31. The supplement was apparently not published. See Muntner, op. cit., p. 412.

32. H. Friedenwald, *The Jews and Medicine* (Baltimore: Johns Hopkins Press, 1944), pp. 99–145.

33. S. R. Kagan, "The Bibliography of Ancient Jewish Medicine," *Bulletin of the History of Medicine* 22 (1948): 480–485.

34. S. Shunami, *Bibliography of Jewish Bibliographies* (Jerusalem: Magnes Press, 1965), pp. 313–318.

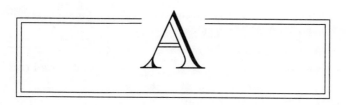

ABDOMEN—Abdomen is referred to as *beten* (Numbers 5:21; Job 40:16) and *keres* (Jeremiah 51:34; *Baba Batra* 7a; *Rosh Hashanah* 25a). *Beten* also refers to uterus (Genesis 25:23 and 28:27) so that God blesses the fruit of the abdomen (i.e., uterus) (Deuteronomy 7:13). A child emerges naked from its mother's abdomen (Job 1:21) and is the fruit of its parents' abdomen (Micah 6:7). The abdomen of a woman consists of many cavities, coils, and bands (*Leviticus Rabbah* 14:3). In a cesarean section, the baby is delivered through the abdominal wall (*Yebamot* 84a). The word *beten* thus also refers to the abdominal wall (Song of Songs 7:3; Job 40:16).

During menstruation, a woman may feel pain in the abdomen (*Niddah* 9:8). Heat is applied to the abdomen to alleviate pain (*Shabbat* 40b). Alternatively, one rubs the abdomen with oil and wine (*Shabbat* 134a). Abdominal troubles (*Nedarim* 22a) are a divine punishment for wrongdoing (Deuteronomy 28:65). Specific medications are prescribed for abdominal

pain (*Gittin* 69b). The abdomen of a suspected adulteress swells if she is guilty (Numbers 5:21). The abdomen becomes distended after death (*Shabbat* 151b). Abdominal pain in people who overeat (*Sirach* 34:20) may lead to inability to sleep (Ecclesiastes 5:11). If one swallows a leech or withholds urination, one's abdomen swells (*Bechorot* 44b). He who feigns a swollen abdomen is punished (*Tosefta Peah* 4:14).

Abdominal injuries are described following attempted suicide (2 Maccabees 14:39–46; Judges 3:21–22). An abdominal operation was carried out following the use of a soporific potion (*Baba Metzia* 83b–84a). A needle found in the abdominal cavity of an animal may render it unfit for human consumption (*Chullin* 48b). [*See also* STOMACH, NAVEL, INTESTINES, etc.]

ABORTION—Most women carry their pregnancies to term and only a minority of women miscarry (*Yebamot* 119a; *Bechorot* 20b; *Niddah* 18b).

A woman who miscarries three times is confirmed as a habitual aborter (*Yebamot* 65b). Some women miscarry five times (*Tohorot* 4:13) or even more frequently (*Niddah* 38a; *Baba Batra* 166a). Miscarriages before forty days of pregnancy are considered "mere fluid" and exempt the mother from obligations of childbirth such as Temple offerings (*Bechorot* 21b). Early abortuses do not yet have "limbs knit together by nerves" (*Chullin* 89b and 100b). Miscarriages involve male and female fetuses equally (*Bechorot* 20b). A woman can miscarry within weeks after she gives birth (*Pesachim* 3a; *Niddah* 30a; *Eduyot* 4:10). She may also give birth to a stillborn baby (*Niddah* 8b and 66a). A parent grieves for a dead child but not for a miscarriage (*Baba Batra* 111b). The biblical word "pain" (Genesis 3:16) is interpreted to refer to the sufferings of miscarriages (*Genesis Rabbah* 20:6).

Many causes of spontaneous abortion are cited in the Talmud: shock or fright (*Baba Kamma* 56a; *Baba Batra* 93a) such as if a mad dog barks at the pregnant woman (*Shabbat* 63a), the strong aroma of burnt meat (*Avot* 5:5), the blowing of the south wind (*Gittin* 31b), and the evil eye (*Genesis Rabbah* 45:5). A woman who steps over discarded cut finger- or toenails may miscarry (due to fright?); hence such cut nails should be burned or buried (*Niddah* 17a; *Moed Katan* 18a). Accidental abortion due to trauma to the

woman's abdomen is described (Exodus 21:22; *Baba Kamma* 48b; *Sanhedrin* 109b) as is intentional abortion (*Arachim* 7a) and even embryotomy (*Oholot* 7:6).

Groundless hatred is also said to be a cause of spontaneous abortions (*Shabbat* 32b). During times of moral behavior no miscarriages will occur, promises the Lord (Exodus 23:26). One of the miracles in the Temple is that no woman ever miscarried from the odor of the sacrificial flesh (*Avot* 5:5; *Baba Batra* 93a). The men of the priestly watch fasted on Thursday and prayed that women not miscarry (*Taanit* 27b). For thirteen years when Rabbi Judah the Prince studied Torah in the Babylonian synagogue in Sepphoris, no woman in Israel miscarried (*Genesis Rabbah* 33:3 and 96:5). Women wore preserving stones as safeguards against abortion (*Shabbat* 66b).

Women buried their aborted fetuses in small mounds of earth near the town (*Tosefta Oholot* 16:1) or in special burial chambers (*Baba Batra* 101b) or grottos (ibid., 102b). Special burial places where women brought their abortions are described (*Ketubot* 20b). A grave in which an abortion is buried cannot be used for a deceased person (*Sanhedrin* 47b). An abortus conveys ritual uncleanness by overshadowing (*Oholot* 2:1; *Nazir* 50a). Heathen women used to bury their fetuses in their own homes in "menstruation rooms" (*Niddah* 7:4; *Oholot* 18:7). Samaritan women buried their abortions in certain chambers or rooms (*Niddah* 56b). Some abortions were simply thrown into pits and devoured by animals (*Oholot* 16:5).

Abortuses can have varying sizes, shapes, and appearances. Thus, a woman may abort a sandal-like fetus (*Bechorot* 44a), or a bag full of many-colored substances, or something resembling fish or locusts or reptiles or creeping things (*Bechorot* 47b). A miscarriage may have the shape of cattle or beast of chase or bird (*Keritot* 7b; *Chullin* 71a). An aborted fetus may have articulated limbs (*Keritot* 7b) or be dismembered (ibid.), or be a hermaphrodite or of indeterminate sex (*Baba Batra* 127a; *Niddah* 29a). A woman may abort a cut hand or foot (*Niddah* 18a), or a shapeless object (*Niddah* 18b), or an object like rind or hair or earth or like red flies (*Niddah* 21a and 54b). A woman can abort within weeks after a normal birth (*Keritot* 7b; *Pesachim* 3a; *Niddah* 30a) and can even abort twins (*Keritot* 7b). Animals also abort fetuses (*Chullin* 75a; *Bechorot* 43b). These are all discussed at length in talmudic sources as to whether or not such miscarriages constitute valid births requiring the mother to go through the usual process of ritual purification. Preuss discusses the medical conditions that these abortuses might represent.[1] The Jewish attitude toward therapeutic abortion including pregnancy reduction or selective abortion is discussed in detail elsewhere.[2,3,4]

1. F. Rosner (trans.), *Julius Preuss' Biblical and Talmudic Medicine* (Northvale, NJ: Jason Aronson, 1993), pp. 413–418.
2. F. Rosner, *Modern Medicine and Jewish Ethics*, 2nd ed. (Hoboken, NJ, and New York: Ktav and Yeshiva University Press, 1991), pp. 133–162.
3. D.M. Feldman, *Marital Relations, Birth Control, and Abortion in Jewish Law* (New York: Schocken, 1975), pp. 251–294.
4. J.D. Bleich, *Contemporary Halakhic Problems*, vol. 1 (New York: Ktav and Yeshiva University Press, 1977), pp. 325–371.

ABSCESS—An abscess is incised to drain out the pus (*Eduyot* 2:5). It was done in antiquity by physicians (*Tosefta Eduyot* 1:8) and is even permissible on the Sabbath (*Shabbat* 107b; *Ketubot* 6b). Afterward, a cup of wine in soapwort is applied or imbibed (*Gittin* 69b). An abscess is a forerunner of fever and should be opened crosswise (*Abodah Zarah* 28a). Incantations can also be recited to heal boils and abscesses (*Shabbat* 67a). King Hezekiah's illness (2 Kings 20:1ff.; Isaiah 38:1ff.; 2 Chronicles 32:24ff.) is said to have been a leprous abscess, which was softened by the application of figs thereon (Isaiah 38:21). Alternatively, he may have had a throat abscess.[1] Antiochus may have died (2 Maccabees 9:5ff.) from bowel perforation with peritonitis and abscess formation.[2] [*See also* INFLAMMATION].

1. F. Rosner (trans.), *Julius Preuss'*
Biblical and Talmudic Medicine (Northvale, NJ: Jason Aronson, 1993), p. 342.
2. Ibid., p. 184.

ADULTERY—Adultery is prohibited
in the Ten Commandments (Exodus
20:13; Deuteronomy 5:17) and the
death penalty is prescribed for both
partners (Leviticus 20:10). The execution is usually by strangulation
(*Sanhedrin* 84b) except if the adultery
is with one's daughter-in-law, in which
case the penalty is stoning (*Deuteronomy Rabbah* 2:21). Adultery is one
of the seven Noahide laws (*Sanhedrin*
56a; *Abodah Zarah* 2b). A Gentile who
commits adultery is also executed (*Sanhedrin* 57ab). A betrothed maiden who
commits adultery is stoned (Deuteronomy 22:21; *Kiddushin* 9b; *Sanhedrin*
66b) whereas a priest's daughter who
does so is burnt (Leviticus 21:9; *Sanhedrin* 49a). Adulterers are people of
violence (*Numbers Rabbah* 11:1). An
adulterer weakens the power of the
Divine Presence (ibid., 9:1). God does
not grant adulterers a long respite
before punishing them (Malachi 3:5;
Numbers Rabbah 10:2).

Adultery was rampant in biblical
Sodom (*Genesis Rabbah* 41:7). The
curses in the Bible (Deuteronomy
27:15ff) are addressed to sinners including adulterers (*Sotah* 37b). The
phrase "Stolen waters are sweet"
(Proverbs 9:17) refers to adultery and
other illicit sex. The wanton deed of
Achan (Joshua 7:19) is that he committed adultery with a betrothed
maiden (*Sanhedrin* 44a). Joseph withheld himself from an act of adultery
with Potiphar's wife (Genesis 39:7)
when his father's face appeared to him
(*Genesis Rabbah* 87:6–7). Tamar committed an act of fornication with her
father-in-law (Genesis 38:14) and
gave birth to kings (e.g., David) and
prophets (e.g., Amos and Isaiah)
(*Nazir* 23b; *Horayot* 10b). Zimri committed an act of fornication (Numbers
25:14) and on his account many thousands of Jews perished (Numbers
25:9; *Nazir* 23b; *Horayot* 10b).

Jews are not ordinarily suspected of
adultery (*Exodus Rabbah* 1:29). Yet
when adulterers multiplied in Israel,
the ceremony of the bitter waters was
discontinued (*Sotah* 47a). Adultery is
one of the three cardinal sins for which
one must give up one's life rather than
transgress (*Sanhedrin* 74a). Adulterers caught in the act hide or flee
(*Nedarim* 91b). A man who commits
adultery with a married woman de-
scends into Gehenna and does not re-
ascend (*Baba Metzia* 58b). Those who
seduce to adultery are as the spark that
kindles the ember (*Sanhedrin* 100b).
If a married woman commits adultery
she can be divorced (*Kiddushin* 66a).
An adulteress emits a bad mouth odor
(*Numbers Rabbah* 9:21). A woman
only commits adultery due to temporary mental derangement (*Sotah* 3a).
If a man suspects his wife of adultery,
the ceremony of the bitter waters was

implemented (see *SOTAH*). A man suspected of adultery is nevertheless eligible to serve as a witness in a legal proceeding (*Sanhedrin* 26b).

Lustful thoughts such as coveting one's neighbor's wife are also forbidden (Exodus 20:14). He who gazes lustfully at the little finger of a woman is morally equivalent to an adulterer (*Shabbat* 64b). Committing adultery with one's eyes is prohibited (*Leviticus Rabbah* 23:12). To deflect one's temptation one should even grind one's fingernails into the ground (*Shevuot* 18a) as did Joseph. It is forbidden to pray in the presence of a woman with uncovered hair because a covetous look is considered as reprehensible as consummated adultery (*Berachot* 24a). One who thinks of another women while cohabiting with his wife is also morally guilty of adultery (*Nedarim* 20b). If a divorced man marries a divorced woman, four minds are in the marital bed, a figurative double adultery (*Pesachim* 112a). [*See also* INCEST, *SOTAH*, and MARRIAGE]

ALMONDS—Almonds are considered a delicious food (*Taanit* 23a). Almonds can be bitter or sweet, large or small (*Chullin* 25b; *Eruvin* 28b). Some almonds have shells to protect the nuts (*Uktzin* 2:7). Almonds were used to decorate *sukkot* (booths) during the Festival of Tabernacles (*Betzah* 30b). Almond trees are included in the biblical law (Leviticus 19:9–10

and 23:22; Deuteronomy 14:28–29) of leaving a portion of each harvest to the poor (*Peah* 1:5). "And the almond tree shall blossom" (Ecclesiastes 12:5) alludes to Jeremiah's prophecy (Jeremiah 1:11) that an almond tree takes twenty-one days from the time it blossoms until it gives ripe fruit (*Bechorot* 8a), referring to the twenty-one days between the piercing of the walls of Jerusalem and the destruction of the Second Temple (*Lamentations Rabbah Proem*; *Ecclesiastes Rabbah* 12:7:1).

ALOES—An aloe containing a mixture of herbs and medication is said to be efficacious to treat hemorrhoids if applied to the anal area (*Gittin* 69b). A compound made from aloes, myrtle, and violets serves as a depilatory (*Shabbat* 50b). Aloe was also used as a cleansing agent (*Taanit* 13b). Aloe wood is so hard it can be used for making ax handles (*Betzah* 33b).

ALUM—A remedy for jaundice that also serves as a contraceptive potion contains alum (*Shabbat* 109b–100a). Cloaks can be dyed with alum (*Sanhedrin* 44a). Genuine blue dye can be distinguished from imitation blue with a compound mixture containing liquid alum (*Menachot* 42b). Vessels glazed with alum crystals are porous and absorb fluids (*Abodah Zarah* 34a). Glazed vessels are made from earth containing alum crystals (*Shabbat* 16a; *Pesachim* 30b; *Niddah* 17a). Alum crystals come from alum mines (*Ketubot* 79b; *Abodah Zarah* 33b).

AMMI—Rabbi Ammi the physician is cited several times in the Talmud (*Jerushalmi Berachot* 2:4). He said that one should not put coins in one's mouth, nor food under the bed, nor carry bread under the armpits because it is unappetizing (unhealthy?) (*Jerushalmi Terumot* 8:45). He said that Abraham and Sarah had no children for many years because they were *tumtums* (indeterminate or doubtful sex) and had to be "split open" before their sex was confirmed (*Yebamot* 64a). [*See also* MAR SAMUEL, BENJAMIN, and THEODUS]

AMNION—The amnion (*shefir*) is a membrane that forms the sac containing a fetus bathed in amniotic fluid. Twins can be housed in one or two separate sacs, thus distinguishing between identical and fraternal twins, respectively (*Oholot* 7:5). A pregnant woman may expel an amniotic sac full of water or blood or multicolored matter, which may represent an aborted fetus (*Niddah* 24b). Mar Samuel was an expert in the examination of amniotic sacs (ibid., 25a). The biblical phrase "He took his brother by the heel in the womb" (Hosea 12:4) seems to suggest a single amniotic sac

for those twins. [*See also* TWINS, PREGNANCY, and ABORTION].

AMPUTEE—When the Jews received the Torah at Mount Sinai, all physical defects were healed and there were no amputees (*Tanchuma*, Exodus 19:8). Legend relates that the Jews exiled to Babylon after the destruction of the first Temple cut off their thumbs so that they would not have to sing songs of Zion and play musical instruments before Nebuchadnezer (*Midrash Psalms* 137:4; *Yalkut Shimoni*, Psalms 137). Bar Kochba had two hundred thousand soldiers, each of whom cut off one of his fingers to demonstrate his courage (*Lamentations Rabbah* 2:5; *Jerushalmi Taanit* 4:8). The captured King Adoni-Bezek had his thumbs and toes cut off by Judah and Simeon just as he had done to his enemy kings (Judges 1:6–7). Amputation of limbs does not exist as a punishment in Jewish law. The biblical verses "And thou shalt cut off her hand" (Deuteronomy 25:12) and "a hand for a hand" (Exodus 21:24 and Deuteronomy 19:21) are interpreted to refer to monetary compensation (*Sanhedrin* 29a and *Baba Kamma* 83b). The command of King David to amputate the hands and feet of the murderers of Ish-Boshet was after their deaths (2 Samuel 4:12).

The Talmud speaks of surgical amputations (*Gittin* 56a), women amputees (*Yebamot* 105a), and amputation of the hand as a life-saving measure (*Jerushalmi Nazir* 9:58). Lepers used to bury their arms in small earthen mounds near cemeteries (*Ketubot* 20b). An amputation that includes the knee joint is said to be fatal (*Niddah* 24a). Nachum Gamzu was a quadruple amputee, probably secondary to leprosy (*Taanit* 21a). A procedure is described for someone who needs a limb amputated on the eve of Passover and wishes that both he and the physician remain ritually clean by not handling the amputated limb, which is unclean (*Keritot* 15b).

In talmudic law, someone who cuts off the hand of his fellow man must pay a variety of penalties including pain, damages, medical treatment, enforced idleness, and humiliation (*Baba Kamma* 85a). Anesthesia or analgesia for amputations is also described (*Baba Metzia* 83b). A handless person cannot function as a judge (*Jerushalmi Sanhedrin* 8:26) nor can he offer testimony as a witness (*Sanhedrin* 45b). If a man or woman is handless, the prescribed procedure for a suspected adulteress cannot be carried out (*Sotah* 27a). If one sees an amputee one should say "Blessed be the true Judge" (*Berachot* 58b). A person missing some fingers cannot spin flax or silk (*Song of Songs Rabbah* 8:11), even if only one finger is missing (*Midrash Psalms* 8:2).

The Rabbinic decisors discuss at length if and how an amputee dons phylacteries and performs other commandments requiring the presence of hands, such as holding the four species on the Festival of Tabernacles or lifting the hands for the priestly benediction if the amputee is a priest.[1] [*See also* PROSTHESES]

---

1. A. Steinberg, "*Geedem*," in *Encyclopedia of Jewish Medical Ethics*, vol. 1 (Jerusalem: Schlesinger Institute of the Shaare Zedek Medical Center, 1988), pp. 121–125 (Hebrew).

AMULETS—An amulet is called *kemiya* and consists either of a written parchment or of roots (*Tosefta Shabbat* 4:9) or herbs (*Jerushalmi Shabbat* 8b). It is worn on a small chain, in a signet ring, or in a tube. A *kemiya* is considered to be of proven efficacy if it cures a sick person on three different occasions or if it cures three different patients (*Shabbat* 60a). An assurance by a physician who prescribed or wrote such an amulet is accepted as credible without question, for in antiquity amulets were considered part of the legitimate therapeutic armamentarium of the physician.[1]

There is no objection in Jewish religious law to the use of amulets for healing purposes. Amulets are apparently deeply rooted in popular belief. Although a long list of acts falling in the category of idolatrous customs is found in the Talmud (*Tosefta Shabbat*, chs. 7 and 8), anything done for the sake of healing is specifically excluded.

The rabbinic Responsa literature of the past several hundred years is replete with references to amulets as preventives to keep off the "evil eye"; to avert demons; to prevent abortion; and to cure a variety of diseases, such as epilepsy, lunacy, fever, poisoning, hysteria, jaundice, and colic.[2] A distinction is made in Jewish law between the prophylactic and therapeutic use of amulets (*Shulchan Aruch, Yoreh Deah* 179:12).

Amulets were usually pendants worn by the user at all times to prevent or to cure certain ailments. Talismans did not have to be carried or worn at all times. Other objects are also cited in Jewish sources as efficacious against specific complaints. A coin tied to the sole of the foot was worn to prevent or heal bruises. A preserving stone is mentioned in the Talmud (*Shabbat* 66b) and was widely believed in ancient times to protect the wearer against a miscarriage. Moses Maimonides discusses the subject of amulets and preserving stones that were worn for medical purposes and were thought to be efficacious (*Mishneh Torah, Shabbat* 19:13–14).

Contrary to the considerable rabbinic opinion during the Middle Ages that favored the use of amulets to ward off misfortune, sickness, or "evil spirits," Maimonides was strongly opposed to such practices.[3] Perhaps amulets were considered efficacious because of their placebo effect. [*See also* INCANTATIONS, MAGIC, SORCERY, and PRAYER]

1. F. Rosner (trans.), *Julius Preuss' Biblical and Talmudic Medicine* (Northvale, NJ: Jason Aronson, 1993), pp. 146–149.

2. H.J. Zimmels, *Magicians, Theologians, and Doctors* (London: Goldston & Son, 1952), pp. 135–137.

3. F. Rosner, *Medicine in the Mishneh Torah of Maimonides* (New York: Ktav, 1984), pp. 281–283.

ANESTHESIA—Probably the earliest mention of anesthesia is that found in the Bible, in the description of the creation of woman from a rib of Adam. In Genesis 2:21, we find the following statement: "And the Eternal God caused an overpowering sleep [*tardemah*] to fall upon the man and he slept; and He took one of his ribs and shut in flesh instead thereof."

Although this overpowering sleep occurred by divine intervention, it embodies the concept of anesthesia. In fact, some Jewish Bible commentaries specifically interpret the above Pentateuchal phrase to refer to anesthesia. R. Meir Loeb ben Yechiel Michael, known as Malbim, states that *tardemah* is "a deep sleep in order not to feel the pain." The biblical commentary of R. Samson Raphael Hirsch in its English translation interprets *tardemah* as "something like anesthesia." Elsewhere (Genesis 15:12), Malbim interprets *tardemah* to be "a state of deep sleep and cessation of body powers because of mental anguish" (lit., "distress of the heart").

The value of alcohol as an anesthetic is described in the Babylonian Talmud, where we find the following ruling: "When one is led out to execution, he is given a goblet of wine containing a grain of frankincense in order to benumb his senses, for it is written: 'Give strong drink unto him that is ready to perish and wine unto the bitter in soul.' [Proverbs 31:61]" (*Sanhedrin* 43a). Rashi explains that the benumbing of the senses is an act of compassion to minimize or eliminate anxiety of the accused during his execution (loc. cit.). The Talmud also states that the noble women of Jerusalem used to donate the wine and bring it (ibid.). If they did not, it had to be provided from public funds.

Elsewhere the Talmud has a similar pronouncement: "The condemned are given wine containing frankincense to drink so that they should not feel grieved" (*Semachot* 2:9). Maimonides goes one step further by stating that "after the condemned has confessed, he is given a cup of wine to benumb his senses *and to intoxicate him* [emphasis added], and then he is executed by the mode of death prescribed for the offense of which he is guilty" (*Mishneh Torah, Sanhedrin* 13:2).

An unknown anesthetic sleeping potion is also mentioned in the Talmud in relation to an abdominal operation performed upon R. Eleazar, the son of R. Simeon: "He was given a sleeping draught [*samma deshinta*], taken into a marble chamber [perhaps an operating theater], and had his abdomen opened . . ." (*Baba Metzia* 83b). The type of drink used is not indicated, nor do the commentaries on the Talmud specify what it may have been.

There is yet a fourth talmudic mention of an anesthetic: "A man whose arm had, by a written decree of the government, to be taken off by means of a drug, would require that it should be cut off by means of a sword . . ." (*Baba Kamma* 85a).

ANIMAL EXPERIMENTATION— Judaism espouses the concept that everything that was created in this world by Almighty God was created to serve mankind. Animals may thus be used as beasts of burden and for food, providing they are humanely slaughtered. Scientific experiments upon laboratory animals during the course of medical research designed to yield information that might lead to the cure of disease are sanctioned by Jewish law as legitimate utilization of animals for the benefit of mankind. However, wherever possible, pain or discomfort should be eliminated or minimized by analgesia, anesthesia, or other means. Otherwise the pain does not serve to satisfy a legitimate human need and its infliction is prohibited. In addition, animal experimentation is only permissible by Jewish law if its purpose is to obtain practical benefits to mankind and not simply the satisfaction of intellectual curiosity. Furthermore, if alternative means of obtaining the same information are available, such as tissue culture studies, animal experimentation might be considered to fall under the category of unnecessary cruelty to animals and be prohibited. Details are provided in textbooks on Jewish medical ethics.[1,2,3] [*See also* ANIMALS, CRUELTY TO]

1. F. Rosner, *Modern Medicine and Jewish Ethics*, 2nd ed. (Hoboken, NJ, and New York: Ktav and Yeshiva University Press, 1991), pp. 353–373.
2. J.D. Bleich, *Contemporary Halakhic Problems*, vol. 3 (New York: Ktav and Yeshiva University Press, 1989), pp. 194–236.
3. I. Jakobovits, *Jewish Medical Ethics* (New York: Bloch, 1975), p. 294.

ANIMALS—Sows and cows in Alexandria, Egypt were castrated before being exported (*Bechorot* 28b; *Sanhedrin* 93a) to prevent breeding outside of Egypt. Shepherds placed their hands into the womb of an animal to help deliver the fetus (*Chullin* 4:3). If the lower jawbone of an animal is gone, one can keep the animal alive by stuffing food into its gullet (*Chullin* 55b). Jaw bars or receptacles were provided to an injured donkey so that it not turn its head and chafe the wound (*Shabbat* 54b). The talmudic sages correctly recognized that the "knee" joint is the ankle joint of ruminants and that the real knee joint is located very high up. The lower leg, in reality, represents the long, stretched out foot bones (*Chullin* 76a). The breast of slaughtered animals was one of the priestly gifts (Leviticus 7:31) and was excised together with one or two pairs of ribs (*Tamid* 4:3). In birds, the eyes are fixed on the sides of the head (*Niddah* 23a). To and fro ear movements in an animal are a sign of vitality (*Chullin* 38a). It is rare for two hairs to grow from a single hair follicle (*Parah* 2:5).

Characteristics of animals are described. For example, camels chew the cud but have no upper canines (*Chullin* 59a). The rock badger and the hare do have upper canines and chew the cud. Hoofs and horns are also described (ibid., 59b). The incisors of a dog were once removed to prevent it from biting humans (*Shabbat* 63a). A man once removed the tusks from his she-bear so that it not kill his children (*Baba Kamma* 23b). In animals the incisors are distinguished from the bicuspids (*Bechorot* 39a). Animals have a lot of fat around their kidneys (Isaiah 34:6). Animals may rarely be born with one or three kidneys (*Bechorot* 39a).

Observing animals copulate may induce vaginal bleeding in a woman (*Niddah* 20b and 66a). Worm infestation in animals is described in the Talmud (*Chullin* 67b) as are sleep horseflies, which are called "*darnei* of the head" (*Shabbat* 54b). Bloodletting was practiced on animals (*Shabbat* 144a) as it was in humans. Even venesection in birds is mentioned (*Tosefta Moed Katan* 2:11). Growths sometimes form on the pleural membranes of animals (*Chullin* 48a). Animals are said to live simply and are therefore healthy (*Ecclesiastes Rabbah* 1:18).

Cruelty to animals is prohibited (*Abodah Zarah* 13a). A man must feed his animal before he eats (*Berachot* 40a). Animals rest on the Sabbath as do their masters. Almighty God shows pity to all living creatures (*Sanhedrin* 55a). One rabbi even had compassion for weasels (*Baba Metzia* 85a). An animals that falls into a pit on a Festival or on the Sabbath may be hauled up (*Betzah* 26a; *Shabbat* 117b). Rams were fitted with wagonettes to protect their tails from knocking against rocks (*Shabbat* 54b). When ewes are sheared, oil compresses are applied to prevent them from catching cold (ibid.). Hedgehog skins covered cows' udders to protect them (ibid.). Animals suffering under the burden of heavy loads must be helped and unloaded (Exodus 23:5; Deuteronomy 22:45; *Baba Metzia* 31a). The relief of suffering of an animal is a biblical law (*Baba Metzia* 32b). One may assist an animal in giving birth on a Festival (*Shabbat* 128b). Animals in dif-

ficult labor are described (*Chullin* 68a, 69b, and 72a). If its dam dies in childbirth, the animal is an orphan (*Bechorot* 57a). The dam's hide is then stripped from her and placed on the orphan to preserve it (ibid., 57b).

Animals were fed straw as fodder (*Shabbat* 50a), or beans and lentils (*Shabbat* 143a), or corn and carobs (ibid., 155a). Pasture animals constantly graze in the meadow, whereas house (domesticated) animals return home at night (*Shabbat* 45b). The hybridization of heterogeneous animals is prohibited (*Sanhedrin* 56b; *Baba Kamma* 77b). Cattle were sold for slaughter and bought for human consumption (*Bechorot* 33a). In antiquity, animals were mutilated at royal funerals (*Abodah Zarah* 11a and 13a). Cocks were mutilated for pagan worship (ibid., 14b). An animal becomes mutilated by being abused by bestiality (ibid., 24b). He who commits bestiality may be killed (*Sanhedrin* 73a). Lewdness with animals is prohibited (*Abodah Zarah* 22a and 47a). [*See also* BESTIALITY]

ANIMALS, BIRTH—An animal whose mother dies in childbirth is called an orphan (*Bechorot* 9:4). A *ben-pekua* is a live animal found in the uterus of a slaughtered pregnant animal (*Chullin* 74a). An animal newborn may also be delivered by cesarean section (*Chullin* 4:5). The doe has a narrow womb (*Eruvin* 54b); therefore, before delivery, a snake bites her and she then delivers her offspring (*Baba Batra* 16b). To expedite birth, one presses on an animal's abdomen (*Shabbat* 128b). In the case of a lamb, the lips appear first in the vulva, but in the case of a kid, the ears appear first (*Bechorot* 35a).

During difficult labor, the baby may extrude a foot or even the head and then withdraw it. If the delivery cannot otherwise be completed, an animal fetus may be dismembered in its mother's womb (*Chullin* 69b). All animals have a slimy discharge from their vagina during parturition or one day before (*Niddah* 29a). Labor and midwifery in humans differs from that in animals (*Chullin* 68a).

One blows air (or wine) into the nostrils of a newborn animal and places the mother's teat in its mouth to enable it to suckle. If the mother shuns her baby, one places a clump of salt into the mother's vagina and she thereby develops the desire to nurse her offspring. One also sprinkles the "water of the afterbirth" on the newborn animal to encourage its mother to smell and suckle it (*Shabbat* 128b).

ANIMALS, CRUELTY TO—Severing the sinews of one's opponents' horses in wartime was done in antiquity to immobilize the enemy (Joshua 11:6). Dead kings' horses had their Achilles tendons severed to prevent the horses from being used by anyone

else (*Baba Metzia* 31a; *Abodah Zarah* 11a). An angry Arab once cut his camel's sinews and the animal cried from pain until it died (*Yebamot* 120b). All these acts are prohibited in Judaism, which not only forbids cruelty to animals (*tzaar baale chayim*) but requires that we be kind to them and treat them humanely.[1] The biblical prohibitions against muzzling an ox while it is plowing to prevent it from eating (Deuteronomy 25:4), the slaughtering of an animal and its young on the same day (Leviticus 22:28), the eating of a limb cut off from a living animal (Genesis 9:4; *Baba Batra* 20a), and the plowing with an ox and an ass together (Deuteronomy 22:10) are all based in part on Judaism's prohibition of cruelty to animals.

Many additional rules were enacted by the rabbis to guard animals against hunger, overwork, disease, distress, and suffering. Wanton hunting and killing of animals for sport may be prohibited. It is forbidden to inflict a blemish on an animal. Numerous Sabbath laws relating to forbidden acts are waived when such acts are intended to relieve the pain of an animal. A person is not permitted to buy animals unless he can properly care and provide for them. [*See also* ANIMAL EXPERIMENTATION]

1. F. Rosner, *Modern Medicine and Jewish Ethics*, 2nd ed. (Hoboken, NJ, and New York: Ktav and Yeshiva University Press, 1991), pp. 353–373.

ANIMALS, DEFECTS—After the ritual slaughtering of animals (*shechitah*), their internal organs have to be examined before they are declared fit for human consumption (i.e., kosher). Eighteen defects that render an animal nonviable and unfit for human consumption (i.e., *terefah*) are discussed in the Talmud (*Chullin* 3:1). These are: a pierced gullet or a severed windpipe; if the membrane of the brain was pierced; a broken spine or severed spinal cord; an absent liver; a pierced or deficient lung; a pierced abomasum, gallbladder, intestines, or inner rumen; a torn outer covering; an external piercing of the omasum or reticulum; if the animal fell from a roof; if most of its ribs are fractured; or if it was clawed by a wolf or a lion.

The main internal examination of slaughtered animals is concentrated on the lungs, and lengthy discussions of illnesses, malformations, and injuries of the lungs and pleura occur in the Talmud. Perforations of the lung, including the pleura, are life-threatening (*Chullin* 46a–b). A fibrin film or crust on the outer pleura from an infection does not render an animal *terefah* (ibid., 47b). A fistulous communication between two adjacent bronchi is a life-threatening condition (*Chullin* 48b). A needle found in an animal's lung could have been aspirated through the trachea or could have pierced the lung from the outside (ibid.). Lung cavitation (cysts or bronchiectasis or tuberculosis?) is dis-

cussed (*Chullin* 47b). Lung obstruction may be due to an abscess (dangerous) or from non-dangerous atelectasis (ibid.). A lung that looks like a block of wood (i.e., pneumonic consolidation) (*Chullin* 46b), or that crumbles from dryness (caseation?), or is shrivelled up (*Chullin* 55b) may represent a lethal illness from which the animal would have died had it not been slaughtered. Pleural blisters containing air, clear fluid or a honey-like substance, or solid vegetation on the pleura are not life-threatening conditions (*Chullin* 48a–b). Adhesions between lobes of the lung, known as *sirchot*, and color changes of the lungs are discussed at length.[1]

Firstling animals had to be blemish-free to be sacrificed in the Temple as holy offerings. Blemishes include blindness, a cut-off forefoot, or a broken hind leg (*Bechorot* 36b). Nondisqualifying defects in animals include a defective ear (ibid., 37a); a perforated, nipped, or slit eyelid; a cataract or growth on the eye; or a snail- or snake-shaped eye (ibid., 38a). Disqualifying blemishes include white spots on the cornea; constant fluid dripping from the eye (ibid., 38b); a perforated, nipped, or slit nose; a perforated, mutilated, or slit upper lip (ibid., 38a); and broken incisors or torn-out molars (ibid.). Other blemishes are mutilated genitals, mutilated tail bone (ibid., 39b), absent testicles or only one testicle (ibid., 40a), three or five feet, a dislocated hip, a broken hind foot, the lower jaw larger than the upper jaw, double ears, or an abnormal tail (ibid., 40b). The inspectors of animal blemishes in Jerusalem received their wages from Temple funds (*Ketubot* 106a). One rabbi spent eighteen months with a shepherd to study animal blemishes firsthand (*Sanhedrin* 5b).

---

1. F. Rosner (trans.), *Julius Preuss' Biblical and Talmudic Medicine* (Northvale, NJ: Jason Aronson, 1993), pp. 175–178.

ANKLE—The ankle or *karsul* is said to be made up of ten bones (*Oholot* 1:8). God strengthens one's steps so that the ankles do not slip (Psalms 18:37). Rashi interprets *istewara* to refer to the ankle joint (*Menachot* 33a; *Yebamot* 103a). *Afsayim* is also translated as "ankles" (Ezekiel 47:3). *Kashan* is an abnormality in a priest "whose ankles or knees knock together," which disqualifies him from serving in the Temple (*Bechorot* 7:6). Ankle chains or bracelets were worn as adornments (*Shabbat* 63a). The ankle bone reaches down to the ground and connects to the foot (*Yebamot* 103a).

The heel is called *ekev* (Genesis 26:26). The same term is used euphemistically for the vulva, "which is situated opposite the heel" (*Niddah* 20a). A person stands on his heels and toes because the foot is shaped like a bow

or a sickle (*Sukkah* 32a). Injuries to the Achilles tendon in animals can be life-threatening (*Chullin* 76a and ff.). A snake bite to a human heel (Genesis 3:15) can also be dangerous. To lie in wait for one's heels (Psalms 56:7) or to take one by the heel (Job 18:9) has serious negative implications. The heel is also metaphorically representative of the angel of death (*Avot de Rabbi Nathan* 31:2). The Achilles tendon of one's opponent was severed during war to incapacitate him (*Sforno*, Genesis 49:19). One's opponent's horses' Achilles tendons were also severed for the same reason (Joshua 11:6). At a king's funeral, his horse's Achilles tendons were severed so that no one else could use the horse. This practice, however, was designated as cruelty to animals (*Abodah Zarah* 11a) and forbidden. An angry Arab once cut the Achilles tendon of his camel; the latter cried out in pain and died (*Yebamot* 120b).

ANTELOPES—The antelope is one of the seven types of deer fit for human consumption (i.e., kosher) (Deuteronomy 14:5). The *keresh*, a type of antelope, has only one horn (*Chullin* 59b). At New Year, they used to blow with curved *shofars* of rams' horns and on Jubilees with *shofars* of antelopes' horns (*Rosh Hashanah* 26b). A giant antelope is depicted in the Talmud (*Baba Batra* 73b).

ANTS—The ant has three levels in its house and stores its food in the middle level. It gathers wheat, barley, and lentils all summer (*Deuteronomy Rabbah* 5:2). Ants nibble at crops in the field (*Menachot* 71b). They hide grains in their ant holes (*Taanit* 5a; *Chullin* 134a; *Peah* 4:11), including corn (*Maaserot* 5:7). The sages experimented at an ant hill to see if ants have a king (*Chullin* 57b). Ant hills may be destroyed (*Moed Katan* 6b). If one eats an ant one violates five prohibitions (*Eruvin* 28a; *Pesachim* 24a). We can learn modesty from the cat, honesty from the ant, and chastity from the dove (*Eruvin* 100b). Medically, an ant's head left in a seminal duct assists in the closing and healing of the perforation (*Yebamot* 76a).

ANUS—The rectum is the last of the ten organs of digestion (*Ecclesiastes Rabbah* 7:3). The term "opening" is used by the Talmud to denote the anus (*Pesachim* 7:1; *Niddah* 13b; *Shabbat* 151b). God covered man's anus with his buttocks so that he sits in modesty when he defecates (*Genesis Rabbah* 17:6). The possibility of a baby's birth through the rectum and anus is rejected (*Tosafot, Keritot* 76). A newborn infant with an imperforate anus is treated by rubbing the region with oil and cutting the anal skin crosswise with a barley grain (*Shabbat* 134a). Certain folk remedies were applied to the anus or rectum for lower bowel ailments (*Abodah Zarah* 28b, *Gittin* 69b). Wiping one's anus with lime, potter's clay, or previously used pebbles may lead to hemorrhoids (*Berachot* 55a; *Shabbat* 81a). Unnatural intercourse (i.e., anal) is discussed in the Talmud (*Ketubot* 46a). A very hard-boiled egg swallowed whole may pass through the rectum and out the anus (*Nedarim* 50b). King Jehoram, whose bowels fell out (2 Chronicles 21:14–18), may have had rectal prolapse or rectal cancer.[1] When a person died, all his openings, including the anus, were stopped up to delay putrefaction of the body prior to burial (*Semachot* 1:2–4; *Shabbat* 151b). [*See also* DEFECATION, DIARRHEA, HEMORRHOIDS, and INTESTINES]

---

1. F. Rosner (trans.), *Julius Preuss' Biblical and Talmudic Medicine* (Northvale, NJ: Jason Aronson, 1993), p. 183.

APHRODISIACS—In addition to mandrakes, many other aphrodisiacs are cited in ancient Jewish sources. In Deborah's song of praise of Jael concerning the fleeing Siserah, the Bible states that "he asked for water but she gave him milk" (Judges 5:25). The commentaries say she did this so that he would become sleepy and, according to Preuss,[1] to entice him to cohabitation in his weakened condition, bringing him to complete exhaustion and thereby delivering him more easily into the hands of his pursuers. Rabbi Yochanan said that Siserah had seven sexual connections with Jael on that day (*Yebamot* 103a).

Milk, cheeses, fat meat, old wine, pounded beans, eggs, and fish brine are all said to be sexual stimulants (*Tosefta Zavim* 2:2). One withholds certain foods from the High Priest for several days prior to the Day of Atonement to avoid inducing sexual excitement. According to various sages, these include cakes of fine flour, eggs, citron, old wine and fat meat, milk, cheese, soup of pounded beans, fish brine, garlic, pepperwort, purslane, and garden rocket (*Yoma* 18a). One should take advantage of the following five properties of garlic by consuming it on Fridays: It keeps the body warm, brightens the face, increases semen, kills parasites in the bowels, and fosters love and removes jealousy (*Baba Kamma* 82a). The consumption of small fish is said to stimulate propagation and strengthens the whole body (*Berachot* 40a).

Wine is also considered in the Talmud to be a potent sexual stimulant. "One cup of wine is becoming to a woman, two are degrading, and if she has three, she solicits publicly; but if she has four, she solicits even an ass in the street and cares not" (*Ketubot* 65a). The wine from Pethugta seduces men to immorality (*Leviticus Rabbah* 5:3). If a man is drunk with wine, he lusts for intercourse with his wife even if she is menstruating (ibid., 12:1). Other evils of wine imbibition are also enunciated (ibid.). Elsewhere the Talmud states that one who is not conversant with "the way of the world" (i.e., marital intercourse) should take three measures of safflower, grind it, boil it in wine, and drink it (*Gittin* 70a).

The Talmud also recognizes that sexual excitation does not require the ingestion or imbibition of an aphrodisiac food or potion. Gazing at exposed portions of a woman's body can produce the same result (*Berachot* 24a). Even the viewing of obscene pictures can stimulate sexual desire. Legend tells us that Jezebel painted pictures of harlots on King Ahab's chariot that he might look upon them and become sexually aroused, since he had a frigid nature (*Sanhedrin* 39b).

Certain foods and actions produce an antiaphrodisiac or anticonceptive effective. Eight things cause a diminution of semen: salt, hunger, scalls, weeping, sleeping on the ground, lotus, cucumbers out of season (i.e., in the winter), and bloodletting from the lower extremities (*Gittin* 70a). A vivid example of hunger producing a negative effect on sexual potential is described in the Talmud (*Ketubot* 10b). [*See also* MANDRAKES]

---

1. F. Rosner (trans.), *Julius Preuss' Biblical and Talmudic Medicine* (Northvale, NJ: Jason Aronson, 1993), p. 461.

APOPLEXY—Alcimus was paralyzed and could not speak (1 Maccabees 9:55), probably due to a stroke or apoplexy. Philopater also had an apoplectic attack (3 Maccabees 2:22). The death of Nabal (1 Samuel 25:36ff.) is also interpreted to have been due to apoplexy.[1] Apoplexy is more precisely discussed by Maimonides in his medical writings.[2] [*See also* PARALYSIS]

---

1. F. Rosner (trans.), *Julius Preuss' Biblical and Talmudic Medicine* (Northvale, NJ: Jason Aronson, 1993), pp. 306–307.
2. F. Rosner, *Medical Encyclopedia of Moses Maimonides* (Northvale, NJ: Jason Aronson, 1998), pp. 29–30.

APOTHECARY—Physicians in antiquity also served as pharmacists and compounded their own remedies, which they kept in a box (*Jerushalmi Berachot* 5:9) or a metal basket or tower (*Kelim* 12:3 and 15:1). They used ladles (*Kelim* 17:12) to prepare their medications, such as eye salve (*Lamentations Rabbah* 2:15) and the theriac (*Song of Songs Rabbah* 4:5). The biblical incense was prepared by the *rokeach*, an apothecary or perfumer (Exodus 30:35). Priests were sometimes the apothecaries (1 Chronicles 9:30; Nehemiah 3:8). Maidservants also sometimes served in this capacity (1 Samuel 8:13). King Asa was buried in a coffin or bed filled with herbs and spices prepared according to the apothecary's art (2 Chronicles 16:14). [*See also* PERFUME]

APPLES—Apples are considered delicacies (*Song of Songs Rabbah* 2:5), are comforting to lovers (Song of Songs 2:5), and have a pleasant aroma (*Soferim* 16:4). Apple wine was used for medicinal purposes (*Berachot* 38a), sometimes mixed with wine (*Abodah Zarah* 40b). Very old apple wine was used to cure dysentery (ibid.). Jews are compared to an apple tree (Song of Songs 2:3; *Shabbat* 88a). God is also compared to an apple tree (Song of Songs 2:3) because He is sweet and lovely (ibid., 2:16; *Exodus Rabbah* 17:2). An apple tree is said to give fruit sixty days after it blossoms (*Bechorot* 8a).

Pastries were baked in the shape of Cretan apples (*Menachot* 63a). Sorb apple and crab apple trees are also described (*Kilayim* 1:4). The *charoset* food used at the Passover Seder contains apples in memory of the apple tree (Song of Songs 8:5) under which the Israelite women in Egypt gave birth to their children (*Pesachim* 116a; *Sotah* 11b). In the Temple, it was forbidden to leaven the meal offering with apples (*Menachot* 54a). Women used to play with apples on the Sabbath (*Eruvin* 104a). A proverb states that a woman prostitutes herself for apples and then distributes them to the sick (*Exodus Rabbah* 31:17; *Leviticus Rabbah* 3:1).

ARM—The term *zeroa*, for "arm," is often used to portray power and might. God breaks the arm of the wicked (Psalms 10:15). The man of the arm (Job 22:8) is a mighty man. The Lord brought the Jews out of Egypt with an outstretched arm (Deuteronomy 26:8). Women support a woman in labor by her arms (*Shabbat* 129a). A shepherd carries little lambs in his arms (Isaiah 40:11). The Lord is our support (literally: arm) every day (Isaiah 33:2). To cut off the arm means to break the might of a person (1 Samuel 2:31).

Phylacteries are placed on "the hand" (Deuteronomy 6:8), which is interpreted to mean the biceps area of the arm (*Menachot* 37a). The upper arm and forearm are joined at the elbow. The sweat about which the prophet speaks (Ezekiel 44:18) is that at the elbows and lower ribs (*Zevachim* 19a). One should not lean on a Torah scroll with one's elbows (*Soferim* 3:11). The cubit measure (*amma*) refers to the distance from the elbow to the tip of the middle finger (*Ketubot* 5b). The elbow has two bones (*Oholot* 1:8).

Amputation of arms (*Keritot* 3:8) and amputees (*Taanit* 21a) are described in the Talmud. A priest with a broken arm is unfit to serve in the Temple (Leviticus 21:19). Job speaks figuratively about the breaking of his arm (Job 31:21–22). One can break an arm falling out of a wagon (*Leviticus Rabbah* 31:4). Intentionally break-ing someone's arm is a punishable offense (*Baba Kamma* 8:7).

One should not carry bread under the arm because it may become soaked with harmful perspiration (*Jerushalmi Terumot* 8:45). Axillary hair was frequently removed in Jewish women (*Sanhedrin* 2a). Axillary hair is short-lived compared to hair on the head. In elderly obese men it gradually falls out (*Nazir* 59a). [*See also* HAND and FINGERS]

ARTERIES—Cain slew Abel by severing the arteries in his neck (*Sanhedrin* 37b), the same carotid arteries that are severed during the ritual slaughtering of animals (*Chullin* 2:1 and 93b). A man with his arteries cut is mortally wounded (*Yebamot* 120b; *Oholot* 1:6) although cauterization may allow him to survive (*Yebamot* 120b). After cutting arteries for bloodletting, blood gushes forth immediately and, if not stopped, will cause the patient's life to go out (*Keritot* 22a; *Pesachim* 22b; *Sanhedrin* 59a). The slightest perforation in the aorta may be fatal (*Chullin* 45b).

ARTIFICIAL INSEMINATION—Artificial insemination is the instrumental deposition of semen into the female genital tract without sexual intercourse. The semen may be that of the woman's husband (AIH) or a donor (AID). Many moral, legal, and religious issues arise from this procedure including its permissibility; the status of the child concerning paternity, inheritance, support, and custody; the procurement of sperm for fertility testing and insemination; and many more. These issues are discussed in detail in the Jewish medical ethics literature.[1,2,3,4]

The main talmudic source dealing with artificial insemination concerns a case of accidental insemination whereby a maiden became pregnant without cohabitation by sitting in a bathhouse where a man had previously ejaculated sperm (*Chagigah* 14b). Another key source is the thirteenth-century work *Hagahot Semak* (quoted by the Bach in *Tur, Yoreh Deah* 195 and by Taz in *Shulchan Aruch, Yoreh Deah* 195:7), which discusses the possibility of pregnancy occurring by a woman lying on bedsheets upon which a man had previously ejaculated. The procurement of semen for legal reasons without masturbation is described in the Talmud (*Yebamot* 76a).

The conclusion of most rabbinic decisors, based on these and other sources, is that artificial insemination using the semen of a donor other than the husband is considered by most rabbinic opinion to be an abomination and strictly prohibited for a variety of reasons, including the possibility of incest, lack of genealogy, and problems of inheritance. Some authorities regard AID as adultery, re-quiring the husband to divorce his wife and her forfeiture of the *ketubah* or marriage settlement; even the physician and the donor are guilty when involved in this act akin to adultery. Most rabbinic opinion, however, states that without a sexual act involved, the woman is not guilty of adultery and is not prohibited to cohabit with her husband.

Regarding the status of the child, rabbinic opinion is divided. Most consider the offspring to be legitimate, as was Ben Sira, the product of conception *sine concubito*; a small minority of rabbis consider the child illegitimate; and at least two authorities take a middle view and label the child a *sofek mamzer*. Considerable rabbinic opinion regards the child (legitimate or illegitimate) to be the son of the donor in all respects (i.e., inheritance, support, custody, incest, levirate marriage, and the like). Some regard the child to be the donor's son only in some respects but not others. Some rabbis state that although the child is considered the donor's son in all respects, the donor has not fulfilled the commandment of procreation. A minority of rabbinic authorities asserts that the child is not considered the donor's son at all.

There is near unanimity of opinion that the use of semen from the husband is permissible if no other method is possible for the wife to become pregnant. It is permitted by most rabbis to obtain sperm from the husband both for analysis and for insemination, but difference of opinion exists as to the method to be used in its procurement. Masturbation should be avoided if at all possible, and coitus interruptus or the use of a condom seem to be the preferred methods. [*See also* SURROGATE MOTHERHOOD]

1. F. Rosner, *Modern Medicine and Jewish Ethics*, 2nd ed. (Hoboken, NJ, and New York: Ktav and Yeshiva University Press, 1991), pp. 85–99.
2. I. Jakobovits, *Jewish Medical Ethics* (New York: Bloch, 1975), pp. 244–250 and 261–266.
3. J.D. Bleich, *Judaism and Healing* (New York: Ktav, 1981), pp. 80–84.
4. A.S. Abraham, *The Comprehensive Guide to Medical Halachah* (Jerusalem and New York: Feldheim, 1990), pp. 207–208.

ARTIFICIAL RESPIRATION—Among the earliest accounts of the mouth-to-mouth method of resuscitation is the miraculous revival by Elisha the prophet of the son of the Shunammite woman, the boy having collapsed of sunstroke. The method used by Elisha is described in the Bible as follows:

> And he went up and lay upon the child, and put his mouth upon his mouth, and his eyes upon his eyes, and his hands upon his hands . . . and he crouched over him; and the child sneezed seven times, and the child opened his eyes. (2 Kings 4:34–35)

Another nearly identical incident is described wherein Elijah the prophet revived the child of a woman from Zaraphat as follows:

> And he stretched himself upon the child three times, and cried unto the Lord, and said: "O Lord my God. I pray Thee, let this child's soul come back into him." And the Lord hearkened unto the voice of Elijah, and the soul of the child came back into him, and he revived. (1 Kings 17:17–22)

The phrase "There was no breath left in him" is interpreted by Josephus (*Antiquities* 8, 13:3) to mean that he appeared to be dead. Most biblical commentators, however, including Rashi, Ralbag, Metzudat David, and Radak consider the boy to have actually died. Metzudat David remarks that the verse "And he stretched himself upon the child" means that Elijah placed his mouth on the child's mouth and his eyes on the child's eyes just as Elisha did to the son of the Shunammite woman. Radak again states that this was done to breathe onto the boy and warm him with Elijah's natural body warmth. Ralbag also supports this viewpoint, and further remarks that it was as if the prophet wished to transfer the breath of his limbs to the limbs of the child.

These two biblical narratives seem to describe accurately and vividly the mouth-to-mouth method of resuscitation. It seems entirely plausible and reasonable to interpret these anecdotes in this fashion without denying one's faith in the miraculous divine intervention on behalf of the two victims.[1]

1. F. Rosner, "Artificial Respiration in Biblical Times," in *Medicine in the Bible and the Talmud*, 2nd ed. (Hoboken, NJ: Ktav and Yeshiva University Press, 1995), pp. 288–290.

ARTIFICIAL TEETH—Lost teeth were replaced with artificial teeth. The Talmud describes such inserted or extra teeth (*Jerushalmi Shabbat* 8b). Such teeth can be removed at will (*Tosefta Kelim* 3:16) and shown to a friend (*Shabbat* 65a). The Mishnah (*Shabbat* 6:5) speaks of gold teeth and the Gemara speaks of silver teeth (*Shabbat* 65a). The commentaries also mention a wooden tooth (*Korban Ha'edah* on *Jerushalmi Shabbat* 6:8). Maimonides interprets the "gold tooth" to be a gold case or crown that a woman places over a damaged or defective tooth to hide the blemish (*Mishneh Torah, Shabbat* 19:7).

Tooth replacement in antiquity was purely for cosmetic reasons. Therefore, talmudic writings do not mention it at all in regard to men. Furthermore, the Talmud and Codes of Jewish Law discuss this subject in the sections dealing with women's ornaments (*Shulchan Aruch, Orach Chayim* 303). Golden teeth were expensive, but even women of modest means could afford an ordinary artificial tooth (*Jerushalmi Shabbat* 8b). Special craftsmen prepared artificial teeth (ibid.). When a maiden with an ordinary false tooth was provided with a golden tooth, she was able to be married (*Nedarim* 66b). [*See also* DENTISTRY]

ASAFETIDA—Asafetida is an umbelliferous plant used as a resin or as leaves for a spice or for medicinal purposes. Its leaves were eaten (*Abodah Zarah* 40b) and its juice obtained from the root (ibid., 39a). It was used as a foodstuff (*Niddah* 51b) although eating a lot of it loosens the skin and may be dangerous (*Jerushalmi Shabbat* 20:17). If an animal suffering from congestion swallows asafetida, it may die from perforation of its internal organs (*Chullin* 58b). Heaviness of the heart is treated with asafetida dissolved in water and consumed in three consecutive days (*Shabbat* 140a). A parturient woman who catches a cold "on the birthstool" should be given an asafetida-containing mixture of herbs cooked in beer (*Abodah Zarah* 29a). Asafetida may be bought with tithe money (*Uktzin* 3:5).

ASCETICISM—Judaism is generally opposed to asceticism (*Numbers Rabbah* 10:7; 10:15) and considers someone who deprives himself of what he may legitimately enjoy to be a sinner

(*Nazir* 22a; *Nedarim* 10a). This includes a Nazarite who abstains from wine (*Nedarim* 10a) and who must bring a sin offering (*Taanit* 11a). When the Second Temple was destroyed, many Jews became ascetics and ate no meat and drank no wine. The rabbis objected to this asceticism and hardship (*Baba Batra* 60b). He who deprives himself of sleep imperils his life (*Avot* 3:4) because sleep is enforced by nature (*Tamid* 28a). If someone swears not to sleep for three days, he is flogged and his oath is invalid (*Nedarim* 15a). If a woman makes ascetic vows such as to not bathe or use facial makeup, the vows can be invalidated by her husband (Numbers 30:14; *Ketubot* 7:3). Although fasting is a form of asceticism, in times of calamity Jews fast for deliverance (Joel 1:14; Esther 4:16; *Taanit* 1:5; *Baba Metzia* 85a). Private fasts were also practiced in antiquity (Judith 8:6; 1 Maccabees 3:47), although Abaye practiced hunger and developed dropsy (*Shabbat* 33a).

ASKARA—*Askara* (diphtheria) is a disease that affects primarily children (*Taanit* 27b) but also adults (*Sotah* 35a; *Yebamot* 62b). It causes death by asphyxiation (*Leviticus Rabbah* 18:4), which is the hardest death of the 903 types of death that exist. The death throes are vividly portrayed in the Talmud (*Berachot* 8a and 40a) and may represent diphtheritic croup.[1] The biblical *magepha* (Numbers 14:36) is said to refer to *askara* or epidemic croup (*Sotah* 35a). During Temple times, the priestly divisions fasted every Wednesday so that the *askara* should not attack children (*Taanit* 27b). *Askara* is a punishment for the sin of slander and therefore afflicts the mouth and throat (*Shabbat* 33a). Preventive measures include eating lentils, salting all foods, and diluting all beverages with water (*Berachot* 40a). A lengthy philological and etymological discussion of *askara* is found in Preuss' classic book. [*See also* THROAT]

---

1. F. Rosner (trans.), *Julius Preuss' Biblical and Talmudic Medicine* (Northvale, NJ: Jason Aronson, 1993), pp. 157–160.

ASPARAGUS—Asparagus brew, prepared in wine or beer, is good for the stomach (or heart), the eyes, and certainly for the intestines. If one uses it regularly, it is good for the whole body, unless one gets drunk on it (*Berachot* 51a). Asparagus brew combines with other liquors for good and not for harm (*Pesachim* 110b).

ASSES—An ass or a donkey has uncloven hooves (*Bechorot* 40a), a small belly, small hooves, a small head, and a short tail (*Chullin* 60a). An ass's urine is thick and resembles milk (*Bechorot* 7b). Special jaw bars or neck braces were made for injured donkeys (*Shabbat* 54b). Ass meat is recommended by some to cure certain illnesses (*Yoma* 84a). The fetus of an ass is part of a folk remedy for jaundice (*Shabbat* 109b–110a). A she-ass once ate a certain herb and turned blind; she then ate another herb and regained her sight (*Leviticus Rabbah* 22:4). An ass rests on its hind feet (*Shabbat* 93b) and leans on its forelegs (*Zavim* 4:7). It is fastidious and does not drop saliva into its food (*Shabbat* 140b). Asses wear blankets or cushions to protect them from the cold (*Shabbat* 52b). They also wear straps on their legs to prevent them from knocking into each other (ibid., 54b).

Asses are primarily beasts of burden and carry foods, beverages, dainties (*Taanit* 21a), or wine (*Abodah Zarah* 62a) in their saddle bags (*Berachot* 18a), which are attached to their saddles (*Sukkah* 17b; *Yebamot* 120b). They also turn mills (*Moed Katan* 10b). One also rides on asses (*Berachot* 30a; *Eruvin* 64b; *Pesachim* 53b and 11a; *Taanit* 20a; *Chagigah* 14b; *Ketubot* 66b). The Messiah will come riding on an ass (Zechariah 9:9; *Sanhedrin* 98a). The Jews left Egypt with Lybian asses laden with silver and gold (*Bechorot* 5b). Just as an ass bears burdens, so do the Jews bear the burden of Torah (*Genesis Rabbah* 99:10). Asses have saddles, pack saddles, covers and saddle belts, saddle bags, and pack frames (*Kelim* 23:3). The Talmud speaks of young asses (*Baba Batra* 78b), white asses (ibid., 74a), wild asses (*Abodah Zarah* 16b; *Berachot* 9b), and Lybian asses (*Shabbat* 51b and 116b).

Ass drivers are not always trustworthy (*Demai* 4:7; *Kiddushin* 82a; *Ketubot* 24a). Some are wicked and some are righteous (*Niddah* 14a). They engage in conjugal duties once weekly because they are absent from home during the week selling their wares (*Ketubot* 61b). The ass of Rabbi Pinchas ben Yair was stolen, refused to eat, was set free, and returned to its master's house (*Genesis Rabbah* 60:8). The story of Balaam and his ass (Numbers 22:21ff.) is discussed in the Talmud. It is alleged that he committed bestiality with his ass (*Sanhedrin* 105a–b).

A donkey once bit off the hand of a child (*Baba Kamma* 84a). Another donkey once trod on Rav Ashi's foot (*Shabbat* 109a). Having donkey ears means one hears everything (*Genesis Rabbah* 45:7). He who rolls himself on a marble floor behaves like a donkey (*Derech Eretz Rabbah* 10:2). A veterinarian once cauterized a she-ass and she bore an offspring with a brand mark (*Numbers Rabbah* 9:5). [*See also* MULE, HORSES, and GOATS]

ASTROLOGY—The famous Babylonian talmudic sage Mar Samuel was known as *yarchinai* (*Baba Metzia* 85b), meaning "astrologer" or "astronomer." The belief in astrology in the Middle Ages among the Chaldeans, Greeks, and others[1] also gained acceptance among the Jews, although the Talmud frowns upon it (*Pesachim* 113b). Mar Samuel said that people born under the planet Mars were predestined to shed blood (*Shabbat* 156a). According to legend Abraham said: "I have seen in the stars that I will have only one son." God retorted that Jews are not under astrological influences (*Nedarim* 32a). The prophet has already spoken: "Do not dread the signs of heaven, like the heathens, who fear these signs" (Jeremiah 10:2).

The disciples of Rabbi Chanina stated: "It is not the planetary constellation of the day that decides one's fate, but the stars at the moment of birth." Thus is created another particular type of *fatum*. Therefore, neither an illness with which a person is afflicted, nor his death, occurs by chance (*Baba Kamma* 2b). Astrological reasons were especially decisive for the selection of days appropriate for bloodletting, not only in the time of the Talmud (*Shabbat* 129b; *Yebamot* 72a), but also throughout the centuries and millennia until our own times. Pharaoh's astrologers are also cited in the Talmud (*Sanhedrin* 101a).

The work of astrologers was not confined to predicting the future from the stars. They claimed to be able to influence the future by changing misfortune into good fortune. They applied the occult virtues of heavenly bodies to earthly objects. The medicine was an image made by human art with due reference to the constellation. On this principle is based the method of curing disease with figures especially made for this purpose. For example, Rabbi Solomon ben Abraham Adret, known as Rashba, writes that to cure pains in the loins or in the kidneys, people used to engrave the image of a tongueless lion on a plate of silver or gold (Responsa *Rashba* 1:167).

The generally prevalent belief in astrology during the Middle Ages was fully shared by the Jews, many of whom were convinced of the fundamental truth of the power of celestial bodies to influence human destiny. Moses Maimonides was one of the few who not only dared raise his voice against this almost universally held belief, but even branded it as a superstition akin to idolatry and an offense punishable by disciplinary flogging.[2] He categorically rejects astrology and other superstitious practices and beliefs (*Mishneh Torah, Akum* 11:16). [*See also* MAGIC, SORCERY, EVIL EYE, and INCANTATIONS]

---

1. F. Rosner (trans.), *Julius Preuss' Biblical and Talmudic Medicine* (Northvale, NJ: Jason Aronson, 1993), pp. 140–141.

2. F. Rosner, "Astrology," in *Medical Encyclopedia of Moses Maimonides* (Northvale, NJ: Jason Aronson, 1998), pp. 34–35.

AUTOPSY—The sages of the Talmud had an amazing knowledge of human anatomy although references to anatomical dissection or postmortem examinations are very rare in the Talmud. It is likely that animal dissections were frequent and the knowledge obtained therefrom was applied to the human situation. Rabbi Ishmael related that the Alexandrian queen Cleopatra cut open pregnant slaves who were condemned to death and found that a male fetus was completely formed at forty days of gestation and a female fetus at eighty days of gestation (*Tosefta Niddah* 4:17). Another incident concerned the disciples of Rabbi Ishmael who "cooked" the body of a prostitute who had been condemned to death and ascertained the number of "limbs" or bones of the human body (*Bechorot* 45a). The death of Titus, the postmortem examination of his head by the opening of his skull, and the discovery of a brain tumor (acoustic neuroma?) near his ear is described in the Talmud (*Gittin* 56b).

Two other talmudic passages deal with autopsy, although neither deals directly with dissection of the dead for purely medical purposes. One case deals with criminal law wherein an autopsy was requested in a case of murder (*Chullin* 11b). The autopsy was disallowed since the findings would have been irrelevant to the conviction of the murderer and insufficient to acquit him even if the autopsy had been permitted. The second case deals with civil law wherein exhumation of a body was requested to determine whether or not the deceased was a minor, which would invalidate a sale he made before he died (*Baba Batra* 154a). The request was denied, as in the earlier case based on the biblical prohibition against desecrating the dead (Deuteronomy 21:22–23). Other objections to routine autopsy in Judaism include the thwarting of the requirement for prompt burial (ibid.; *Sanhedrin* 46b) and the prohibition against deriving any benefit from the dead (*Abodah Zarah* 29b; *Nedarim* 48a).

The consensus of rabbinic opinion today[1] seems to permit autopsy only in the spirit of the famous responsum of Rabbi Ezekiel Landau (Responsa *Noda Biyehuda*, part 2, *Yoreh Deah* 210), that is, if it may directly contribute to the saving of the life of another patient already afflicted with a life-threatening illness. A case in point would be a person with cancer who died after receiving an experimental drug or drug combination. Postmortem examination to ascertain possible toxicity in order to prevent potential harm to other patients on the same course of treatment, or to obtain information concerning the therapeutic efficacy of the drug or drug combination, would be warranted according to Jewish law when such information is deemed to be essential in the treatment of other patients already suffering from the same illness. Another situation where autopsy may be sanctioned or even mandated is in the case of a mysterious infectious or contagious illness such as Legionnaire's disease where numerous deaths have occurred. Autopsy would probably have been permitted to discover the organism (now known) and treatment (now available) to save the lives of other Legionnaires who were dying of the same illness. The dominant consideration in permitting an autopsy is the immediacy of the constructive application of the findings in keeping with the "here and now" principle first enunciated by Rabbi Landau. Routine autopsy in Judaism is prohibited.

---

1. F. Rosner, "Autopsy," in *Modern Medicine and Jewish Ethics* (Hoboken, NJ: Ktav and Yeshiva University Press, 1991), pp. 313–333.

AYLONIT—A congenitally sterile woman is called an *aylonit* (*Yebamot* 119a; *Ketubot* 11a). The signs and symptoms of such a woman are that she has no breast development, suffers pain during copulation, has a deep voice like a man's, has no pubic hair even at age twenty years, and is incapable of procreation (*Yebamot* 8ab). Most young girls turn out not to be affected by this condition (ibid., 61a–b). A priest may not marry a woman incapable of procreation (*Yebamot* 61a). One should not marry a woman who has never menstruated because she is probably an *aylonit* (*Niddah* 12b). A marriage can be annulled if the wife turns out to be an *aylonit* unless the husband knew about it in advance (*Ketubot* 101b). Seduction or rape of an *aylonit* is punishable (Exodus 22:15) but the man is exempt from marrying her (Deuteronomy 22:28). [*See also* CHILDLESSNESS, MARRIAGE, and PROCREATION]

B

BALDNESS—Anterior baldness is called *gabe'ach* and posterior baldness is called *ker'ach* (Leviticus 13:40–41; *Tosefta Negaim* 4:9; *Negaim* 10:10). A bald-headed man was the subject of ridicule in antiquity (*Sotah* 46b) as was the case with the prophet Elisha (2 Kings 2:23). Immorality of women may be punished by the divine infliction of baldness (Isaiah 3:17). Sorceresses are referred to as bald-headed (*Pesachim* 110a). "Baldheaded buck" is an abusive term for a castrate (*Shabbat* 152a). A curse is to wish baldness on someone (*Jerushalmi Shabbat* 20:17). A bald-headed priest is disqualified from serving in the temple (*Bechorot* 7:2) because of his unsightly appearance (*Bechorot* 43b). A bald man, on the other hand, does not have to worry about dust or sand flying into his hair (*Genesis Rabbah* 65:15). A treatment for baldness is discussed in the Midrash (*Ecclesiastes Rabbah* 1:8). For men to pluck out their white hairs, as was practiced by some women, is forbidden (*Shabbat* 94b) since it might eventually lead to baldness (*Baba Kamma* 60b). Female war captives shaved their heads as a sign of mourning for their relatives killed in the war (Deuteronomy 21:12). The prophet Micah exhorts the people to shave their heads as a sign of mourning for their children taken into captivity (Micah 1:16).

Causes of baldness include illnesses such as leprosy (Leviticus 13:42); an act of God; the use of a depilatory caustic substance (*Negaim* 19:10); severe emotional trauma such as fright upon seeing a snake (*Exodus Rabbah* 24:4); shearing off the scalp hair as a sign of mourning, an act prohibited to Jews (Deuteronomy 14:1), especially priests (Leviticus 21:5), as a heathen custom; or the forbidden plucking out of one's hair as a sign of mourning (Ezra 9:3). [*See also* HAIR, BEARD, and DEPILATORIES]

BALL PLAYING—Ball playing or tossing is described in the Bible (Isaiah 22:18). A midrashic interpretation of a biblical phrase (Ecclesiastes 12:11) compares the words of the sages to the ball playing of young maidens (Midrash *Tanchuma Beha-aloscha* 15). A girl's ball (*kaddur banot*) is thrown from hand to hand without falling to the ground (*Ecclesiastes Rabbah* 12:11), a sport perhaps similar to present-day volleyball. Playgrounds (Proverbs 8:31) and playstreets (Zechariah 3:5) are also cited.

A talmudic commentary describes walking and ball playing on the Sabbath and Jewish holidays (*Tosafot, Betzah* 12a s.v. *hocho garsinon*). The ball was thrown from hand to hand (*vide supra*) or against the wall (*Jerushalmi Sukkah* 5). According to some, playing ball on the Sabbath is a desecration of the day, meriting divine punishment (*Jerushalmi Taanit* 4:5). [*See also* EXERCISE]

BALM OF GILEAD—Gilead is described in the Bible as pasturage land (Numbers 2:1; Jeremiah 50:19; Micah 7:14) and was known for spices (Jeremiah 8:22 and 46:11). The famous medicinal balm of Gilead is first mentioned in the Bible in relation to Joseph and his brethren: "And they sat down to eat bread, and they lifted up their eyes and saw, and, behold, a company of Ishmaelites came from Gilead with their camels bearing spicery and balm and labdanum, going to bring it down to Egypt" (Genesis 37:25). Rashi explains the balm to be a resin that exudes from the wood of the balsam tree and that it is the same resin that is enumerated among the ingredients of the incense used in the Tabernacle as described in the Bible (Exodus 30:34) and the Talmud (*Keritot* 6a).

The Hebrew word for balm is *tzori*, which is first mentioned by the Patriarch Jacob when he offered his children prudent counsel: "Take of the best fruits in the land . . . a little balm and a little honey, spices and labdanum, nuts and almonds" (Genesis 43:11). Balm as an aromatic resin used for medicinal purposes is also mentioned in the books of the prophets. For example: "Take balm for her pain; perhaps she will be healed" (Jeremiah 51:8). The commerce between Judah and Israel included "balsam and honey and oil and balm" (Ezekiel 27:17).

The best and most famous medicinal balm was the balm of Gilead, which the prophet Jeremiah cites by name twice: "Go up into Gilead and take balm, O virgin daughter of Egypt; in vain dost thou use many medicines" (Jeremiah 46:11) and "Is there no balm in Gilead? Is there no physician there? Why then is not the health of the daughter of my people recovered?" (ibid., 8:22) The latter scriptural quotation is interpreted by most biblical commentators to be a metaphor or parable as if to say: Are there no prophets and righteous men among them to heal their spiritual sickness? The phrase "Is there no balm in Gilead?" has become proverbial. Nonetheless, the commentators also agree that Gilead was famous for its balm from early times and that this balm is the resin used as one of many ingredients in the preparation of the incense for the Tabernacle. In addition, however, the balm of Gilead had marvelous medicinal qualities.

The exact botanical identification of the balm of Gilead is a matter of considerable controversy. The various possibilities are discussed elsewhere.[1]

_____

1. F. Rosner, "The Balm of Gilead," in *Medicine in the Bible and the Talmud*, 2nd ed. (Hoboken, NJ: Ktav and Yeshiva University Press, 1995), pp. 132–135.

BALSAM—The biblical verse "I will plant . . . an oil tree" (Isaiah 41:19) is said to refer to the balsam tree (*Rosh Hashanah* 23a; *Baba Batra* 80b). Balsam sap is considered to be the tree's fruit (*Niddah* 8a–b) and therefore the sabbatical year laws apply to balsam trees (*Sheviit* 7:6). Balsam oil is fragrant but volatile (*Shabbat* 25b). Pure balsam was used for anointing kings (*Horayot* 11b). Cinnamon and balsam were dainties found in the Garden of Eden (*Song of Songs Rabbah* 1:15:4). The balm of Gilead (Jeremiah 8:22) is a form of balsam used to treat wounds in biblical times. A mixture of old wines, clear water, and balsam was used as a cooling drink when people emerged from a hot bath (*Abodah Zarah* 30a; *Shabbat* 140a). For ear pain, wicks soaked in balsam wood oil were placed in the ear (*Abodah Zarah* 28b).

Women in talmudic times bought perfumes, cosmetics, and balsam from peddlers (*Avot de Rabbi Nathan* 18:1). "The daughters of Zion are haughty . . . they make a tinkling sound with their feet" (Isaiah 3:16) means that they place vials of myrrh and balsam in their shoes. When young men passed by, the girls would step on the vials, thereby crushing them and spurting the balsam on the young men whose passions were thus aroused (*Shabbat* 62b; *Yoma* 9b).

BANDAGES—In biblical times, wounds were bandaged (Isaiah 1:6). Wool tufts or wool flocks were used as bandages on wounds (*Shabbat* 50a). Chewed wheat kernels (*Ketubot* 103a) and caraway (*Shabbat* 133a) were bandaged on wounds including circumcision to help them heal. A priest had a reed grass bandage wrapped around his wounded finger (*Eruvin* 103b). A universal bandage was once publicized causing some physicians to fear that their medical practice might decrease (*Shabbat* 133b). [*See also* WOUNDS]

BARBER—Barbers in antiquity and medieval times also served as bloodletters (*Baba Metzia* 97a). The barber puts a sheet or wrap over the client before beginning the haircut (*Shabbat* 9b; *Moed Katan* 18a). Barbers do not cut their own hair (*Leviticus Rabbah* 14:9). The town barber (*Baba Metzia* 97a and 109b) used barbers' scissors (*Betzah* 35b; *Kelim* 13:1), barbers' shears (*Baba Metzia* 116a), barbers' towels (*Moed Katan* 14a), and barbers' tools (*Leviticus Rabbah* 28:6). The wicked Haman was a barber (*Megillah* 16a; *Leviticus Rabbah* 28:6; *Esther Rabbah* 10:4). Barbers charged high fees for special coiffures (*Shabbat* 9b) and only rich people could afford them (*Nedarim* 51a). After a bath, the barber tended to peoples' hair (*Esther Rabbah* 10:4). Alternatively, a hairdresser did so (*Tosefta Baba Metzia* 9:14) or people combed their own hair (*Shabbat* 41a). A barber once discussed a remedy for hair falling out (*Ecclesiastes Rabbah* 1:8). One should not go to a barber for a haircut close to the time for afternoon prayers lest the time for prayer pass one by (*Shabbat* 9b). [*See also* HAIR, HAIRCUTTING, and HAIRCUTTING INSTRUMENTS]

BARLEY—Barley cakes streaked with fresh sauce and washed down with dilute wine is a remedy for "heaviness" of the heart (*Gittin* 69b). Barley, safflower, and salt is a remedy for biliary diseases (*Shabbat* 110a; *Pesachim* 42b). Heavy, large-kerneled barley, cooked like beef, is good for "sick patients" (*Nedarim* 41b). A certain type of barley grain was used to treat abnormal vaginal bleeding (*Shabbat* 14:3). Bar-

ley flour in honey was consumed for stomach pains (*Yoma* 83b). Pregnant women eat barley groats (*Yoma* 47a). On the other hand, eating barley bread with fish pie and date wine can lead to diarrhea (*Shabbat* 108a). Barley is a sexual stimulant and may cause pollution (*Yoma* 18a). One interpretation of the aphrodisiac *dudaim* that Reuben gave to his mother Leah (Genesis 30:14) is barley (*Genesis Rabbah* 72:2). Eating very hot barley gruel may produce the illness *tzafdina* (*Yoma* 84a). Excessive barley bread consumption can be dangerous and even fatal (*Yebamot* 64b; *Sanhedrin* 81b).

Barley is a food staple that a husband must provide for his wife even if he does not live with her (*Ketubot* 64b). Barley grain is washed before grinding to moisten the grain (*Pesachim* 40a and 42a) but one should not do so on Passover. Barley can be hulled and eaten raw (*Betzah* 13b). Unripe barley was used as an herb (*Eruvin* 28b) and as cattle feed (*Betzah* 14b). Barley from Edom is of inferior quality (*Ketubot* 64b). Both wheat and barley are needed by mankind but the former more than the latter (*Genesis Rabbah* 36:4). Wheat exhausts the soil more than barley; therefore, if one leases a field to sow barley, he may not sow wheat (*Baba Metzia* 106b). Certain nonmedicinal beverages contained barley water (*Pesachim* 42b), barley meal (*Jerushalmi Pesachim* 3:29), or barley beer (*Baba Batra* 96b). Barley bread is preferable to wheaten bread (*Shabbat* 140b). Rich men eat wheat bread and poor men eat barley bread mixed with coarse bran (*Shabbat* 76b). Homiletically, the Philistines came tall like barley and departed lowly as lentils (*Ruth Rabbah* 5:1).

Legally, barley is one of the five species of cereals subject to the law of *Challah* (Numbers 15:17–21), which relates to the portion of the dough assigned to the priests (*Challah* 1:1). Barley of the first fruits of the harvest was offered in the Temple (Leviticus 23:10). Some barley from each harvest had to be given to the poor (*Peah* 8:5). Barley and oats mixed together are not considered forbidden mixed species (*Kilayim* 1:1). Farm laborers who stole barley were disqualified from acting as witnesses in legal proceedings (*Sanhedrin* 26b). Barley was used to pay the poll tax (*Baba Batra* 55a).

BASTARDY—Several definitions of "bastard" (Deuteronomy 23:2) are given in the Talmud. The accepted one is the offspring of any union the penalty for which is extinction at the hands of heaven (*karet*) (*Yebamot* 49a and 69b). A bastard (*mamzer*) and all of his or her descendants may never marry an Israelite (Deuteronomy 23:3) but may marry a convert or another *mamzer*. Bastards are eligible to serve as judges in civil suits (*Sanhedrin* 36b). No man cohabiting with his wife should think of another woman, lest the children figuratively be like bastards (*Nedarim* 20b). Numerous laws pertaining to a bastard are discussed in the Talmud (*Yebamot*), where a method of purifying such a person is also described (*Yebamot* 78a).

BATHHOUSE—Bathhouses were originally private enterprises and called *merchatz* or *bet hamerchatz* (*Shabbat* 33b), as opposed to public baths (*Moed Katan* 20b; *Yoma* 11a), which are called *demosia* (*Jerushalmi Sanhedrin* 7:15). The hot springs of Tiberias are considered public baths. Some bathhouses had statues and other adornments (*Abodah Zarah* 44b) and were used by both Jews and Gentiles (*Machshirin* 2:5). Public funds were used to build bathhouses (*Abodah Zarah* 1:7). One should not reside in a city that does not have public baths (*Sanhedrin* 17b) that belong to its citizens (*Betzah* 39b). Dwellers in huts and desert travelers have no bathhouses (*Eruvin* 55b). Travelers arriving in a city go straight to the bathhouse (*Abodah Zarah* 5:4). When Rabbi Simeon ben Yochai left his hiding place after many years, he went first to a bathhouse (*Shabbat* 33b). The Israelite tribes each had their own public baths (*Leviticus Rabbah* 5:3). Rome had three thousand bathhouses (*Megillah* 6b).

The medieval bathhouse had three rooms: the bathing room where everyone was naked, the dressing room where some people were dressed and others naked, and the post-bath resting room (*Tosefta Berachot* 2:20; *Kiddushin* 33a). Holes or windows could be closed to keep the steam in (*Shabbat* 40a). Clothes were stored in niches in the wall (*Tohorot* 7:7) but were occasionally switched accidentally (*Chagigah* 20a). Bath water was drawn from ponds through pipes (*Baba Batra* 4:6) and heated with portable ovens (*Mikvaot* 6:10). After use the water flowed into a trench, which was covered with boards (*Leviticus Rabbah* 28:6). The boards sometimes rotted and people fell into the trench (*Berachot* 60a). Fuel for the ovens or stoves consisted of charcoal (*Betzah* 32a), wood (*Jerushalmi Shabbat* 3:6), or straw and stubble (*Sheviit* 8:11). Hot springs were naturally heated (*Shabbat* 39a). Bathhouse benches and their legs were made of stone or of wood (*Kelim* 22:10).

An entrance fee or token (*asimon*) was paid to gain entrance to the bathhouse (*Baba Metzia* 47b; *Sheviit* 8:5; *Meilah* 5:4). A special prayer was recited on entering and leaving a bathhouse (*Berachot* 60a). At night it was closed but used as a hiding place (*Kiddushin* 39b). It was thought to be inhabited by demons at night (ibid.). One can rent a bathhouse on a monthly or annual basis (*Baba Batra* 105a). One should not study Torah in a bathhouse (*Shabbat* 150a; *Zevachim* 102b). Bathhouses cannot be used for ritual ablution (*Niddah* 66b). Proceeds from

the sale of a synagogue cannot be used to build a bathhouse (*Megillah* 27b). [*See also* BATHING, WASHING, and OIL EMBROCATIONS]

BATHHOUSE ATTENDANTS— The bath attendant brings the bath laundry with the bath (*Shabbat* 147b) and takes the clothes of the bathers (*Tohorot* 7:7; *Jerushalmi Berachot* 2:4). He uses special baskets for this purpose (*Kelim* 17:1). He has a special place to sit (*Kelim* 8:8; *Zavim* 4:2). He is also asked to provide soap and combs (*Shabbat* 41a) and towels (*Shabbat* 147b; *Eruvin* 88a). Attendants who worked at public baths (*Moed Katan* 11b) were paid for their services (*Sheviit* 8:5).

Other personnel in the bathhouse included the *ballan* or manager (*Tosefta Baba Metzia* 9:14), the *sappag* or orderly who attended to the bathers' sponging or drying (*Kilayim* 9:3), the *sappar* or barber (*Esther Rabbah* 10:4), and the *chappan* or hairdresser (*Tosefta Baba Metzia* 9:14). Haman is said to have been a bathhouse attendant (*Leviticus Rabbah* 28:6; *Esther Rabbah* 10:4). [*See also* BATHING, WASHING, and OIL EMBROCATIONS]

BATHING—Bathing rejuvenates people (*Shabbat* 33b) and they revel in bathing (*Abodah Zarah* 2b). Bathing in a river may be for pleasure or cleansing (Exodus 2:5) or for therapeutic purposes (*Exodus Rabbah* 15:21; Ezekiel 47:9). The Syrian general Naaman cured his leprosy by bathing in the Jordan River (2 Kings 5:14). Bathing in the Euphrates River was thought to prevent leprosy in Babylon (*Ketubot* 77b). Bathing in the hot mineral springs of Tiberias is therapeutic for patients with *chatatin* or skin boils (*Shabbat* 109b). These may develop from not drying oneself after bathing (*Leviticus Rabbah* 19:4). The hot springs of Tiberias, however, are so hot and so high in minerals that skin disorders such as *shechin* can develop from bathing there (*Negaim* 9:1). Nevertheless, many sages bathed there (*Jerushalmi Peah* 8:21). If one drinks those waters, one may develop diarrhea (*Machshirin* 6:7). The hot springs of Emmaus (*shamta*) have pleasant and soothing waters (*Ecclesiastes Rabbah* 7:7) that can cure bulimia (ibid., 7:11). Therapeutic baths are popular for several weeks between Passover and Pentecost (*Shabbat* 147b).

Some people take steam baths instead of tub or pool baths (*Shabbat* 40b). The sweat of a bath is very healthy (*Avot de Rabbi Nathan* 41:4). One drinks water while taking a hot bath to compensate for perspiration losses (*Shabbat* 41a). Special cooling drinks were also consumed (ibid., 140a). The vapor of the bathhouse is harmful to the teeth; thus, some people do not talk in a bathhouse (*Jerushalmi Abodah Zarah* 3:42).

After the bath, cold or tepid water is poured over the bather (*Tosefta Shabbat* 3:4). Alternatively one can stand under a drain to be rinsed off like a modern shower (*Machshirin* 4:4). The bath is followed by an oil embrocation and the drinking of a glass of wine (*Genesis Rabbah* 10:7).

Bathing is dangerous for patients with fever from a wasp sting, the prick of a thorn, an abscess, a sore eye or an inflammation (*Abodah Zarah* 28b), and after bloodletting (ibid.). Bathing the hands and feet in hot water every evening is healthy (*Shabbat* 108b). People wash and bath on Sabbath eve (*Shabbat* 9b and 25b). Townspeople bathe often (*Niddah* 48b). Bathing is prohibited on Yom Kippur (*Yoma* 8:1) and on most fast days (*Taanit* 12b and 30a; *Pesachim* 54b). Mourners do not bathe but may wash their hands and face (*Moed Katan* 15b). One should not study Torah in the bath (*Shabbat* 150a; *Zevachim* 102b). More details about bathing in classic Jewish sources are found elsewhere.[1] [*See also* BATHHOUSE, WASHING, and OIL EMBROCATIONS]

1. F. Rosner (trans.), *Julius Preuss' Biblical and Talmudic Medicine* (Northvale, NJ: Jason Aronson, 1993), pp. 524–544.

BATHING, RITUAL—For ritual purification, the Bible prescribes immersion in a ritual bath of "living [i.e., flowing] water" (Numbers 19:17) from a well or cistern or gathering of water (Leviticus 11:36). These waters can be collected in a reservoir of at least forty *seahs* (about eight hundred liters), corresponding to the forty references to "well" in the Bible (*Numbers Rabbah* 18:21), for immersion of a full grown person (*Eruvin* 4b; *Pesachim* 109a; *Rosh Hashanah* 13a; *Chagigah* 11a). Rainwater can be led through a pipe to the immersion pool or *mikveh* (*Mikvaot* 4:1, *Yebamot* 15a). Drawn water, however, is not usable by itself for ablution and may in fact disqualify a *mikveh* (*Terumot* 5:6; *Eduyot* 1:3; *Parah* 5:7). An entire tractate of Talmud (*Mikvaot*) is devoted to this subject.

The ritual bath is a religious ceremony and not a hygienic or medical procedure. He who uses it as a regular bath is considered abominable (*Tosefta Mikvaot* 5:14). A ritual bath is called *tevilah* (immersion), as opposed to a cleansing bath, which is called *rechitzah* (washing). The body is first physically cleansed with soap and water before the ritual immersion because no interposition, including dirt, is allowed between the body and the water (*Mikvaot* 9:2). Ritual baths are secluded and surrounded by gates for privacy (*Berachot* 20a), although rivers (*Nedarim* 40b) and oceans (*Parah* 8:8) can also be used for ritual ablutions. Solomon made one hundred and fifty ritual baths (*Eruvin* 14a). A synagogue may not be sold to build a ritual bath (*Megillah* 27b).

There were several ritual baths in the Temple, one for the High Priest on the Temple Mount (*Parah* 3:7), and one for lepers (*Negaim* 14:8). Jews performed ritual ablutions before eating the Paschal lamb (*Yebamot* 71b). The High Priest takes several ritual baths on the Day of Atonement (Leviticus 16:24). Every woman after menstruation or confinement takes a ritual bath (*Niddah* 66b–67b). The same applies to people who eat forbidden foods (Leviticus 17:15) or touch a corpse (ibid., 11:32; Numbers 19:17), after cohabitation (Leviticus 15:18) or nocturnal pollution (Deuteronomy 23:12), and to patients with gonorrhea (Leviticus 15:13; *Berachot* 26a) and leprosy (Leviticus 14:8; *Yoma* 6b). [*See also* PURITY AND IMPURITY, BATHING, and WASHING]

BEANS—Joseph gave his brothers the "best of the land of Egypt" (Genesis 45:18), which is interpreted to mean split beans, which were highly esteemed (*Genesis Rabbah* 94:2). The Bible considers beans and lentils to be nutritious substances (2 Samuel 17:29; Ezekiel 4:9). Beans can be pounded and consumed raw or cooked (*Peah* 8:3). Raw beans are fit for chewing (*Betzah* 26b). Edible beans are separated from non-edible ones (*Shabbat* 142b). A bean dish improves as it continues to be cooked and shrinks (*Shabbat* 38a). Beans were made into grist (*Chullin* 6a) or mashed (*Tohorot* 3:1). Cooked beans were used as a bread spread (*Tevul Yom* 2:5). Vinegar on hot split beans spoils them, but vinegar on cold split beans improves their flavor (*Abodah Zarah* 67a). Various types of beans are described, including white beans (*Pesachim* 53a), black beans (*Tevul Yom* 1:5), green beans (*Eruvin* 28b), kidney beans (*Kilayim* 1:1), and Egyptian beans (*Shabbat* 85b; *Abodah Zarah* 38b).

Beans are a food staple that a husband must provide his wife even if he does not live with her (*Ketubot* 5:8). Bean soup is an aphrodisiac (*Yoma* 18a) and eating beans may lead to sexual arousal (ibid.). Eating bean gruel may lead to pollution (*Tosefta Zavim* 2:5). Panicles of beans and lentils are food for animals (*Shabbat* 143a). Beans may be efficacious against spiritual torment (*Niddah* 9:9; *Genesis Rabbah* 94:2). A paste made from crushed beans was used as part of a cleansing mixture (*Niddah* 61b; *Sanhedrin* 49a).

The Rabbis who gathered to intercalate the month ate only wheat bread and beans (*Sanhedrin* 70b). A blood stain the size of a bean on a woman's undergarments renders her ritually unclean (*Niddah* 58b; *Chullin* 55a). Two beans long and one bean wide is the size of a leprosy spot legally needed to render a house ritually unclean (*Sanhedrin* 71a and 87b; *Niddah* 11a). Carrying two seeds of Egyptian beans into a public domain on the Sabbath violates biblical law (*Shabbat* 90b). A leprosy spot less than the size of a split bean on a person is of no consequence (*Negaim* 1:5). More than that size renders a person ritually unclean (*Negaim* 4:6 and 6:2–3).

BEARD—A beard (*zakan*) on a man is an ornament but on a woman it is a blemish (*Jerushalmi Ketubot* 7:31). A castrate or eunuch is beardless (*Yebamot* 80b). A person with a fully grown beard is qualified to act as the representative of the community (*Chullin* 24b). The beard is defined as the hair below the ears (*Tosefta Negaim* 4:12). The presence of a beard is proof that a male is an adult and obligated to fulfill all Torah commandments (*Baba Metzia* 39a). Some people, such as Rabbi Nachman, have only a few bristles of hair on their beard and can be mistaken for eunuchs (*Yebamot* 80b). A thin-bearded man is said to be very wise (*Sanhedrin* 100b). Rav Huna did not allow a thin-bearded man to recite the priestly blessing (*Jerushalmi Taanit* 67b).

Leprosy can affect the beard (Leviticus 13:29). It is an insult to cut off the beard (1 Chronicles 19:4–5) or especially only half the beard (2 Samuel 10:4–5). It is impertinent to threaten to cut off someone's beard

(*Berachot* 11a). Incessant stroking of the beard can cause it to part (*Sanhedrin* 100b). A grave robber, caught in the act, held Abaye's beard so tightly that he had to get scissors and cut it off (*Baba Batra* 58a). Cutting off the corners of the beard is biblically prohibited (Leviticus 19:27; *Kiddushin* 35b; *Makkot* 20a). This applies to a razor. It is permitted to cut one's beard with scissors or to use a depilatory substance. A razor is specifically required, however, to shave the head and beard of a leper after his quarantine period (Leviticus 13:33) and of Levites at the first consecration for Temple service (Numbers 8:7). A Nazarite shaves only his head (Numbers 6:18).

Cutting off the beard is a heathen practice of mourning (Isaiah 15:2; Jeremiah 48:37). Some Israelites may also have done so (Jeremiah 41:5). During mourning, one covers the moustache (Ezekiel 24:17–22). A leper must cover his moustache (Leviticus 13:45). Moustache trimming was done free as part of a haircut for which a fee was charged (*Shabbat* 129b). A beard can be dyed to make a person look younger (*Baba Metzia* 60a). [*See also* HAIR, BALDNESS, DEPILATORIES, HAIRCUTTING, and HAIRCUTTING AND WASHING]

BEER—Median beer (*Pesachim* 42a) and Egyptian beer (*Berachot* 38a) are barley beers used for medicinal purposes or as an ordinary beverage (*Shab-bat* 156a). Hops are used to brew beer (*Moed Katan* 12b). Barley beer (*Shabbat* 139b; *Baba Batra* 96b) was prepared for every meal (*Abodah Zarah* 8b). Date palm beer was the most common beverage in Babylon (*Baba Batra* 96b) and was stored there (*Pesachim* 8a). Beer drinking in Babylon resulted in the absence of leprosy in that country (*Ketubot* 77b). Other beers are made from figs and blackberries (*Pesachim* 107a). Asparagus beer is good for the stomach, eyes, and bowels except if consumed in large amounts that intoxicate (*Berachot* 51a). Fresh date beer increases bowel movements, bends the stature, and dims one's eyesight (*Pesachim* 42a–b). Beer also neutralizes the harmful effects of eating small salted fish (*Berachot* 44b). Beer acts as a purgative (*Shabbat* 108a).

Fresh beer is better than old beer (*Baba Batra* 91b). If one drinks the froth of beer, one may develop catarrh. The remedy is to drink water (*Chullin* 105b). The "cup of roots" contraceptive potion is prepared in grape wine or beer (*Shabbat* 110a). For a heart (or stomach) ailment, a mixture of herbs in wine is recommended; for a breathing disorder, the same mixture in beer (*Abodah Zarah* 29a). For liver worms, one remedy is to drink thorns cooked in beer (*Shabbat* 109a). A remedy for puerperal illness is a mixture of herbs cooked in beer (*Abodah Zarah* 29a). The gall of a white stork in beer was given to a child bitten by a scorpion (*Ketubot*

50a). Drinking date palm beer or wine causes the hair to grow and the flesh to thicken (*Moed Katan* 9b). An ox with a toothache drank a whole barrel of beer, became intoxicated, and was relieved of its pain (*Baba Kamma* 35a). For forty years in the desert, the Israelites drank no wine or beer (Deuteronomy 29:5) even though wine gladdens the heart of man (Psalms 104:15). [*See also* WINE and DRUNKENNESS]

BEES—The honey of the bee is sweet but its sting is sharp (*Deuteronomy Rabbah* 1:6). To hornets and bees, we say: "Neither your honey nor your sting" (*Numbers Rabbah* 20:10). Evils and troubles (Deuteronomy 31:17) refer to bee stings and scorpion bites (*Numbers Rabbah* 10:2). God can accomplish His purpose by means of a hornet (Exodus 23:28). He destroyed the Amorites (Amos 2:9) by means of the hornet (*Numbers Rabbah* 18:22). Jews who sin may also perish from hornet stings (Deuteronomy 7:20). Swarms of hornets are like a plague and are a cause for alarm (*Taanit* 14a). Bee stings can be fatal. Wasp stings on the head (*Shabbat* 80b) or on the penis (*Moed Katan* 17a) can also be fatal. A hornet sting in the eye or on the testicle can produce blindness or sterility, respectively (*Sotah* 36a–b). Hornets can devastate whole armies (Exodus 23:28; Joshua 24:12), perhaps by blinding them (*Sotah* 36a).

Bee stings are treated with palm tree creepers in water (*Ketubot* 50a), cold compresses (*Abodah Zarah* 28b), or strong vinegar (*Gittin* 70a). An antidote for a hornet sting consists of squashed flies applied to the sting site (*Shabbat* 77b). Prayers are recited for people stung by hornets (*Baba Kamma* 80b). Bees can be sterilized by feeding them mustard (*Baba Batra* 80a). Bees die after they sting a person (*Numbers Rabbah* 17:3). One who swallows a wasp may die and should drink strong vinegar (*Abodah Zarah* 126). Fever following a wasp sting is a bad sign (ibid., 28b). Forty-day-old wine is helpful for a wasp sting (*Shabbat* 109b). It is dangerous to bathe after a wasp sting since cold things are good for wasp bites (*Abodah Zarah* 28b).

Bees, like all insects, are "unclean" animals but their honey is permitted. Wasp and hornet honey, however, is considered to be a type of saliva or body product and therefore prohibited (*Bechorot* 7b). If a man eats a hornet, he violates six biblical commandments (*Eruvin* 28a; *Pesachim* 24b). A haughty woman is called a "hornet" (*Megillah* 14b).

BEETS—Beets are considered a symbol of fertility and, hence, eaten on Rosh Hashanah (*Keritot* 6a). Partially cooked beets are unhealthy (*Eruvin* 29a) but well-cooked beets are beneficial for the heart, the eyes, and the bowels (ibid.). When cooked with other food, beets impart a sharp flavor (*Terumot* 10:1). Young shoots of beets are not neutralized when mixed with other vegetables (*Yebamot* 81b). Beets are good for cold shivers (*Abodah Zarah* 28b) and are one ingredient in a compound used to treat internal inflammation (*Gittin* 69b). Eating beets protects Babylonians from the illness *raatan* (leprosy?) (*Ketubot* 77b). Scabs on the face are washed with beet juice (*Shabbat* 134a). Beets are consumed salted or unsalted (*Nedarim* 49b) and can be eaten as vegetables on the night of Passover (*Pesachim* 114b). King Solomon was sustained (1 Kings 5:7) with beets in the summer and with cucumbers in the winter (*Deuteronomy Rabbah* 1:5).

BENJAMIN—Benjamin the physician, also known as Minyami the physician, said that all kinds of fluids are detrimental to the ears, but fluids from goat kidneys are therapeutic for people with earaches (*Abodah Zarah* 28b). He left Machoza when his medical practice was in danger of becoming smaller (*Shabbat* 133b). His family is mentioned (*Sanhedrin* 99b–100a). Unfortunately, his children became disbelievers or Epicureans (ibid.). [*See also* MAR SAMUEL, AMMI, and THEODUS]

BESTIALITY—Bestiality is biblically forbidden (Exodus 22:18; Leviticus 18:23 and 20:15–16). A person who commits such an act is cursed (Deuteronomy 27:21) and is executed (*Sanhedrin* 53a). Noahides are also forbidden to practice bestiality (ibid., 60a). The animal with whom bestiality is performed is also killed and cannot be used as a Temple sacrifice (*Temurah* 6:1). "All flesh is corrupted on the earth" (Genesis 6:12) is interpreted to refer to bestiality. The generation of the Flood even wrote formal marriage contracts between men and beasts (*Genesis Rabbah* 26:5). Legend relates that Balaam committed bestiality and copulated with his ass (*Sanhedrin* 105a). King Artaxerxes had a bitch with him on his throne (*Rosh Hashanah* 4a).

A heathen once sodomized a goose, then slaughtered and ate it (*Abodah Zarah* 22b). A similar incident is described about a side of beef (ibid.). Cases of bestiality with a hunting dog (*Yebamot* 59b) and an ape (*Derech Eretz* 1:55) are also described. Cattle should not be given to heathen shepherds because they are suspected of committing bestiality (*Abodah Zarah* 2:1). Jews are not suspected of bestiality (*Sanhedrin* 27b). Nevertheless, unmarried Jewish shepherds should not tend cattle (*Kiddushin* 82a). Righteous people remain distant from animals (ibid., 81b). A woman should not rear dogs lest she be suspected of immoral practices (*Abodah Zarah* 22b). If a woman becomes intoxicated, she might even solicit an ass in the street (*Ketubot* 65a).

A cow less than three years old is

thought to become sterile if raped by a man (*Abodah Zarah* 24b). No pregnancy can result therefrom (*Tosefta Niddah* 4:6). No animal can become pregnant from a human nor the reverse (*Tosefta Bechorot* 1:9). Man and wife become one flesh (Genesis 2:24) but animals cannot become one flesh with man (*Sanhedrin* 58a). [*See also* HOMOSEXUALITY, LESBIANISM, and RAPE]

BEVERAGES—Water is the most important beverage. The fear of snake poison led to a rabbinic prohibition from drinking water that was left uncovered overnight. If one nevertheless did so, one should quickly drink a cup of strong wine (*Gittin* 68b). One should not drink water from rivers and streams at night (*Pesachim* 112a). Mar Samuel drank only water that was boiled (*Jerushalmi Terumot* 8:45). If spice roots are added to water, it is rendered harmless (*Chullin* 84b). Snow mixed with red wine is a good beverage (*Negaim* 1:2). Sparkling wine is considered to be a superior drink (*Abodah Zarah* 30a). *Anomalin* is a drink of wine, honey, and pepper. *Alontit* is a mixture of old wine, clear water, and balsam, used as a cooling drink in the bathhouse (ibid.). *Shatika* is a beverage made from roasted flour and vinegar to lessen its sweetness (ibid., 38b). Another beverage is cooked dates (ibid.), which may be intoxicating (ibid., 48a).

For medicinal purposes the following beverages were used: milk, apple wine and other fruit juices (*Berachot* 38a), Babylonian *kutach* and Edomite vinegar in barley water (*Pesachim* 42b), Egyptian *zythom* (a type of barley beer), Medean beer to which barley meal was added, and seasoned Roman vinegar (*Shabbat* 156a). These were used as universal remedies. Barley beer (*Baba Batra* 96b) was consumed at every meal (*Abodah Zarah* 8b). In Babylon, the most common beverage was date palm wine (*Baba Batra* 96b). Asparagus brew is good for the eyes, the stomach (or heart), and certainly the bowels (*Berachot* 51a). Other beverages were made from figs, blackberries, and other fruits (*Pesachim* 107a).

One should not drink while lying on one's back so as not to choke (*Pesachim* 108a). Whoever drinks to the accompaniment of four musical instruments (Isaiah 5:11ff.) brings five punishments to the world (*Sotah* 48a). Jews eat and drink on the Sabbath and Festivals (*Megillah* 12b). [*See also* MILK, BEER, and WINE]

BILE—Although the liver is said to be the source of anger, if a drop of gall falls into the liver, the anger is assuaged (*Berachot* 61b). The gall is the seat of jealousy (*Leviticus Rabbah* 4:3). Eighty-three illnesses arise from bile (*Baba Kamma* 92b; *Baba Metzia* 104b). A remedy for biliary disease includes barley, safflower, and salt

(*Shabbat* 110a; *Pesachim* 42b). The gall of a white stork in beer should be given to a child bitten by a scorpion (*Ketubot* 50a). The gall of a fish applied to white spots on the eyes restored the vision of the patient (Tobit 6:2ff. and 11:7ff.). The angel of death lets a drop of gall fall into a person's mouth and thus accomplishes his purpose (*Abodah Zarah* 20b). [*See also* GALLBLADDER, LIVER, and *YERAKON*]

BIRDS—Anatomical features of birds include eyes fixed on the sides of the head (*Niddah* 23a), scales on the legs like the scales of fish (*Chullin* 27b), sixteen tendons (*Chullin* 76b), lungs like rose petals situated immediately beneath the wings (*Chullin* 57a), and spinal cords that extend to the point opposite the lower extremity of the wings (*Chullin* 46a). Birds digest food rapidly (*Oholot* 11:7). Clean (i.e., kosher) birds such as chickens, geese, hens, ducks, turkeys, and doves have an extra toe, a crop, and a gizzard that can be peeled (*Chullin* 59a). The eagle has none of these and is, therefore, an unclean bird (*Chullin* 61a). There are twenty-four species of unclean birds (Leviticus 11:13–19; *Chullin* 61b). Kosher birds require ritual slaughtering (*Chullin* 4a, 27a, and 16b) except for pigeons or turtle doves consecrated for Temple sacrifices, which had the backs of their necks nipped (*Chullin* 19b).

Injuries to birds include a broken leg, a dislodged femur, and a broken skull (*Chullin* 57a). Pigeons that can only hop (*Baba Batra* 23b) and emaciated birds (*Niddah* 19b) are mentioned, as are mythical giant birds (*Baba Batra* 73b) and the phoenix, a legendary immortal bird (Job 29:18). Birds are hunted (*Abodah Zarah* 19a), either outdoors or in tower traps (*Betzah* 24a). Bird traps, bird cages, and bird baskets (*Kelim* 23:54; *Chullin* 57a) are all described in the Talmud, as are pigeon cotes (*Baba Batra* 23a) and dove cotes (*Betzah* 24a). Birds use twigs to build their nests (*Abodah Zarah* 42b). Geese and fowl make their nests in an open field, in a house (*Chullin* 138b), or on top of a tree (*Abodah Zarah* 42b). Doves live in nests, lofts, or pits whereas geese and hens live in orchards (*Betzah* 25a). Young birds need the care of their mother (*Abodah Zarah* 42b). Birds eat up crumbs from people's yards (*Pesachim* 8a), eat fallen dates (*Pesachim* 56b), or nibble on figs (*Chullin* 9a). Even birds recognize stingy people and avoid them (*Sotah* 38b). Hawks claw their prey (*Chullin* 52b). Many birds can swim (*Chullin* 51b). Even venesection in birds is mentioned (*Tosefta Moed Katan* 2:11).

Poetically, after death the soul flies heavenward like a bird (*Sanhedrin* 91a). An old man sleeps lightly; even a bird wakes him (*Shabbat* 152a). When Titus died, his skull was opened and something like a dove was drawn forth (brain tumor?) (*Gittin* 56b). The law of sending the mother bird from the nest (Deuteronomy 22:627), the law of covering the blood (Leviticus 17:13), and other laws pertaining to birds are discussed in detail in the Talmud (*Chullin* 138b and ff.) [*See also* CHICKENS, GEESE, PIGEONS, and DOVES]

BIRTH DEFECTS—Cohabitation with a menstruating woman was thought to result in malformed or leprous infants (*Leviticus Rabbah* 15:5). Hermaphrodites and newborns of indeterminate sex are discussed elsewhere in this encyclopedia [*See* TUMTUM and HERMAPHRODITE]. Babies born circumcised need to be carefully examined for true congenital absence of the foreskin (*Abodah Zarah* 27a; *Yebamot* 71a). Other congenital abnormalities of the external genitalia are discussed by Preuss.[1] Physical blemishes of the eyes including congenital blindness are discussed in the section entitled EYES, BLEMISHES. A variety of abnormal births are described in the section entitled ABORTION. Half-human, half-goat-like newborns are cited in the Talmud (*Niddah* 23b), as well as newborns with facial disfigurement, anencephaly (ibid., 24a), webbed hands and feet (ibid.), absence of the lower half of the body, or fusion of the lower limbs (ibid.). A newborn child with wings or with very long hair (*Niddah* 24b; *Eruvin* 100b), with two

backs or spinal columns (*Niddah* 24b), or with a hunchback (*Bechorot* 43b) or crooked spine (*Niddah* 24a) can survive into adulthood.

The Bible speaks of a giant with six fingers and six toes (2 Samuel 21:20). A thirty-day-old child with two heads is the subject of a talmudic legal discussion (*Menachot* 37a). A *sandal* is a flat "squashed" fetus, or fetus papyraceus,[2] that resembles a flat sole fish (*Niddah* 25b) and is delivered together with a normal newborn child (ibid., 26a). It was thought that superfetation, whereby a pregnant woman became pregnant again and the younger fetus was squashed by the earlier one (*Tosefta Niddah* 2:6), is possible. To prevent this occurrence, a pregnant woman should use an absorbent tampon during cohabitation (*Yebamot* 12b).

---

1. F. Rosner (trans.), *Julius Preuss' Biblical and Talmudic Medicine* (Northvale, NJ: Jason Aronson, 1993), p. 246.
2. Ibid., p. 418.

BLADDER—The Talmud speaks metaphorically about a woman's genitalia and describes her chamber (uterus), antechamber (vagina), and upper chamber (urinary bladder) (*Niddah* 17b). Also discussed are catarrh of the bladder (*Mikvaot* 8:2–4), blood from the bladder (cystitis?) in the urine (*Niddah* 59b), and strangury caused by bladder stones (*Baba Metzia*

85a). Rabbi Judah the Prince suffered for thirteen years from bladder stones and his screams of pain were heard at great distances (ibid.). Various folk remedies for bladder calculi are discussed in the Talmud (*Gittin* 69b). [*See also* URINE, URINATION, and KIDNEYS]

BLEEDING—Exsanguination following circumcision in several siblings or first cousins was recognized by the talmudic sages as a hereditary bleeding disorder for which circumcision in subsequent siblings must be postponed or omitted (*Yebamot* 64b) [*See* HEMOPHILIA]. Some bleeding is essential for ritual circumcision to be valid [*See* CIRCUMCISION]. Bleeding gums are caused by the chill of cold wheat food or the heat of hot barley food as well as the remnant of fish hash and flour (*Abodah Zarah* 28a). The cure is to spread the ashes from burnt and pulverized unripe olives on the gums (ibid.). Spitting up blood (hemoptysis) is described as well (*Yebamot* 105a). Bleeding from hemorrhoids is also a serious problem (*Nedarim* 22a). If one strikes one's friend to cause subcutaneous or internal bleeding, it is defined as a wound (*chabura*) and the striker is liable (*Shabbat* 107b). The bleeding of defloration is also called a wound (*Tosefta Ketubot* 1:1). The blood of a slain person who was stabbed gushes out (*Nid-*

dah 71a), whereas the blood of a corpse oozes out drop by drop (*Oholot* 3:5). [*See also* BLOODLETTING]

BLEMISHES—A series of physical defects that disqualify priests from serving in the Temple is cited in the Bible (Leviticus 21:17). These include a head in the shape of a basket or slice of turnip or resembling a mallet, or which is angular, or with a neck that is sunken or long and thin (*Bechorot* 43a–b). Also a hunchback, baldheadedness, dwarfism, and bleary eyes (ibid.). Additional blemishes include eyes as large as a calf's or as small as those of a goose, a body unduly large or small for its limbs, auricles that are very small or resemble a sponge, lips overlapping each other (ibid., 44a), large breasts like those of a woman (gynecomastia), a swollen abdomen (ascites?), a projecting navel or being subject to epileptic or asthmatic spells (ibid., 44b). Yet more blemishes include legs or ankles that knock against each other during walking (bowleggedness?), extra toes or fingers (polydactyly), fingers grown together (web hands), or feet as wide as those of a goose (ibid., 45a). The Bible describes a man with polydactyly (2 Samuel 21:20), which may be an advantage or the subject of ridicule (*Bechorot* 45b). An extremely tall person (acromegaly), one black like an Ethiopian, a deaf mute, an imbecile, or an intoxicated person (ibid., 45b) is considered blemished. These are medically discussed at length by Preuss.[1]

The same defects in a woman can nullify a marriage (*Ketubot* 72b). Additional defects that disqualify women are excessive perspiration, an unsightly mole, and offensive breath. Some Rabbis also include a keloid, a harsh voice, and very large breasts (ibid., 75a). If a man betroths a woman on condition that she has no bodily defects and she is found to have such defects, her betrothal is invalid (*Ketubot* 72b). If he married her without making any conditions and she is found to have bodily defects, she may be divorced and does not collect her *ketubah*, or marriage settlement (ibid.).

Neither dwarf nor giant may serve as a priest in the Temple. An abnormally tall man should not marry an equally tall woman, lest their offspring be like a mast. A male dwarf should not marry a female dwarf, lest their offspring be like "a thimble" (*Bechorot* 45b). A priest with a defect on his hands or feet should not recite the priestly benediction because people would gaze at him (*Megillah* 4:7). Walking on the back of one's feet (*Yebamot* 103a) may refer to clubfoot. One Rabbi's foot became "reversed" (*Moed Katan* 25b).

---

1. F. Rosner (trans.), *Julius Preuss' Biblical and Talmudic Medicine* (Northvale, NJ: Jason Aronson, 1993), pp. 206–207 and 231–233.

BLINDNESS—The Bible cites a number of people who were blind or had serious visual acuity problems. These include Isaac (Genesis 27:1), Jacob (Genesis 48:10), Balaam (Numbers 24:3), Shimshon (Judges 16:12), Eli (1 Samuel 3:2), Achiya (1 Kings 14:4), and Zedekiah (2 Kings 25:7; Jeremiah 52:11). In Jerusalem, during the reign of the Jebusites, there were blind "people" (i.e., idols) (2 Samuel 5:6). When the Jews received the Torah at Mount Sinai, all blind people were cured of their blindness (*Mechilta*, Exodus 20:15; *Leviticus Rabbah*, 18:4; *Numbers Rabbah* 7:1 and 18:18).

In the Talmud, Nachum Gamzu was blind and otherwise afflicted as punishment for not feeding a starving man who died of hunger (*Taanit* 21a). Rabbi Dosa ben Harkanos was blind from old age (*Yebamot* 16a). Rav Joseph and Rav Sheshet were blind talmudic scholars (*Baba Kamma* 87a). Baba ben Buta was blinded by Herod (*Baba Batra* 4a). Reasons given for blindness include heavenly punishment for specific sins such as the taking of bribes (Exodus 23:8; Deuteronomy 16:19; *Ketubot* 105a), feigning blindness (*Peah* 8:9; *Tosefta Peah* 4:14; *Avot de Rabbi Nathan* 3:1), neglecting one's eyes (*Taanit* 21a), improper behavior during cohabitation (*Nedarim* 20a), mocking one's religion (*Numbers Rabbah* 4:20), gazing at the priests' hands during benediction (*Chagigah* 16a), faulty education (*Tan-*

chuma, Tetze 4), faulty nutrition (*Leviticus Rabbah* 22:4; *Eruvin* 5:8), Sodomite salt (*Eruvin* 17b), Babylonian *kutach* (*Pesachim* 42a), wine from the barrel (*Pesachim* 111b), nuna fish (*Nedarim* 54b), external poisons (*Niddah* 54b), touching the eyes with unclean hands (*Shabbat* 108b), combing one's hair when it is dry and putting on shoes while the feet are still damp (*Pesachim* 111b), a hornet's sting (*Sotah* 35a), scabs on the head (*Nedarim* 81a), dirty water (*Gittin* 69a), old age (*Shabbat* 152a), looking intently at wicked people (*Megillah* 28a), excessive crying (*Shabbat* 151b), taking giant steps (*Shabbat* 113b; *Pesachim* 113a; *Ketubot* 111a), trauma (*Leviticus Rabbah* 8:1 and 31:4), and a blow to the brain, which controls vision (*Tosefta Baba Kamma* 9:27).

A blind person's other senses are increased. A blind infant recognizes its mother's breast by the smell and the taste of her milk (*Ketubot* 60a). A blind man recognizes his wife by her voice (*Gittin* 23a). Rav Joseph recognized his mother's footsteps (*Kiddushin* 31b). Rav Sheshet felt the king's presence (*Berachot* 53a). A blind person uses a cane for assistance in walking (*Betzah* 25b; *Baba Kamma* 31b).

Judaism views the blind with compassion and kindness. The Torah commands that one not place a stumbling block before the blind (Leviticus 19:4; *Tosefta Baba Kamma* 2:10). Cursed is he who leads the blind astray (Deuteronomy 27:18). Even the wicked demon king Ashmodai had mercy on a blind man (*Gittin* 68b). One should show the blind the way (*Yebamot* 121a). Many sages went to visit the blind (*Chagigah* 5b).

The lot of a blind person is sad. He is as good as dead (*Nedarim* 64b). After Samson was blinded he was embarrassed by being led by the hand by a young lad (Judges 16:26). A blind public official is led about by his wife as a beggar (*Jerushalmi Ketubot* 11:34). Legal rules and regulations relating to the blind in terms of fulfilling biblical commandments and rabbinic precepts are discussed at length elsewhere.[1,2] [*See also* EYES and VISION]

---

1. F. Rosner (trans.), *Julius Preuss' Biblical and Talmudic Medicine* (Northvale, NJ: Jason Aronson, 1993), pp. 274–276.
2. A. Steinberg, "Eever," in *Encyclopedia of Jewish Medical Ethics*," vol. 5 (Jerusalem: Schlesinger Institute of the Shaare Zedek Medical Center, 1996), pp. 202–251.

BLOOD—Blood is equated with life (Deuteronomy 12:23), and the draining of blood from a person is associated with the departure of the soul (*Sanhedrin* 59a; *Pesachim* 16b). The consumption of blood is prohibited (Deuteronomy 12:23–25) even though man's soul loathes blood (*Makkot* 23b). Blood from living animals is also forbidden (*Sanhedrin* 59a). Liver substitutes in nutritional value for blood

(*Chullin* 109b) since the liver is the source of blood (*Bechorot* 55a). The spleen is permitted (*Chullin* 111a) but not the blood that flows from the hilum (*Keritot* 21b). So, too, the liver is permitted but not its blood (ibid.).

Man is composed of equal portions of blood and water. If either gains over the other, illness results (*Leviticus Rabbah* 15:2). An excess of blood was thought in antiquity to cause many illnesses (*Baba Batra* 58b), including *schechin* (boils) (*Bechorot* 44b). People and animals overcome by blood are placed in cold water to cool off (*Shabbat* 53b). For blood rushing to the head and for nose, mouth, or lung bleeding, several remedies are cited (*Gittin* 68b–69b). Through fasting one's blood becomes diminished (*Berachot* 17a). Anemia or lack of blood is cause to postpone circumcision (*Shabbat* 134a).

Blood has various shades and colors (*Niddah* 19a). Black blood is really red blood turned black by disease (ibid.; *Chullin* 49b). No person's blood is redder than that of another (*Pesachim* 25b). Menstrual blood can be red, black, bright crocus-colored, like earthy water, or like diluted wine (*Niddah* 19a). Bat blood is used to paint the eyes (*Shabbat* 78a). [*See also* BLEEDING, BLOODLETTING, MENSTRUATION, and PLETHORA]

BLOODLETTING—Nebuchadnezzar chose for himself young people

"without blemish" (Daniel 1:4), which the Talmud explains: "There was not even a lancet puncture on their bodies" (*Sanhedrin* 93b)—that is how rare it was to find a person without venesection scars. The sages teach that a learned man should not live in a town that has no bloodletter (*Sanhedrin* 17b). In Judaism, a physician is considered to be a scholar, whereas a bloodletter is an artisan. Sometimes he is called *garea* (*Kiddushin* 82a; *Kelim* 12:4; *Derech Eretz Zutta* 10:2), which is the exact connotation of the Latin term *minutor*. The bloodletter also sometimes served as a circumciser (*Shabbat* 130a and 139b) but had no other occupation. Few complimentary things are said about bloodletters in the Talmud. He may not be appointed as a leader of a community nor as an administrator (*Derech Eretz Zutta* 10:2). He may not be elected king or high priest—not because he is inherently unsuited, but because his profession was held in low esteem for a variety of reasons (*Kiddushin* 28a). Naturally, there were exceptions to this rule. The Talmud clearly describes the merit of a bloodletter named Abba (*Taanit* 21b), who not only had separate rooms for men and women, but who also insisted that women wear a special garment that was slit at the shoulder so that only the site of the bloodletting was exposed.

The Talmud discusses bloodletting for asphyxia (*Yoma* 84a). Fever present for two days is an indication for venesection (*Gittin* 67b). At the height of fever, however, bloodletting is dangerous (*Abodah Zarah* 29a). Phlebotomy for pain in the eyes may also be dangerous (ibid.). Venesection was not without pain. The deceased Rabbi Nachman appeared to Raba in a dream and told him that in dying he had no greater pain than during venesection (*Moed Katan* 28a). The daughter of Rabbi Hisda described the pain of defloration to her husband with the same words (*Ketubot* 39b). If someone dreamed of venesection, it was considered to be a propitious sign (*Berachot* 57a). The color of venesected blood is described in the Talmud (*Niddah* 19b; *Machshirin* 6:5ff.).

The Bible prohibits cutting into the skin (Leviticus 19:28). Rabbi Bibi bar Abin therefore considers venesection to be a transgression of this biblical prohibition (*Makkot* 21a). Maimonides considers venesection necessary but hazardous and therefore rules that, before bloodletting, the patient should pray to God (*Mishneh Torah, Berachot* 10:12).

Venesection is harmful if excessive but useful if performed in an appropriate way (*Gittin* 70a). Mar Samuel advises that blood be let at twenty-day intervals. Later in life, one should decrease the frequency (*Shabbat* 129b). The minimum amount of blood necessary to sustain human life is one quarter log (approximately four ounces) (*Shabbat* 31b). Therefore, it is considered dangerous to bleed down to this limit because then even a minor stimulus such as a chill, which is ordinarily not harmful, might bring the person's life to an end (*Shabbat* 129a).

Many factors influence the decision as to which days are suitable for bloodletting. It seems appropriate not to perform this operation on a cloudy day if one can equally well carry it out by the light of a clear day (*Yebamot* 72a). One can also understand that days when certain wind directions prevail might be dangerous for bloodletting (*Shabbat* 129b; *Yebamot* 72a). The correct time for bloodletting is on a Sunday, Wednesday, or Friday but not on other days (*Shabbat* 129b). Samuel further stated: a fourth day of the week (i.e., a Wednesday) that is the fourth, fourteenth, or twenty-fourth of the month—as well as a Wednesday that is less than four more days from the end of the month—is dangerous for bloodletting. On the first and second days of the month, bloodletting causes weakness; on the third day, it is dangerous. On the eve of a festival, it causes weakness. On the eve of Pentecost it is dangerous and, therefore, bloodletting was prohibited on the eve of every festival.[1] These talmudic passages dealing with bloodletting reflect a mixture of astrology, medicine, and religion. The hours and the months of the year were thought to stand under the influence of the planets.

The Talmud describes a *kusilta* or lancet, a small knife to cut the skin.

The skin wound produced by the *kusilta* is called *ribda*. Another instrument is a *masmar* (literally, "nail") or pointed instrument (*Kelim* 12:4). The blood was allowed to flow onto the ground, where birds came to drink it (*Baba Batra* 12a), or onto old rags (*Baba Batra* 20a). Alternatively, the blood was collected in a vessel called a *kaddin* (*Leviticus Rabbah* 10:5), in a potsherd (*Gittin* 69a), or in a dirty earthenware vessel that was otherwise unusable (*Baba Batra* 20b). A scab that develops at the site of the venesection is at first soft and firmly adherent to the skin. From the third day on, however, it begins to become loosened from the underlying tissue (*Niddah* 67a).

Dietary factors and nutrition are important in relation to bloodletting. The consumption of vinegar, small fish, and cress prior to bloodletting is considered dangerous (*Abodah Zarah* 29a). One should wait a little after bloodletting before eating but may drink immediately after venesection (*Shabbat* 129a–b). One should avoid drafts (ibid.). Nourishing food after bloodletting includes meat and red wine (ibid.). The blood-rich spleen is also recommended. Eating fowl or fish after bloodletting is not recommended (*Meilah* 20b). Also contraindicated are milk, cheese, onions, and cress (*Nedarim* 54b; *Abodah Zarah* 29a; *Taanit* 25a). One should not exert oneself or indulge in cohabitation shortly before or after bloodletting (*Gittin* 70a; *Niddah* 17a).

In summary, bloodletting was considered in antiquity to be a panacea to cure nearly all ailments. Mar Samuel and other talmudic sages also advocated prophylactic venesection to avert illness. Mar Samuel correctly points out that excessive phlebotomy is harmful and can endanger a person's life. He also advises a person to eat a little prior to and after bloodletting, to rest for a while after bloodletting, and to decrease the frequency of blood donation as one becomes older, particularly when past sixty years of age. All these suggestions are perfectly reasonable and applicable to this very day. Many of Mar Samuel's assertions regarding bloodletting seem to have no scientific merit at all. For example: If one is bled and then eats fowl, his heart will palpitate like a fowl's (*Nedarim* 54b). So, too, the passages dealing with bloodletting that reflect a mixture of astrology, medicine, and religion.

1. F. Rosner, "Bloodletting," in *Medicine in the Bible and the Talmud*, 2nd ed. (Hoboken, NJ: Ktav and Yeshiva University Press, 1995), pp. 150–161.

BLOODLETTING IN ANIMALS— Just as in human beings, venesection was also practiced on animals (*Shabbat* 144a). Even venesection in birds is mentioned (*Tosefta Moed Katan* 2:11). Although it is ordinarily strictly forbidden to injure a firstborn animal and to thereby render it unfit to be offered as a sacrifice, it is specifically decreed that such an animal may be phlebotomized if the intent is to help the animal (*Tosefta Bechorot* 3:17). The amount of blood withdrawn from an animal was normally not very great. As a rule, one did not let the blood flow until one came down to the last blood that was sustaining life (i.e., the soul), as was no doubt done in human beings.

BOILS—The biblical *shechin* and *ababuot* (Exodus 9:8–11) may represent boils, blisters, or perhaps a form of eczema.[1] The moist form is curable; the dry one is not (*Bechorot* 41a). Other biblical skin afflictions (Deuteronomy 28:27) may also refer to boils.[2] Different types of boils, quick flesh, burning, and their like are described in the Talmud (*Negaim* 1:5ff.). A boil and a burning are obviously different (*Chullin* 8a).

Nachum was blind and his body was covered with boils because he once postponed giving food to a poor person and the latter died of hunger (*Taanit* 21a). A man was once healed of his boils and scabs by a "magical" formula (*Kiddushin* 39b). A levir was once afflicted with boils (*Yebamot* 4a). A man with boils may be forced to give his wife a divorce (*Ketubot* 77a). A folk remedy for boils is described in the Talmud (*Shabbat* 67a). [*See also* SKIN]

1. F. Rosner (trans.), *Julius Preuss' Biblical and Talmudic Medicine* (North-

vale, NJ: Jason Aronson, 1993), pp. 339–347.
2. Ibid., pp. 154–155.

BONES—The body has between 200 and 280 bones (*Tosefta Oholot* 1:7). The usual number in the Talmud is 248 (*Oholot* 1:8). These are discussed in depth by Preuss.[1] In the creation of a child, the father's sperm contributes the bones (*Niddah* 31a). "May your bones rot" is a curse (*Genesis Rabbah* 10:3, 28:3, and 78:1; *Exodus Rabbah* 5:18). Job cursed himself by wishing that his arm bone be broken (Job 31:22). He also complained of nighttime bone pain (Job 30:17) and that his bones cleaved to his skin and flesh (Job 19:20). Fire in the bones (fever?) is milder than generalized body pain (*Eruvin* 54a). Snakes have little bones (*Pesachim* 112b). Human bones are white like the color of whitewash (*Baba Kamma* 69a). The thigh bone of a biblical giant (Deuteronomy 3:11) was gargantuan (*Niddah* 24b). A man carrying human bones should not sit on them because this is disrespectful (*Berachot* 18a). A man once left a barrel of bones as an inheritance (*Baba Batra* 58a). Rabbi Yochanan carried with him a bone (tooth) of his tenth son, who died, when going to comfort those who mourned the loss of a child (*Baba Batra* 116a).

On postmortem examination, the bones of one who drinks undiluted wine or who drinks more than he eats are burned. The bones of one who drinks wine excessively diluted or who eats more than he drinks are transparent and dry, but the bones of one who drinks wine properly mixed and eats and drinks properly are full of marrow (*Niddah* 24b). The Hebrew word for both bone marrow and the brain is *moach* (*Chullin* 93a). Bones were gathered from disinterments for reburial elsewhere (*Moed Katan* 8a; *Yebamot* 100b; *Semachot* 12:49). The dry bones in Ezekiel's prophecy (Ezekiel 37:14) came back to life (*Sanhedrin* 92b). Based on the Bible (Numbers 19:14), bones from corpses transmit ritual defilement (*Sukkah* 6a; *Oholot* 2:3; *Kelim* 1:4; *Niddah* 55a). A bone crusher was used to reduce the size of bones for transport for burial (*Shekalim* 8:2). The bones of Saul and his sons were buried under a tree in Jabesh (1 Samuel 33:13).

The verse "And He will strengthen your bones" (Isaiah 58:11) is interpreted both literally and figuratively (*Yebamot* 102b). Broken bones are set even on the Sabbath (*Shabbat* 148a). Bone fractures may protrude (*Chullin* 77a), both above or below the knee (ibid., 76b). The paschal lamb's bone may not be broken (Exodus 12:46) and must be burned (*Pesachim* 83a). An animal with a broken leg is unfit to be offered in the Temple (*Bechorot* 6:8). An animal with a compound fracture can be saved if the wound is cauterized (*Tosefta Chullin* 3:6). A priest with a broken arm or leg is un-

fit to serve in the Temple (Leviticus 21:19). A variety of foot or hand deformities (*Bechorot* 45a) may represent healed fractures. Other bone abnormalities are also described in the Talmud.[2] Eli the priest fell backward and broke his neck (1 Samuel 4:18), as did a young man who fell off a ladder in the dark (*Kallah Rabbati* 9:54). In olden days, people occasionally broke an arm or leg falling out of a coach (*Leviticus Rabbah* 31:4).

---

1. F. Rosner (trans.), *Julius Preuss' Biblical and Talmudic Medicine* (Northvale, NJ: Jason Aronson, 1993), pp. 60–62.

2. Ibid., p. 232.

BRAIN—The inner and outer membranes of the brain (pia and dura mater) are discussed in the Talmud. The former is called the bag in which the brain lies (*Chullin* 45a). All the substance (literally: marrow) in the skull is called the brain. When it begins to elongate it is the spinal cord (ibid.). The two bean-shaped protuberances that lie at the base of the skull (occipital condyles) demarcate the brain from the spinal cord (ibid., 45b). A baby's skull is soft and pulsates at the anterior fontanel, which overlies the brain (*Menachot* 37a). Embalming in ancient times included the removal of the brain [*See also* EMBALMING].

Craniotomy was performed in ancient times (*Leviticus Rabbah* 22:3).

When Titus died, they opened his skull and found a brain tumor resembling a dove (*Gittin* 56b; *Genesis Rabbah* 10:7). One interpretation of *raatan* is "brain tumor,"[1] since its therapy consists of trepanning and removing it with a pair of tweezers (*Ketubot* 77b). A blow to the brain can cause blindness (*Tosefta Baba Kamma* 9:27). If a bird is struck on the head and the brain oozes out, the bird is nonviable since the brain membrane was perforated (*Chullin* 56a). Perforation of the dura mater is a life-threatening defect (ibid., 45a). Striking one's head in a bathhouse fall may produce a temporary concussion (ibid.). Softening of the brain (gelatinous degeneration?) is also described (ibid.). To have no brains in the head (*Yebamot* 10a) means a person is stupid. [*See also* SKULL and SPINAL CORD]

---

1. F. Rosner (trans.), *Julius Preuss' Biblical and Talmudic Medicine* (Northvale, NJ: Jason Aronson, 1993), pp. 347–350.

BRAN—Bran is an ingredient in a remedy for a gum or mouth abscess (*Gittin* 69a). Bran in water is fed to a person recovering from hunger or starvation to slowly expand the intestines (ibid., 56a). Bran bread (*pat kiber*) was black (pumpernickel?) and sold outside bakeries (*Song of Songs Rabbah* 1:6). Prisoners were fed this type of bread (Jeremiah 37:21). Coarse black bran bread increases bowel movements, bends the stature, and diminishes one's eyesight (*Pesachim* 42a). One may not soak bran for fowls nor may a woman make a bran paste on Passover because it turns leaven (ibid., 39b). [*See also* BREAD]

BREAD—Bread is regarded as food par excellence (*Berachot* 12a). Bread is baked in ovens (*Shabbat* 4a) and forms a crust on its surface (*Shabbat* 19b). Taking bread out from the oven requires skill (*Rosh Hashanah* 29b). Dough baked in a cavity in the ground is considered to be merely a thick mass of regular bread or "bread of affliction" (*Berachot* 38a). Bread is either homemade (*Yebamot* 81a) or baked by bakers (*Baba Batra* 93b; *Machshirin* 2:8). Some bread dealers had exclusive rights to sell bread to the public (*Demai* 5:4). Bread can be kneaded with fruit juice (*Machshirin* 3:2) and be well-kneaded or not well-kneaded (*Shabbat* 62b). Bread is consumed both hot and cold (*Demia* 5:3). Bread is sometimes spongy (*Uktzin* 2:8). Bread can become moldy (*Baba Batra* 95b) or crumble (*Shabbat* 50b). Bread crumbs are swept off the table after a meal (*Berachot* 52b). Bread soaked in wine is forbidden to Nazirites (*Pesachim* 44b). Dough placed in cold water does not ferment (ibid., 46a).

Bread can be made from wheat, barley, rice, millet, spelt, lentils, or beans (*Eruvin* 81a; *Chagigah* 20a). As a rule bread was eaten with a relish such as turnips (*Negaim* 13:9), olives, or onions (*Eruvin* 29a). Babylonian *kufach*, a preserve made of bread crusts and sour milk, was also spread on bread as a relish (*Pesachim* 44a). The poor break their fast with bread (*Sanhedrin* 35a). During times of famine, bread was baked with human dung (Ezekiel 4:12). Without relishes during times of need, bread was consumed with salt (*Berachot* 2b; *Yebamot* 15b) or vinegar (Ruth 2:14). Hungry people can faint or even die from the odor of fresh-baked bread (*Baba Batra* 91b). The Babylonians who ate "bread with bread," i.e., without relish, are called fools (*Betzah* 16a).

Coarse black bread (i.e., bran bread) was sold outside bakeries (*Song of Songs Rabbah* 1:6). Prisoners received this type of bread as their daily ration (Jeremiah 37:21). Coarse black bread increases one's bowel movements, bends one's stature, and diminishes one's eyesight (*Eruvin* 55b–56a; *Pesachim* 42a). Samuel gave Rav barley bread to eat and the latter developed diarrhea (*Shabbat* 108a). One cupful of water with a loaf of bread prevents intestinal ailments (*Berachot* 40a). On the other hand, white bread decreases intestinal activity, straightens the stature, and gives light to the eyes (*Pesachim* 42a). White bread is defined as bread made from fine meal (ibid., 42b). Coarse bread, unfit for normal sale in bakers' shops (Jeremiah 37:21), is blacker than coarse barley bread (*Song*

of Songs Rabbah* 1:6:4). Eating hard bread can cause the gums to bleed (*Keritot* 21b). Scurvy is also caused by eating very hot wheaten bread (*Yoma* 84a). Barley flour is said to give rise to worms (*Berachot* 36a).

Bread strengthens the heart (*Genesis Rabbah* 48:11) as confirmed in the Pentateuch (Genesis 18:5), the Prophets (Judges 19:5), and the Hagiography (Psalms 114:15). That is why Abraham served bread to his guests (Genesis 18:5). Wheat bread and beans is considered a meal (*Sanhedrin* 70b). A person should not break bread for guests unless he eats with them (*Rosh Hashanah* 29b). The biblical *manna* tasted like bread to young men and like honey wafers to old men (*Exodus Rabbah* 5:9). Bread soaked in wine serves for eye compresses (*Shabbat* 108b).

Four things were said with reference to bread: Raw meat should not be placed on bread; a full cup should not be passed along over bread lest some liquid spill on the bread; bread should not be thrown; and a dish should not be propped up on bread (*Berachot* 50b). A loaf of bread upon which roast meat was cut may not be eaten because of the blood that the bread absorbs (*Chullin* 112a). The Talmud states that many illnesses can be mitigated by eating one's morning bread with salt and drinking a jug full of water (*Baba Metzia* 107b). Furthermore, thirteen things were said about morning bread: It is an antidote against heat and cold, winds, and demons; it instills wisdom into the simple; it causes one to triumph in a lawsuit; it enables one to study and teach the Torah, to have his words heeded, and to retain scholarship; he who partakes thereof does not perspire, lives with his wife, and does not lust after other women; and it kills the worms in one's intestines. Some say it also expels jealousy and induces love (ibid.).

A popular proverb says that sixty runners speed along but cannot overtake him who breaks bread in the morning (*Baba Metzia* 107b). Another proverb says: If one give's bread to a child, inform his mother (*Numbers Rabbah* 19:33). The verse "Cast thy bread upon the waters" (Ecclesiastes 11:1) is explained to refer to a man who threw bread into the sea daily. One day he bought a fish and found a valuable object therein and people said of him "His bread stood him in good stead" (*Ecclesiastes Rabbah* 11:1:1). The verse "He that serves the land is satisfied with bread" (Proverbs 12:11) refers to one who becomes a slave to the land, continually toiling therein, and who is satisfied with bread (*Sanhedrin* 58b). He who leaves no bread for the poor on the table at the end of a meal will never see a sign of blessing (*Sanhedrin* 92a). In talmudic times, Jewish villages had to supply bread for passing troops (*Betzah* 21a).

One may not bake thick bread on Passover lest the dough become leavened (*Betzah* 22b). Unleavened bread must be consumed by men and women alike on the Passover Festival (*Shabbat* 131b; *Eruvin* 27a). The unleavened bread of Solomon, made of the finest flour, is equally valid as "bread of affliction" as that made from coarse flour (*Pesachim* 36b). "Bread of affliction" (Deuteronomy 16:3) is interpreted several ways in the Talmud (*Pesachim* 115b). Decrees were issued by the rabbinic sages against consuming bread from Gentiles (*Shabbat* 17b). One may not buy bread from Gentiles in cities as a safeguard against intermarriages (*Abodah Zarah* 35b), but it is allowed to buy bread from a private Gentile (ibid., 13b). Whoever eats the bread of a Jew enjoys the taste of bread (*Sanhedrin* 104b). It is permitted to derive benefit from a Gentile's leavened bread after the Passover Festival (*Eruvin* 64b).

During the time of the Temple, bread loaves accompanied certain sacrifices (Leviticus 7:12–13; *Pesachim* 63b; *Rosh Hashanah* 5b). The "shewbread" (Exodus 25:30; Leviticus 24:5–7) was changed weekly on the Sabbath (*Avot* 5:3). The "two loaves" were baked of the first fruits of the wheat harvest and offered on the Pentecost Festival (Leviticus 23:15ff.). Warm barley bread applied to a man's genitalia can induce ejaculation to determine whether a priest has a blemish on his penis, which disqualifies him from serving in the Temple (*Yebamot* 76a).

Hands are washed before eating bread (*Berachot* 43a). Eating wheaten bread where barley bread would suffice (*Shabbat* 140b) violates the biblical precept of "Thou shalt not destroy" (Deuteronomy 20:19). Only the rich eat wheat bread. The poor eat barley bread, possibly mixed with coarse bran (*Shabbat* 76b). Foods made from fine flour and eggs soften the stool but stimulate the sexual drive (*Yoma* 18a). A person who commits murder without witnesses is incarcerated and fed meager bread until his stomach bursts (*Sanhedrin* 81b). If a man swears not to eat wheat bread, barley bread, and spelt bread, and he eats, he is liable for each one (*Shevuot* 22b). Bread can be used to prepare an *eruv* to enable people to walk beyond the town boundary by an extra two thousand cubits, or to enable residents in a courtyard to carry to and fro in their courtyard on the Sabbath (*Eruvin* 39a).

BREASTS—The female breast is vividly portrayed in the Bible (Song of Songs 4:5). With puberty, the breasts become fashioned (Ezekiel 16:7) together with other body changes (*Kiddushin* 16b). The age of puberty and breast development varies (*Baba Batra* 155b). The signs of puberty in a girl are the appearance of a wrinkle when the breast is raised, the breast juts forward, and the nipple darkens (*Niddah* 47a). The right breast develops before the left in rich girls because it rubs against their scarves, which hang down tightly against the body (*Leviticus Rabbah* 2:4). In poor girls, the left breast develops first because they carry water jugs and their younger siblings on the left side (*Niddah* 48b). Breasts in a man are considered a defect that renders him unfit to serve in the Temple if he is a priest (*Bechorot* 7:5). Excessively large and pendulous breasts in a woman are unsightly (*Ketubot* 75a). Human breasts are well situated (compared to animals) so that the newborn does not face the mother's genitals when it nurses (*Midrash* Psalms 103:3). Breast-feeding is discussed in the section LACTATION.

A sterile woman has no breast development (*Yebamot* 80b). The skin illness *tzaraat* (leprosy?) can affect the nipples of the breasts (*Negaim* 6:7). Women carry bundles of fragrant herbs "between their breasts" (Song of Songs 1:13). The breast and shoulder of slaughtered animals in the Temple belonged to the priests (Leviticus 7:29ff.; *Chagigah* 7b; *Chullin* 130a).

BREATHING—The nose is the site of respiration or breathing (*Yoma* 85a; *Ecclesiastes Rabbah* 12:2). God breathes the breath of life into the nostrils (Genesis 2:7) and it remains in the nose as long as the soul is in a person's body (Job 27:3). One also breathes through the mouth (Job 15:30) and yawns with the mouth (*Berachot* 24a–b; *Niddah* 9:8). A mouth deformity known as *balum* may make breathing difficult

(*Bechorot* 40b). A woman in labor may have difficulty in breathing (Isaiah 42:14). God did not let Job catch his breath (Job 9:18). The illness *rucha* (defective breathing) can be treated with specific remedies (*Abodah Zarah* 29a). Breathing differs in different people: Some people have long breathing whereas others have short breathing (*Leviticus Rabbah* 15:2). [*See also* LUNGS]

BURIAL—It is a commandment in Judaism to bury the dead in the ground (*Sanhedrin* 46b). God buries the dead (Genesis 8:13; *Ecclesiastes Rabbah* 7:2:3). Abraham buried his wife Sarah (Genesis 23:19). A man must provide for his wife's burial (*Ketubot* 46b). Even dead infants are buried (*Moed Katan* 24b). Women used to bury their aborted fetuses and lepers their amputated limbs in earthen mounds near cemeteries (*Ketubot* 20b). Burial is intended to avert disgrace by the disintegration of the body and as a means of atonement (*Sanhedrin* 49b). Even executed criminals were buried (ibid., 46a). It is best to be buried in the land of Israel (*Genesis Rabbah* 96:5; *Ketubot* 111a), preferably under a tree (*Niddah* 57a). Deborah, the wet nurse of Rebecca, was buried under an oak or tamarisk tree (Genesis 35:8). Assisting at burials is very praiseworthy (*Ketubot* 72a; *Baba Metzia* 30b; *Moed Katan* 28b). Burial society members occupied themselves with visiting the sick and burying the dead (*Moed Katan* 27b).

Burial sites have to be at least fifty cubits from the town limit (*Baba Batra* 2:9). Burial was not allowed in walled cities (*Kelim* 1:7). No corpse or pile of bones could be kept overnight in Jerusalem (*Tosefta Negaim* 6:2). Only members of the royal family of King David are buried in Jerusalem (ibid.; *Semachot* 14:10). Soldiers in wartime are buried where they are killed (*Eruvin* 17a). During epidemics, bodies are buried wherever possible (*Semachot* 14:4ff.), preferably near relatives (2 Maccabees 12:39). Enemy corpses were at least thrown into a pit (Jeremiah 41:9).

Burial of Jewish bodies occurs as soon as possible, preferably the same day (Deuteronomy 21:23) unless necessary funeral arrangements need more time (*Sanhedrin* 4:5). Burial garments (*Shabbat* 114a; Deuteronomy 9:5) are white or black shrouds (*Genesis Rabbah* 96:5 and 100:2). Shovels and spades were used to dig graves (*Taanit* 21b). Money was contributed in each town for burials of the dead (*Baba Batra* 8a; *Shekalim* 2:5). Any surplus funds were used to erect tombstones over the graves (*Shekalim* 2:5; *Sanhedrin* 48a; *Genesis Rabbah* 82:10). Family burial plots (*Sanhedrin* 6:6) and family burial chambers are described in some detail (*Baba Batra* 101b; *Sotah* 44a).

A burial site is inviolable forever and is therefore called a *bet olam*, meaning "house of eternity" (Ecclesiastes 12:5).

A grave is opened only to transfer the bones to a place of honor. In addition, a grave that is harmful to society may be moved to another site (*Sanhedrin* 47b). Exhumation is otherwise not allowed even to provide evidence in court (*Baba Batra* 154a; *Semachot* 4:12). The prophet (1 Samuel 12:15) warns against the exhumation of the dead (*Yebamot* 63b). [*See also* COFFIN, CORPSE, GRAVE, and MOURNING]

BURNS—A burn wound is called a *keviya* or *michva* (Leviticus 13:23). Such burns or granulating leprosy lesions are described in detail elsewhere.[1] If a person burns his hand while cleaning an oven, he puts his finger in his mouth (*Kelim* 8:10). A red-hot stove fell on the leg of a woman and she died as a result (*Chagigah* 4b). Red-hot coals placed on the chest or abdomen can lead to a person's death (*Baba Kamma* 27a). As a child, Moses put a hot coal in his mouth and burned his tongue (*Exodus Rabbah* 1:26).

---

1. F. Rosner (trans.), *Julius Preuss' Biblical and Talmudic Medicine* (Northvale, NJ: Jason Aronson, 1993), pp. 327–334.

BUTTER—The word *chemah* in modern Hebrew means "butter." However, in biblical Hebrew *chemah* probably refers to either butter, curd, buttermilk, or cream. According to Rabbi Chani-nah, the best butter is made from a hundredth part of the milk (i.e., from the creamiest part of its cream), medium quality from a fortieth part, and inferior butter from a twentieth (*Genesis Rabbah* 48:14). When David and his followers were languishing from hunger and thirst, they were given "honey and *chemah* and cheese of kine" (2 Samuel 17:29) in addition to flour and vegetables, suggesting a solid substance such as butter or curd. A solid substance also seems to be implied in the scriptural phrases "*Chemah* and honey shall he eat" (Isaiah 7:15) and "Smoother than *chemah* were the speeches of his mouth" (Psalms 55:22). However, in the Song of Deborah, when the exhausted Sisera asked for water, she gave him milk and *chemah* in a lordly bowl (Judges 5:25); and concerning Job, it is related that he bathed his feet in *chemah* (Job 29:6) and that there were "flowing streams of honey and *chemah*" (ibid., 20:17), implying that *chemah* is a liquid substance. Abraham treated his guests to *chemah* and milk (Genesis 18:8). Elsewhere, the Bible also speaks of "*chemah* of kine and milk of sheep" (Deuteronomy 32:14), and the "churning of milk which brings forth *chemah*" (Proverbs 30:33). At least some of these references probably refer to a refreshing artificially soured milk drink popular in ancient and medieval times, made by shaking milk in the skin-bottle in which it was stored and fermenting it with the stale milk adhering to the skin from previous processes.

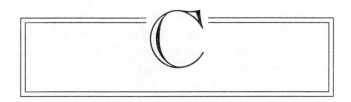

CABBAGE—Cabbage consumption is one of six things that help the sick to recover from illness (*Berachot* 44b and 57b; *Abodah Zarah* 29a). The white outer leaves of the cabbage are edible (*Uktzin* 2:7), as is the aftergrowth (*Shabbat* 51b), but not the roots of the cabbage (*Yebamot* 81b). When a cabbage grows, its tuber diminishes in size (*Lamentations Rabbah* 1:16:51). Cabbages are not considered wild vegetables (*Ecclesiastes Rabbah* 10:8:1; *Sheviit* 9:1). Cabbage stew shrinks and improves as it cooks (*Shabbat* 38a). Cabbage stalks were used for making crude whiskey (*Betzah* 3b; *Zevachim* 72b).

Farmers left cabbages in the corners of the fields for the poor (*Pesachim* 56b). Cabbage stalks do not contract nor impart ritual uncleanness (*Uktzin* 1:4). Cabbage stalks can be extremely large (*Ketubot* 111b).

"Cabbage head" is an expression for a dull or ugly person (*Yebamot* 118b; *Ketubot* 75a).

CALF—A calf embryo was once observed like a bean in its amniotic sac (*Jerushalmi Nazir* 7:5b). The kidney from a three-year-old calf (*Shabbat* 119b) and the leg from a third-born calf (*Megillah* 7a; *Taanit* 12b) are considered special delicacies. Abraham served his guests tender calf meat (Genesis 18:7). Two sages created a third grown calf by means of the "Book of Creation" and ate it (*Sanhedrin* 65b). A calf once ran away from the slaughterer (*Baba Metzia* 85a). Calves of bulls not used for breeding are sold for slaughtering (*Baba Metzia* 90b). Cheese is made by coagulating milk directly in the stomach of a calf (*Chullin* 8:5).

In antiquity, calves were used in idol worship (*Sanhedrin* 63b). King Jeroboam introduced calf worship (1 Kings 12:28). The Jews in the desert created the Golden Calf (Exodus 32:1ff.; Deuteronomy 9:16ff.).

CAMELS—The camel is not a kosher animal for human consumption (Leviticus 11:4; Deuteronomy 14:7). It chews its cud and has only canines for upper teeth (*Chullin* 59a). Its milk is forbidden for humans (*Bechorot* 66) but is good for their own young (*Yebamot* 114a). Camel hair was used to make garments (*Shabbat* 27a). The urine of camels is very dilute (*Bechorot* 7b). The camel's hump is well described (*Chullin* 9:2). The camel is modest when it copulates (*Genesis Rabbah* 76:7) but can become ferocious and kick other male camels close by (*Baba Batra* 93a; *Sanhedrin* 37b; *Shevuot* 34a). Epilepsy does not afflict camels (*Ecclesiastes Rabbah* 1:6), although a she-camel is described as blind in one eye, pregnant with twins, and carrying two barrels (*Lamentations Rabbah* 1:1:12; *Sanhedrin* 104b). Dead camels were flayed for their skins (*Chullin* 123b).

Camels were sometimes used as theater or circus performers (*Lamentations Rabbah, Proem* 17; 3:13; and 14:5). An Arab once performed magic with a camel (*Sanhedrin* 67b). Mostly, however, camels carried burdens such as flax or bundles of vine rods (*Baba Batra* 27b) and even coffins (*Moed Katan* 25b). Camels had pack saddles (*Kelim* 23:2) that produced sores by chafing. Rancid honey was applied on the sores and wounds (*Shabbat* 154b). Cutting a camel's tendons is forbidden as cruelty to animals (*Yebamot* 120b). One may not stuff or force-feed camels on the Sabbath but may put food in their mouths (*Shabbat* 155b). It is said that camels on the Sabbath have short tails because they walk on thorns and a long tail would become entangled in the thorns (*Shab-*

bat 77b). Thorns and thistles in the fields of Arabia were left there for camel fodder (*Shabbat* 144b; *Baba Batra* 156b).

Homiletically, "Many an old camel is laden with the hides of younger ones" means that many an old man survives the young (*Sanhedrin* 52b). "The ear of a camel is valuable" means that even a small part of a valuable object is valuable (*Shevuot* 11b). Passing under a camel or between two camels adversely affects one's study (*Horayot* 13b). A man never dreams of a camel going through the eye of a needle (*Berachot* 55b). Abraham's camels were always muzzled so they should not graze on other people's land (*Genesis Rabbah* 59:11). The "flying camel" (*Yebamot* 116a; *Makkot* 5a) perhaps refers to very fast traveling camels.

Camel drivers are suspected of immorality and of robbery (*Niddah* 14a). They often ride without saddles and therefore "warm their flesh" (ibid.). One should not, therefore, teach one's son to become a camel driver (*Kiddushin* 82a) like Pishon the camel driver (*Yebamot* 107b). Camel drivers travel in groups (*Sanhedrin* 112a). Since they are constantly traveling, they copulate with their wives only once in thirty days (*Ketubot* 61b).

Legally, the laws of firstlings do not apply to camels (*Bechorot* 5b). Camel drivers should not work on the intermediate days of the Festivals (*Moed Katan* 11b). A camel may be led out on the Sabbath with a pad tied to its afterbirth (*Shabbat* 54a) but not with a pad tied to its tail (ibid.). It may go forth with a bit, however (ibid., 51b). Camels are led by pulling their reins (*Eruvin* 35a), whereas an ass can be driven from behind (ibid., 52a).

CAPITAL PUNISHMENT—Capital punishment was very rarely carried out in Judaism because of very strict legal requirements such as premeditation and warning. A court that imposed it once in seventy years was branded a murderous tribunal (*Makkot* 7a). In the absence of the Sanhedrin, capital punishment cannot be implemented. However, he who would have been sentenced to strangulation either drowns or dies of suffocation or is strangled by heathens (*Ketubot* 30ab). Pestilence comes to the world as a death penalty at a time when Jewish tribunals cannot enforce capital punishment (*Avot* 5:8).

The punishment for adultery is the death of both partners by strangulation (Leviticus 20:10; *Sanhedrin* 11:1). Incest is punished by stoning or burning (Leviticus 20:11–12). A priest's daughter who plays harlot is sentenced to death by burning (Leviticus 21:9; *Sanhedrin* 52b). Murder and idolatry are capital offenses (*Sanhedrin* 15b and 60b). Adultery (ibid., 85), bestiality (ibid., 10a), and homosexuality are all capital offenses (Leviticus 20:13–16). A man called Yakim subjected himself to all four modes of execution (*Genesis Rabbah* 65:22).

A pregnant woman sentenced for a capital crime is executed immediately to spare her the agony of a long wait (*Arachin* 7a). If a person incurs two death penalties, he is executed by the more severe (*Sanhedrin* 81a). Capital cases require inquiry and examination (*Sanhedrin* 31b). A majority of at least two of the twenty-three judges must vote for a capital sentence (ibid.). [*See also* DEATH]

CARAWAY—Caraway is an ingredient of a compound mixture used to treat a cardiac or stomach disorder (*Abodah Zarah* 29a). It is also an ingredient in a remedy for a woman with puerperal infection (ibid.).

CASTRATION—Castration of men is biblically prohibited (Leviticus 22:24). This prohibition may also include women (*Shabbat* 110b–111a) although women during a certain generation were sterilized (*Yebamot* 17a). Orchiectomy is one form of castration (*Kiddushin* 25a). It is said that Ham emasculated his father Noah (Genesis 9:20–24; *Genesis Rabbah* 36:7; *Sanhedrin* 70a). Noahides are forbidden to practice castration (*Baba Metzia* 90b). One may not perform another act of castration on a castrate (*Tosefta Bechorot* 3:24).

The castration of animals is also biblically forbidden (Leviticus 22:24) and constitutes a punishable offense (*Tosefta Makkot* 5:6). Castrated animals may not be offered in the Temple (Leviticus 22:24). In Alexandria, cows and sows were castrated prior to being exported to prevent them from propagating abroad (*Sanhedrin* 93a; *Bechorot* 28b). One can castrate a cock by cutting off its crest (*Shabbat* 110b). Bees are sterilized by feeding them mustard (*Baba Batra* 80a). A hornet sting in the testicles can sterilize a man (*Sotah* 36a). [*See also AYLONIT*, EUNUCH, and STERILITY]

CATS—Eating food from which a cat has eaten makes one forget one's studies (*Horayot* 13b). Cats kill snakes and eat them (*Pesachim* 112b) and are, therefore, said to be immune to snake poison (*Shabbat* 128b; *Abodah Zarah* 30b). Cats also kill mice (*Baba Metzia* 97a) and may, therefore, be bred because they help to keep the house clean (*Baba Kamma* 80a). White cats are dangerous whereas black cats make good housepets (ibid., 80b). Weasels and cats occasionally team up to find prey (*Sanhedrin* 105a), which they claw (*Chullin* 52b). Only rarely do cats devour large hens (*Ketubot* 41b). Duck entrails are a delicacy for cats (*Betzah* 3a; *Shabbat* 142b).

A cat gives birth after fifty-two days (*Bechorot* 8a; *Genesis Rabbah* 20:4). We should learn modesty from the cat

(*Eruvin* 100b). The placenta of a black cat was once used for a demonic exorcism (*Berachot* 6a).

CAUTERIZATION—Cauterization of a wound can cause it to heal (*Tosefta Yebamot* 14:4). A man with cut arteries may survive if his wound is cauterized (*Yebamot* 120b). An animal with a compound bone fracture can be saved if the wound is cauterized (*Tosefta Chullin* 3:6). A veterinary surgeon once cauterized a she-ass and the baby was born with a brand mark on it (*Numbers Rabbah* 9:5).

CEDAR—Cedar wood, hyssop, and scarlet were added to the ashes of the red heifer (Numbers 19:6; *Parah* 3:10) and used for the purification of ritually unclean people. The same ingredients were used for the purification of lepers (*Exodus Rabbah* 17:1). A remedy for plethora, or an excess of blood, contains *shurbina*, a type of cedar (*Gittin* 68b).

The cedars of Lebanon are famous for their large size and symbolize strength and power (Judges 9:15; Isaiah 2:13; Psalms 29:5). Some cedar trees are wider than a wagon (*Bechorot* 57b). The cedar is the tallest of all trees and the hyssop is the smallest (*Numbers Rabbah* 19:3; *Exodus Rabbah* 17:2). Cedars have no crooked curves or excrescences (*Genesis Rabbah* 41:1). It is sinful to cut down the cedars of Lebanon (ibid., 24:11), although Noah planted cedars and cut them down (*Genesis Rabbah* 30:7). When the wicked Nebuchadnezzar died, the cedars of Lebanon rejoiced (*Lamentations Rabbah* 1:3:30). There are either ten types of cedar trees (*Taanit* 25b; *Baba Batra* 80b; *Rosh Hashanah* 23a) or twenty-four kinds of cedars, of which seven are especially fine (*Genesis Rabbah* 15:1; *Exodus Rabbah* 35:1). The cedar tree does not grow by the wayside, its stock does not grow new shoots, its roots are not many, but it offers resistance to the wind (*Taanit* 20a; *Sanhedrin* 106a). Cedar trees are converted to lumber (*Shabbat* 157a) and long poles were made of cedar wood (*Rosh Hashanah* 22b). The cedar does not yield fruit (*Taanit* 25b) other than its cones or pines (*Abodah Zarah* 14a; *Song of Songs Rabbah* 7:3:3).

CELIBACY—Celibacy is contrary to Judaism because Jews are commanded to procreate (Genesis 1:28). Even the High Priest must be married (*Yoma* 1:1). Eunuchs are consoled because of their inability to procreate (Isaiah 56:4). Rabbis and religious scholars are specifically instructed never to be without a wife (*Yoma* 18a). The biblical prophets Samuel (1 Samuel 8:2), Isaiah (Isaiah 8:18), Ezekiel (Ezekiel 24:18), and Hosea (Hosea 1:2) all had wives, as did Moses, the father of all prophets (Exodus 2:21). In the Tal-

mud, a single rabbi was celibate, excusing himself because he was totally immersed in and in love with Torah (*Yebamot* 63b). [*See also* ASCETICISM]

CESAREAN SECTION—The term "cesarean section" is derived from the fact that Julius Caesar or another Caesar was born by being extracted from his dead mother's abdomen. Postmortem cesarean section is discussed in the Talmud, where it is advocated in trying to save an unborn child (*Arachin* 1:4) even on the Sabbath. It was assumed that the fetus usually dies before the mother except following the violent death of an otherwise healthy pregnant woman (*Arachin* 7a). The Hebrew term for cesarean section is *yotzeh dophen* (literally: "exits from the wall").

A variety of laws relate to a baby born by cesarean section. Such a baby boy is not considered to be a firstborn in regard to inheritance and in regard to the obligation of redeeming the firstborn (*Bechorot* 8:2). Since the infant was not "born" in the normal manner (Deuteronomy 21:15), it is not entitled to a double portion of inheritance (ibid., 21:17). The baby is also not the "opener of the womb" (*peter rechem*) and is therefore exempt from being redeemed as a firstborn (Exodus 13:12). A baby born by cesarean section does not render its mother ritually unclean as in the case of a vaginal birth (*Leviticus Rabbah*

27:10; *Niddah* 5:1). Such a baby is not circumcised on the Sabbath. A baby extracted by cesarean section cannot become consecrated, nor can it cause consecration (*Bechorot* 42a; *Temurah* 17a).

Similar laws apply to animals extracted by cesarean section. Such animals are not considered to be firstborn (*Bechorot* 19a and 47a) and are not included in animal tithing (ibid., 57a). Such animals do not become holy nor cause holiness (*Temurah* 11a). Such animals are unfit for the altar (ibid., 28a) and disqualified from the sanctuary (*Zevachim* 71b, 84a, and 112b; *Bechorot* 45b). Valuations of animals born by cesarean section are also discussed in the Talmud (*Arachin* 18b).

Some talmudic commentators describe *yotzeh dophen* as a situation in which a woman's abdomen is opened by means of a caustic substance or a knife (Rashi, *Abodah Zarah* 28a; Rashi, *Chullin* 69b; R. Gersom, *Bechorot* 19a). The uterus then heals and the patient becomes pregnant again. Maimonides categorically dismisses this possibility since all such women died from the surgery (*Mishnah Commentary, Bechorot* 8:2). Preuss suggests that the Talmud may be referring to abdominal rather than uterine pregnancy with survival of both mother and child.[1]

---

1. F. Rosner (trans.), *Julius Preuss' Biblical and Talmudic Medicine* (Northvale, NJ: Jason Aronson, 1993), pp. 420–426.

CHAMOMILE—Dried chamomile has a purgative effect (*Chullin* 69b). Chamomile also heals some human sicknesses (*Berachot* 57b).

CHASTITY—Chastity is said to be a biblical requirement (*Tosefta Kiddushin* 1:4) based on the prohibition against fornication (Leviticus 19:29). A fence against sexual immorality leads to sanctity (*Leviticus Rabbah* 24:6). Jewish women in Egypt were rewarded for their chastity (*Numbers Rabbah* 9:14). The women of the generation of the wilderness were chaste (*Leviticus Rabbah* 2:1). Long before the Egyptian bondage of Jews, the matriarch Sarah and Joseph went to Egypt and guarded themselves against immorality (*Song of Songs Rabbah* 4:12:1). Israelites were also chaste and virtuous in the war of Midian (*Song of Songs Rabbah* 6:6:1). "The mandrakes give forth fragrance" (Song of Songs 7:14) is interpreted to refer to the youths of Israel who never felt the taste of sin (*Song of Songs Rabbah* 7:14:1; *Eruvin* 21b).

The Lord hates unchastity (*Sanhedrin* 93a). Conversing much with women may lead to unchastity (*Nedarim* 20a). The dove is the symbol of chastity (*Eruvin* 100b). The virgins of Israel reserve themselves for their husbands (*Pesachim* 87a). "Tamar put ashes on her head" (2 Samuel 13:19) means that she set up a great fence about chastity (*Sanhedrin* 21a). One should be careful to avoid even unchaste thoughts (ibid., 45a). One must struggle against one's desires and take preventive measures, if necessary, to avoid unchastity (*Moed Katan* 17a). Early marriage is a deterrent to illicit sexual relations. [*See also* MASTURBATION, VIRGINITY, INCEST, ADULTERY, and MARRIAGE]

CHEEK—To strike someone on the cheek is an insult (Job 16:10). The term "full cheeks" or "a mouthful" (*melo lugmav*) refers to the amount of fluid one holds in one cheek or in half of the mouth (*Jerushalmi Yoma* 8:44) or to a full mouthful (*Yoma* 80a). The word *nashak*, or "kiss," can refer to a kiss on the cheek (Ibn Ezra, Song of Songs 1:1). Human facial features include fully formed cheeks (*Niddah* 23b). The nose and the cheeks can be sufficient to identify a mutilated corpse (*Jerushalmi Yebamot* 16:15). The cheekbones become prominent in old age (*Ecclesiastes Rabbah* 12:2). The cheeks also darken in the elderly (*Shabbat* 151b). Priestly gifts prescribed in the Bible (Deuteronomy 18:3) include the shoulder, the cheeks, and the maw of slaughtered animals (*Yebamot* 99b). [*See also* JAWS]

CHEESE—Cheese was prepared by curdling milk with rennet (*Abodah Zarah* 35a), and if one sets milk and makes cheese on the Sabbath one transgresses the prohibition against performing work on the Sabbath (*Shabbat* 95a). The making of cheese on Festivals is also forbidden (*Shabbat* 135a; *Pesachim* 65a). Cheese was also prepared by coagulating milk directly in the stomach of an animal (*Chullin* 116a), and if a man curdles milk with the skin of the stomach of an animal that was validly slaughtered and it imparts its flavor to the milk, it is forbidden because of the prohibition of milk and meat (*Chullin* 116a). Milk was also curdled in the sap of the leaves or the root of fruit trees (*Orlah* 1:7; *Niddah* 8b), such as the sap of unripe figs (*Abodah Zarah* 35b).

The Midrash and the Talmud both state that it is impossible to tell whether "white" cheese came from the milk of a white or black goat (*Lamentations Rabbah* 1:1:9; *Bechorot* 8b). Liquid milk can turn solid (*Tohorot* 3:1). The serum watery part of milk that is separated from the coagulable part or curd in the process of making cheese (i.e., whey) is called *mey halav* (*Machshirin* 6:5) and *nisyube dechalba* (*Baba Metzia* 68b), which literally means "milk water."

The milk water is considered to be one of the ingredients of *kutach* or *kameka*, which is a "sour spicy side dish" used by many Oriental peoples. In the Talmud, Babylonian *kutach* is mentioned as a distinctive specialty: "It closes up the stomach [or the heart] because of its content of whey; it blinds the eyes because of its salt content [into which Sodom salt might easily have become admixed]; and it weakens the entire body because of the mold of the flour that is also contained therein" (*Pesachim* 42a). Occasionally, it also incorporated small pieces of sourdough. When Rabbi Gaza came to Palestine and prepared some Babylonian *kutach*, all the invalids from Palestine asked him for it (*Shabbat* 145b).

The biblical phrase "and bring these ten cheeses" (1 Samuel 17:18) can be understood literally, but the following statement of Job probably refers to the formation of the embryo within the womb: "Hast Thou not poured me out as milk and curdled me like cheese?" (Job 10:10). An interesting parable about the creation of the world in which milk and cheese are prominently mentioned is cited three times in the Midrash (*Genesis Rabbah* 4:7 and 14:5; *Leviticus Rabbah* 14:9).

The cheese of heathens is prohibited because they smear its surface with rennet (*Chullin* 116b; *Song of Songs Rabbah* 1:2:1) or with fat of swine (*Abodah Zarah* 35b; *Makkot* 21a; *Betzah* 28b; *Ketubot* 61n) or because it is curdled with sour wine, which is forbidden (*Abodah Zarah* 35b). Similarly, Bithynian cheese is forbidden because the majority of Bithynian calves are slaughtered as sacrifices to idols and the rennet of these calves is used in preparing the cheese (*Abodah Zarah* 34b). It is not proper to buy wine, milk, cheese, and certain other products in Syria

unless it be from a reliable dealer, lest the product was adulterated (*Abodah Zarah* 39b).

CHEWING—Clean (i.e., kosher) animals chew their cud and have cloven hoofs (Leviticus 11:3; Deuteronomy 14:6). The teeth are hard and serve for biting and chewing (*Abodah Zarah* 28a). We are told to chew well with the teeth, i.e., to eat slowly (*Shabbat* 152a).

CHICKEN SOUP—Although the Bible and Talmud do not discuss the therapeutic efficacy of chicken soup, Moses Maimonides states that boiled chicken soup neutralizes body constitution and is an excellent food.[1] Chicken soup is a medication for the beginning of leprosy and fattens the body substance of the emaciated and those convalescing from illness. Turtledoves increase memory, improve intellect, and sharpen the senses. The consumption of fowl, continues Maimonides, is beneficial for feebleness, hemiplegia, facial paresis, and the pain of edema. It also increases sexual potential. House pigeons that graze in the streets increase natural body heat. Soup made from the bird called *kanaber* loosens cramps of colic. Maimonides further states that chicken testicles provide excellent nourishment for a weakened or convalescent individual. Pigeon eggs are good aphrodisiacs, especially when cooked with onion or turnip. Finally, soup made from an old chicken is of benefit against chronic fevers that develop from white bile, and it also aids the cough that is called asthma. Maimonides also advises the consumption of lean chicken meat for sufferers of asthma. Other small fowl, such as the turtledove, are also useful. The soup of chickens or fat hens is said to be an effective remedy for asthma. The method of preparation of the chicken soup and the ingredients are also described. An enema with sap of linseed, fenugreek, or both, with oil, chicken fat, and an admixture of beet juice, is strongly endorsed for the treatment of asthma. Maimonides further recommends the meat of hens or roosters (or chickens or pullets) and their broth, because this type of fowl has the property of rectifying corrupted humors, especially the black humor (i.e., black bile, an excess of which was thought to cause melancholy), so much so that physicians mention that chicken broth is beneficial in leprosy. It thus seems evident that Maimonides, in the twelfth century, gave scientific respectability to what the proverbial Jewish mother has always known: that chicken soup can help cure a variety of ailments.[2]

---

1. R. Rosner, *Medical Encyclopedia of Moses Maimonides* (Northvale, NJ: Jason Aronson, 1998), pp. 55–56.
2. F. Rosner, "Therapeutic Efficacy of Chicken Soup," *Chest*, vol. 78 (1980), pp. 672–674.

CHICKENS—The hen or chicken is a clean (i.e., kosher) bird and requires ritual slaughtering (*Chullin* 4a, 16b, and 27a). If a brooding chicken leaves its nest, its heat remains intact for three more days (*Pesachim* 55b). Chicken is usually less expensive than beef (*Chullin* 84a). The specially prepared "chicken of Rav Abba" was good for him but not for others (*Shabbat* 145b). Chickens are found in chicken houses (*Pesachim* 55b). Hen feces are not harmful to man if accidentally ingested (*Chullin* 3:5; *Tosefta Chullin* 3:19). One should not eat chicken excessively lest one develop a greedy appetite for it (*Pesachim* 114a). An egg can hatch chickens but not an egg found in the hen (*Betzah* 6b). Eggs found in a hen slaughtered on a Festival may also be consumed on the Festival (*Betzah* 6b). [*See also* BIRDS, GEESE, DOVES, and PIGEONS]

CHILDBIRTH—The divine curse on Eve resulted in women having pain in giving birth (Genesis 3:16). Thus labor pains are variously described by the prophets as pangs (Isaiah 13:8), pain (ibid., 27:7), moaning (Jeremiah 4:31), gasping (Isaiah 42:14), and crying out (Isaiah 26:17). A woman kneels to give birth (*Berachot* 34b) and presses her heels against her thighs (*Yebamot* 103a). She also presses her hands against her hips (Jeremiah 30:6). This kneeling position of both humans (1 Samuel 4:19) and animals (Job 39:3) is mentioned both in the Bible and in the Talmud (*Shabbat* 54b; *Niddah* 31b; *Baba Batra* 16a). Mountain goats deliver this way without pain (Job 39:3). Only rarely does a woman deliver without pain (Isaiah 66:7). More often, she cries out one hundred times during labor (*Leviticus Rabbah* 27:7) and sometimes suffers agonizing pains during childbirth (*Yebamot* 65b). The pains of a female birth are more intense than those of a male birth because a female baby emerges by turning her face upwards (*Niddah* 31a).

When a woman bends to deliver her child, her thighs grow cold like stone (*Sotah* 11b). A woman in difficult labor may not be able to walk and needs to be supported under the armpits (*Oholot* 7:4). Soothing words by another woman present at the delivery are offered to help the parturient woman during childbirth (*Sotah* 11b; *Deuteronomy Rabbah* 2:11). Some women sat on a *mashber*, or birthstool, to give birth (*Shabbat* 129a; Isaiah 37:3; *Arachin* 7a). Even an animal sat on a birthstool (*Midrash Psalms* 42:1). Another term for birthstool is *ovnayim* (Exodus 1:16). Other meanings of this word are discussed by Preuss.[1] Birth on a birthstool or on one's knees is described in the Bible (Genesis 30:2 and 50:23; Job 3:12).

Normally, birth is accompanied by bleeding although, rarely, a dry birth may occur (*Keritot* 10a; *Niddah* 42b). A woman in labor is in danger (*Ecclesiastes Rabbah* 3:2) and therefore a fire

may be made (*Eruvin* 79b) and oil procured on the Sabbath (*Shabbat* 28b) on her behalf. Women may die in childbirth (*Moed Katan* 28a) as a result of a variety of causes (*Shabbat* 31b; *Ecclesiastes Rabbah* 3:2). In fact, there was a much greater chance of a woman dying than surviving childbirth in ancient times (*Exodus Rabbah* 46:2). If the fetus is endangering the mother during difficult labor, one performs an embryotomy to try to save her life (*Oholot* 7:6). Three famous women in the Bible experienced hard labor and died in childbirth: Jacob's wife Rachel, the wife of Phinehas, and Saul's daughter Michal (*Genesis Rabbah* 82:7). Queen Esther is also said to have died in childbirth (*Megillah* 13a). If a woman dies in childbirth, one performs a postmortem cesarean section to try to save the baby (*Arachin* 7a). Midwives helped deliver women in labor (Exodus 1:15).

A newly delivered woman is ritually unclean (Leviticus 12:1–8) and must undergo a process of purification (*Negaim* 14:3; *Yebamot* 74b). She used to bring bird sacrifices to the Temple (*Sheviit* 8:8; *Shekalim* 2:5) even for a doubtful birth (*Niddah* 54b; *Nazir* 29a). Her blood after childbirth conveys ritual uncleanness (*Eduyot* 5:4; *Niddah* 34a, 35b, and 36a). She also brought a burnt offering (*Menachot* 48b and 91b; *Chullin* 41b; *Temurah* 14b). The reason she brings a sin offering of birds is because during her labor pains, she may have sworn impetuously never again to cohabit with her husband (*Niddah* 31b). If a woman brought her sin offering after childbirth and then died, her heirs must bring her burnt offering (*Kiddushin* 13b; *Zevachim* 5a). For the first three days after childbirth, a woman is considered dangerously ill and the Sabbath must be desecrated, if necessary, on her behalf (*Shabbat* 129a). She may also wear shoes on Yom Kippur (*Yoma* 78b) and wash her clothes on the intermediate days of Festivals (*Moed Katan* 14a).

Twin births are described in the Talmud (*Yebamot* 98b), including the birth of one live and one dead twin (*Oholot* 7:5). Rapid severance of the umbilical cord is necessary to prevent twins from endangering each other (*Shabbat* 129b). The Israelite women in Egypt gave birth to sextuplets (*Exodus Rabbah* 1:8). So did the wife of Oved-Edom (*Berachot* 63b). Premature births after six months of pregnancy can be viable (*Yebamot* 42a). An eight-month pregnancy was thought to produce a nonviable child (*Tosefta Shabbat* 15:5), which is now known to be untrue. Protracted labor can continue for three or even up to forty or fifty days (*Niddah* 36b). Pains may cease while bleeding continues or both may cease for a day or longer and then recur (*Niddah* 37b).

1. F. Rosner (trans.), *Julius Preuss' Biblical and Talmudic Medicine* (Northvale, NJ: Jason Aronson, 1993), p. 394.

CHILDLESSNESS—Infertility is a curse and fertility is a blessing (Exodus 23:26; Deuteronomy 7:14). A person without children is considered as if excommunicated by heaven (*Tosafot, Pesachim* 113b). A barren woman might prefer death to childlessness (Genesis 30:1). A childless man is regarded as if dead (*Nedarim* 64b; *Abodah Zarah* 5a; *Genesis Rabbah* 71:6; *Exodus Rabbah* 5:1). The key to childbirth is one of three keys that God Himself administers and does not entrust to an emissary (*Taanit* 2a; *Sanhedrin* 113a). A number of barren women are described in the Bible, all of whom eventually had children: Sarah (Genesis 11:30), Rebecca (Genesis 25:21), Rachel (Genesis 29:31), the wife of Manoach (Judges 13:2), Hannah (1 Samuel 1:2), the woman from Shunam (2 Kings 4:14), and Ruth (*Ruth Rabbah* 7:13). The sages say that these women were at first barren because God desires the prayers of the righteous (*Yebamot* 64a). A number of additional reasons for the matriarchs' barrenness are also cited (*Song of Songs Rabbah* 2:21). Male barrenness is also recognized (*Nedarim* 91a).

Abraham used to pray for barren women and they conceived (*Genesis Rabbah* 39:11). God remembers barren women as he did for Sarah (*Leviticus Rabbah* 27:14), Hannah (*Numbers Rabbah* 14:1), and the woman from Shunam (*Deuteronomy Rabbah* 10:3). God blesses the Jews (Deuteronomy

7:14) by saying there shall be no male or female barren among them (*Deuteronomy Rabbah* 3:6). The Lord also opens His good treasure (Deuteronomy 28:12), which means He will keep the key to barrenness locked up (*Deuteronomy Rabbah* 7:6). Just as God makes barren women fertile, so the righteous can make barren women fertile (*Song of Songs Rabbah* 1:4:2). The prophet sings about barrenness (Isaiah 54:1), although one weeps and mourns for a person who died childless (*Moed Katan* 27b). Childless women are like prisoners in their houses because of the disgrace they feel to be so afflicted (*Genesis Rabbah* 71:1). Childless couples may have marital relations even in years of famine to help them overcome their childlessness (*Taanit* 11a). If a man lives with a wife for ten years and she bears him no children, he should take another wife (*Yebamot* 64a), although male infertility could be the cause; polygamy was then allowed. Manoach and Hannah disagreed among themselves as to who was the infertile partner in their childless marriage (*Numbers Rabbah* 10:5). Some rabbinic scholars became impotent because of long scholarly discourses (*Yebamot* 64b). The wife of a man who dies childless must be married by the deceased husband's brother in a levirate marriage to preserve the name of the deceased (Deuteronomy 25:5–6).

CHILLS—If one has chills following bloodletting, one should make a fire to warm oneself (*Shabbat* 129a). Chills may lead to a person's death (ibid.). For a chill, one should eat fat meat broiled on the coals with undiluted wine (*Gittin* 67b).

CINNAMON—Cinnamon is a very fine spice (Song of Songs 4:14) and is used as a perfume (Proverbs 7:17). Cinnamon placed in the mouth makes the breath pleasant (*Shabbat* 65a). Cinnamon was one of the ingredients Moses used to prepare the anointment oil (Exodus 30:23). Cinnamon grew so abundantly in the land of Israel that goats and deer used to eat it (*Genesis Rabbah* 65:17; *Esther Rabbah* 3:4; *Song of Songs Rabbah* 4:14:1). The cinnamon tree provided logs for Jerusalem fires that, when lit, emitted fragrance throughout the land (*Shabbat* 63a).

CIRCUMCISION—Since ancient times, circumcision (*brit milah*) has been a holy precept, as important as all the other commandments combined (*Nedarim* 32a). The term *brit*, or covenant (between God and Abraham), occurs thirteen times in the seventeenth chapter of Genesis. Circumcision is an everlasting covenant (Genesis 17:7) for which Jews martyred themselves during times of persecution (*Shabbat* 120a). Abraham is not called "complete" until after his circumcision (*Tosefta Nedarim* 2:5). Lack of circumcision represents an imperfection. Hence, the phrases "uncircumcised lips" (Exodus 6:12), referring to a poor speaker, and "uncircumcised ears" (Isaiah 6:10) and "uncircumcised heart" (Leviticus 26: 41). To "circumcise the foreskin of the heart" (Deuteronomy 10:16; Jeremiah 4:4) means to abandon evil and imperfection. "Uncircumcised" also means "contemptible" or "profane" (Judges 14:3; 1 Samuel 17:26; Ezekiel 31:18; Isaiah 52:1). A newly circumcised boy is called a bridegroom (Exodus 4:25; *Nedarim* 5:3 and 32a), a feast is held to celebrate the joyous occasion (*Ketubot* 8a; *Deuteronomy Rabbah* 9:1), and special benedictions are recited (*Tosefta Berachot* 7:12).

God commanded Abraham to circumcise every male child on the eighth day of life (Genesis 17:10ff.). At age ninety-nine years he circumcised himself, his thirteen-year-old son Ishmael (Genesis 17:23–27) and, a year later, his eight-day-old son Isaac (Genesis 21:4). The obligation of circumcision rests primarily on the father although women are allowed to do so (*Shabbat* 134a) as exemplified by Zipporah, wife of Moses (Exodus 4:25). In ancient Egypt, according to legend, only the tribe of Levi practiced circumcision (*Exodus Rabbah* 19:5). Joshua later circumcised all those born in the desert (Joshua 5:2–8) in order for them to be able to eat the paschal

offering, since no uncircumcised person can eat it (Exodus 12:48).

The Bible does not discuss the technical aspects of *milah*, or ritual circumcision, but the nineteenth chapter of tractate *Shabbat* in both the Babylonian and Jerusalem Talmuds is replete with details. The three parts of *milah* are the removal of the foreskin (*chittuch*), the uncovering of the corona (*periyah*) by the tearing of the inner preputial membrane (established by Joshua—*Yebamot* 72b), and the sucking of the wound (*metzitzah*). The first two acts are essential. If the third is omitted, the circumcision is still valid. Circumcision instruments include a stone (Exodus 4:25), *sakkin* or large knife (*Abodah Zarah* 26b; *Arachin* 7a), *izmel* or small knife (*Jerushalmi Shabbat* 19:16), a sharp stone or knife (Joshua 5:2; *Genesis Rabbah* 31:8) or any sharp-edged object except a reed (*Chullin* 16b). The Talmud speaks of a street of circumcisers (*Jerushalmi Eruvin* 5:22) and Rabbis Judah and Judan, who were ritual circumcisers (*Shabbat* 130b; *Jerushalmi Rosh Hashanah* 3:59; *Jerushalmi Megillah* 1:71). Nowadays, a double-edged knife is often used. After the circumcision, a bandage (*ispelanit*) with ground caraway is applied to the wound. The baby is washed or bathed before and after the circumcision and again on the third day. The normal timing of circumcision is on the eighth day (Leviticus 12:3), even if it falls on the Sabbath, except for a baby born by cesarean section, who is then circumcised on Sunday, the ninth day (*Shabbat* 136a). The circumcision is preferably done in the morning (Genesis 22:4), but not before sunrise (*Megillah* 2:4). The child must be healthy for circumcision to be performed. The procedure is postponed if the baby has fever (*Shabbat* 137a), jaundice (ibid., 134a), or a bleeding disorder whose genetic transmission is accurately depicted in the Talmud (*Yebamot* 64b). Further details about circumcision are available elsewhere.[1,2] [*See also* HEMOPHILIA and EPISPASM]

------

1. F. Rosner (trans.), *Julius Preuss' Biblical and Talmudic Medicine* (Northvale, NJ: Jason Aronson, 1993), pp. 240–248.
2. C. Roth (ed.), *Encyclopedia Judaica*, vol. 5 (Jerusalem: Keter, 1971), pp. 567–576.

CITRON—Lemons and citrons have aphrodisiac properties and were not consumed by the High Priest on the eve of the Day of Atonement, to prevent sleep and a nocturnal emission (*Yoma* 18a–b). Lemonade can cure a patient of dysentery (*Leviticus Rabbah* 37:2). A citron tree is considered as a tree for certain laws (e.g., fourth-year fruit or *orlah*) and as a vegetable for other laws (e.g., tithes) (*Bikkurim* 2:6; *Rosh Hashanah* 14b). A citron tree grows by means of all waters (*Kiddushin* 3a). A citron is cut with a knife for consumption (*Abodah Zarah* 76b).

The citron or *etrog* is one of the four species carried together on the Tabernacles Festival (Leviticus 23:40). The *etrog* is a goodly fruit (ibid.; *Sukkah* 31a), meaning the taste of the tree and the fruit is identical, the fruit remains on the tree from year to year, and the tree grows near the water (*Genesis Rabbah* 15:7; *Leviticus Rabbah* 30:8; *Sukkah* 43a). The fruit of the tree of knowledge that Adam and Eve ate is said to be the citron or *etrog* (*Genesis Rabbah* 15:7 and 20:8). One can purchase an *etrog* (*Betzah* 29b) or receive one as a gift (*Baba Batra* 137a; *Bechorot* 31b). A stolen or withered *etrog* is invalid for Holiday use (*Sukkah* 34b). A swollen, decayed, pickled, boiled, black (Ethiopian), white, or speckled *etrog* is also invalid (*Sukkah* 36a). After the Holiday, the *etrog* is consumed (ibid., 46b; *Betza* 30b; *Leviticus Rabbah* 37:2). A heretic was once pelted with *etrogs* (*Sukkah* 48b).

CLIMATOTHERAPY—Changing one's place of residence averts misfortune (*Genesis Rabbah* 44:12). The city of Sephoris is recommended for its clean air since it is located at a high altitude (*Ketubot* 103b). An open town with gardens and parks and fresh air is healthier than the big city (*Genesis Rabbah* 64:3). A similar statement is made by Maimonides in his *Treatise on Asthma*,[1] where he describes the various climates of the Middle

East. He asserts that the dry Egyptian climate is efficacious for people who suffer from asthma. He also states that "the concern for clean air is the foremost rule in preserving the health of one's body and soul."[2]

---

1. F. Rosner, *Moses Maimonides' Treatise on Asthma* (Haifa: Maimonides Research Institute, 1994).

2. Ibid., p. 109.

COFFIN—The biblical *aron*, or coffin (Genesis 50:26), and the talmudic *aron* (*Oholot* 9:15) may not refer to coffins in the modern sense. A wooden coffin (*Moed Katan* 8b) and a stone coffin (*Jerushalmi Moed Katan* 1:80) are described. Joseph was placed in a bronze coffin that sank in the Nile river (*Sotah* 13a). Corpses were first placed in caves; when the flesh decomposed, the bones were placed in a box of cedar wood (*Jerushalmi Moed Katan* 1:80). A coffin and shrouds are prepared to bury the deceased (*Shabbat* 151a). These may be donated or purchased (*Yebamot* 74a). Burial may be postponed overnight in order to prepare a coffin (*Sanhedrin* 47a). Coffins may be broad below and narrow above (*Oholot* 9:15). A body is sometimes transported from one place to another for burial (*Moed Katan* 25a; *Sanhedrin* 68a). Coffins of people placed in a ban have a large stone put on them by order of the court (*Moed Katan* 15a; *Pesachim* 64b; *Berachot* 19a; *Eduyot* 5:6).

At a funeral, mourners line up about the coffin (*Sanhedrin* 68a). Coffins are borne by bier bearers (*Berachot* 17b). Others follow the bier (ibid., 42b). A king may follow the bier of his deceased relative (*Sanhedrin* 20a), but not too closely (ibid., 18a). Coffin bearers should not tie their shoelaces (*Genesis Rabbah* 96). The public is distressed when they see a bier (*Moed Katan* 24b). [*See also* BURIAL, CORPSE, DEATH, and GRAVE]

COHABITATION—Cohabitation is a conjugal right of a Jewish wife (Exodus 21:10). A man may not vow to deny her that right (*Ketubot* 61b), nor should she refuse him sexual intercourse (ibid., 63b). One should not cohabit while fully clothed (ibid., 48a); out in an open field (*Sanhedrin* 46a); while one is intoxicated (*Nedarim* 20b); in a sitting or standing position; near a light; during the daytime (*Niddah* 17a; *Pesachim* 112b; *Gittin* 70a; *Shabbat* 86a; *Genesis Rabbah* 64:5); or after bloodletting (*Gittin* 70a), for it can be dangerous (*Niddah* 17a; *Shabbat* 129b). Cohabitation immediately after defecation (*Gittin* 70a) or bloodletting (*Leviticus Rabbah* 16:1) results in epileptic or leprous children (*Ketubot* 77b). So, too, if parents cohabit with their young child in the room (*Pesachim* 112b). Young married couples taste the pleasure of cohabitation (*Sanhedrin* 19b). It is most pleasurable in the month of Tevet (approximately December) (*Megillah* 13a).

Cohabitation, unlike food and beverage, is not absorbed by the body but the body derives pleasure therefrom (*Berachot* 67b). It is beneficial in small amounts but harmful in large amounts (*Gittin* 70a). Cohabitation is preferred at night (*Genesis Rabbah* 64:5; *Ruth Rabbah* 2:16). One should cohabit near sunrise (*Leviticus Rabbah* 4:3). Excessive indulgence in coitus weakens the body (*Berachot* 57b), accelerates the deterioration of body powers (*Ketubot* 7:10), and causes premature aging (*Shabbat* 152a). Cohabitation is harmful during the first trimester of pregnancy but beneficial during the last trimester (*Niddah* 31a). It is also harmful to cohabit immediately upon returning from a journey, after bloodletting or rising from an illness, and on being released from prison (*Avot de Rabbi Nathan* 34:7). One should, however, cohabit with one's wife before setting out on a journey (*Yebamot* 62b). Cohabitation with one's wife is permitted naturally (vaginally) or unnaturally (anally) (*Ketubot* 46a), but children born from the latter may be defective (*Nedarim* 20a; *Kallah Rabbati* 1:13). A man should not compel his wife to cohabit with him. If he does, he will have unworthy children (*Eruvin* 100b).

Cohabitation is prohibited during the week of mourning for a close relative (*Moed Katan* 24a), during the days of leprosy quarantine (*Negaim* 14:2), during a famine (Genesis 41:50; *Genesis Rabbah* 31:12), and on the Day of Atonement (*Yoma* 8:1). It is forbidden to cohabit with one's menstruant wife (Leviticus 18:19 and 20:18). It is an immoral heathen practice (ibid., 18:3) and if a Jew does so, he is flogged (*Makkot* 3:1). Such cohabitation results in leprous children (*Leviticus Rabbah* 15:5). Cohabitation is also biblically prohibited with a variety of relatives (Leviticus 18:1–5) and others. Noah was forbidden to cohabit in the Ark (*Genesis Rabbah* 31:12 and 34:7). To have forbidden sexual relations is to "uncover a woman's nakedness" (Leviticus 18 and 20).

Three women use an absorbent tampon during cohabitation to prevent conception: a minor, a pregnant woman, and a nursing woman (*Yebamot* 12b). Fetal sex is determined at the time of cohabitation and depends on whether the man or his wife emits seed first.[1] He who desires male offspring should cohabit twice in succession (*Eruvin* 100b). During cohabitation, the penis can become entangled in the woman's pubic hair (*Gittin* 6b; *Sanhedrin* 21a). A sterile woman (*aylonit*) may suffer pain during cohabitation (*Yebamot* 80b). For coitus interruptus, see ONANISM and CONTRACEPTION. [*See also* ADULTERY and MARRIAGE, FORBIDDEN]

---

1. F. Rosner, *Medicine in the Bible and the Talmud*, 2nd ed. (Hoboken, NJ: Ktav and Yeshiva University Press, 1995), pp. 248–253.

COLLYRIA—Remedies for eye disorders described in the Talmud include collyria, which are pastes, usually mixed with a liquid and rubbed into an ointment (*Chullin* 111b). The liquid can be water (*Shabbat* 8:1 and 77b) or a liquid with healing properties such as wine (*Niddah* 19b; *Shabbat* 109b); human spittle (*Baba Batra* 126b), especially from a fasting person (*Shabbat* 108b); human milk (*Tosefta Shabbat* 8:8); dew (*Jerushalmi Shabbat* 8:11), or eggwhite (*Shabbat* 77b). The ingredients of the paste or basic collyrium are not listed in the Talmud, which only mentions that a collyrium to which flour was added does not have to be destroyed before the Passover festival (*Tosefta Pesachim* 2:3) as does all other sourdough. A collyrium that contains bitter substances is described (*Chullin* 111b). One may steep a collyrium on the eve of the Sabbath and place it upon the eyes on the Sabbath (*Shabbat* 108b) and the salve heals all day (ibid., 18a). The famous collyrium with which Mar Samuel healed Rabbi Judah the Prince's eye ailment is known by its name only (*Shabbat* 108b; *Baba Metzia* 85b). Some heathens tasted collyria before applying them to the eyes (*Jerushalmi Abodah Zarah* 2:40). Others added poisons to collyria (*Niddah* 55b). [*See also* EYES]

COMPRESS—Warm compresses are applied to a wound after a splinter is removed (*Abodah Zarah* 28b). They are also applied to the site of a scorpion bite (ibid.) and on the abdomen for abdominal pain (*Shabbat* 40b). Eye compresses using green leaves of certain herbs are applied to an inflamed eye even on the Sabbath (*Shabbat* 109a). Some eye compresses are made from bread soaked in wine (*Shabbat* 108b). A compress of fig cakes was applied to King Hezekiah's skin disease and he recovered (Isaiah 38:21). After their wool is shorn off, ewes have compresses saturated in oil placed on their foreheads so that they do not catch cold (*Shabbat* 54b). [*See also* BANDAGE, COLLYRIA, and PLASTERS AND POULTICES]

CONSTIPATION—The Talmud states that a citron, rash, and egg yolk are very constipating (*Shabbat* 108b). An Egyptian concoction made of barley, safflower, and salt acts as a laxative for those with constipation and as a binding agent for those with diarrhea (*Shabbat* 110a; *Pesachim* 42b). Dropsy arises from the withholding of one's bowels (*Berachot* 25a). [*See also* LAXATIVES and DIARRHEA]

CONSUMPTION—The biblical *schachefet* (Leviticus 26:16; Deuteronomy 28:22) refers to consumption or phthisis (tuberculosis). The biblical commentary known as *Sifra* (loc. cit.) states that with this illness, the body dries out completely. A patient with consumption was treated with warm animal milk (*Baba Kamma* 80a). If the lungs of a slaughtered animal became so dry that they crumble between the fingers (caseation?), the animal is not fit for human consumption (*Chullin* 46b).

CONTRACEPTION—Suckling of a newborn for two years or more is an ancient method of contraception alluded to in the Bible (Hosea 1:8). Another method described in the Talmud is an oral permanent sterilizing potion (*Tosefta Yebamot* 8:4; *Yebamot* 65b) whose exact ingredients are detailed (*Shabbat* 110a). This potion was used to cure jaundice and gonorrhea (*Shabbat* 109b). The modern diaphragm is known in the Talmud as *moch*, or absorbent tampon, and was used by minors, pregnant women, and nursing women to prevent conception (*Yebamot* 12b). Two other contraceptive methods described in the Talmud are twisting movements following cohabitation (*Ketubot* 37a) and the rhythm or safe period method (*Niddah* 31b). A woman is said to play harlot if she "turns over" following coitus to prevent conception (*Ketubot* 37a). A woman is entitled to receive her marriage settlement (*ketubah*) if her husband imposes a vow on her to produce violent movements immediately after intercourse to avoid conception (*Ketubot* 72a).

The Jewish legal attitude toward contraception is discussed in detail elsewhere.[1,2] Essentially, contraception is not allowed unless a medical or psychiatric threat to the mother would ensue from her becoming pregnant. The duty of procreation, coupled with the wife's conjugal rights, militates against the use of the condom, coitus interruptus, or abstinence. Where pregnancy hazard exists and where rabbinic sanction for the use of birth control is obtained, oral contraceptives or the diaphragm are the preferred methods.

1. F. Rosner, *Modern Medicine and Jewish Ethics* (Hoboken, NJ: Ktav and Yeshiva University Press, 1991), pp. 69–83.
2. D.M. Feldman, *Marital Relations, Birth Control, and Abortion in Jewish Law* (New York: Schocken, 1974).

CORPSE—Contact with a corpse ritually defiles a person (Numbers 19:11; *Shabbat* 83b; *Pesachim* 14a; *Yoma* 6b; *Betzah* 10a). A priest may not touch a corpse except when burying his close relative (Leviticus 21:1–3). A corpse found in the field is buried by the people of the closest city (Deuteronomy 21:1ff.), who are considered responsible for the death. If a corpse is burned (*Niddah* 28a) or decomposes in water (*Lamentations Rabbah* 4:17), the skeleton remains. A corpse was once boiled to ascertain the number of bones in the human body (*Bechorot*

45a). The nose and face may be sufficient to identify a mutilated corpse (*Baba Metzia* 27b; *Yebamot* 120a). Other body identification marks may also be seen (*Genesis Rabbah* 65:20 and 73:5; *Leviticus Rabbah* 33:5). After three days, a corpse putrefies and can no longer be identified (*Yebamot* 120a). A corpse becomes offensive when it begins to putrefy (*Pesachim* 54b). Incense was put under corpses to neutralize the odor (*Moed Katan* 27b; *Tosefta Niddah* 9:16). They were placed on sand to slow their putrefaction (*Jerushalmi Shabbat* 4:6). For the same reason they were placed face down (*Abodah Zarah* 20a) and all their orifices were stopped up (*Semachot* 1:1ff.).

Corpses were washed and anointed (*Shabbat* 23:5). They were guarded to prevent weasels and mice from feeding on them (*Shabbat* 151b; *Genesis Rabbah* 24:12). The pale color of corpses (*Ketubot* 103b; *Abodah Zarah* 20b) contrasts with the green color of a person who suddenly sees a corpse (*Shabbat* 129a). Corpses may be moved on the Sabbath from the sun to the shade (*Shabbat* 43b) and from the middle to the side of the road (*Eruvin* 17b). Shrouds and a coffin are prepared for a corpse (*Shabbat* 150b). Corpses are buried the same day as death, if possible, and not kept overnight unless proper funeral arrangements take longer (*Sanhedrin* 46a–47a). Corpses were first placed in caves

until the flesh decomposed, at which times the bones were gathered and put in a cedar box (*Jerushalmi Moed Katan* 1:80). Even corpses of one's enemy were at least thrown into a pit (Jeremiah 41:9). The decomposition of corpses including the flesh, hair, and bones is detailed in the Talmud (*Nazir* 50a; *Oholot* 2:1; *Semachot* 4:12; *Niddah* 24a). [*See also* BURIAL, COFFIN, DEATH, and GRAVE]

COSMETICS—Eye makeup and eye cosmetics are discussed in the section entitled EYES, COSMETICS. It is not clear whether women used facial makeup in biblical times (see Isaiah 3:16).[1] It is alleged that cosmetics came down from heaven to Israel together with manna (*Yoma* 75a). In talmudic times women fixed their hair, applied makeup, and painted their eyes, particularly before the Sabbath or a Festival (*Moed Katan* 9b; *Tosefta Shabbat* 9:13). Cosmetic pastes were applied by young Jewish maidens as depilatories (*Moed Katan* 9b; *Pesachim* 43a). A prominent woman enjoys the scent of her cosmetics (*Ketubot* 71b).

A man should not force his wife who is in mourning to paint her eyes or her face (*Moed Katan* 20b). A man must provide food and clothing as well as cosmetics for his wife (*Ketubot* 48a and 107a). Some menstruating women do not apply makeup to their eyes or faces so as not to entice their husbands, although it is allowed so that they not become repugnant to their husbands (*Shabbat* 64b). The rouge is applied directly to the face with the hand or with a cloth (*Shabbat* 95a). A husband can nullify the vow of his wife if she renounces the use of makeup or cosmetics (*Ketubot* 7:3 and 71a).

It is forbidden to deceive someone by applying makeup. Thus an old person should not apply makeup to make others think that she is young (*Baba Metzia* 60a). A widowed woman may adorn herself and apply cosmetics prior to seeking another mate (*Ketubot* 54a). Makeup can be applied to hide small blemishes (*Shabbat* 34a). [*See also* PERFUME and OIL EMBROCATIONS]

---

1. F. Rosner (trans.), *Julius Preuss' Biblical and Talmudic Medicine* (Northvale, NJ: Jason Aronson, 1993), pp. 369–370.

COUGH—One coughs to clear sputum from the mouth (*Genesis Rabbah* 67:4). Coughing may be a sign that heralds the onset of menstruation (*Niddah* 63b). Goat's milk is recommended for coughing (*Tosefta Baba Kamma* 8:12). Noah is said to have coughed up blood in the Ark because of cold (*Genesis Rabbah* 32:11). Coughed up blood is usually mixed with sputum (*Yebamot* 105a). [*See also* LUNGS, SALIVA, and SPUTUM]

CREMATION—The Talmud describes the Roman practice of crema-

tion in reference to Titus, who said, "Burn me and strew my ashes over the sea" (*Gittin* 56b). The allegation that Jews practiced cremation is based on an erroneous interpretation of the word "burning" in relation to death (e.g., Joshua 20:14 and 21:9). Biblical passages cited in relation to cremation refer to the deaths of King Asa, King Zedekiah, and King Saul and his sons. King Asa was laid in a bed filled with herbs and spices (2 Chronicles 16:13–14). The "great burning" refers either to the fragrant spices that were burned to a powder and then sprinkled on Asa or to the customary funeral pyre of the bed and other personal articles of the deceased king, which were burned as a sign of honor to him (Rashi and others). The same honor was paid to the Patriarchs, and the greater the value of the things burned, the greater the honor (*Abodah Zarah* 11a). The same interpretation of "burning" is offered by the biblical commentators in regard to King Zedekiah (Jeremiah 34:5; *Abodah Zarah* 52b), King Jehoram (2 Chronicles 21:19) and King Saul and his sons (1 Samuel 31:12–13). Such burnings for kings are specifically allowed by Maimonides (*Mishneh Torah, Avel* 14:26) and Karo (*Shulchan Aruch, Yoreh Deah* 345:1) in their codes of Jewish law.

The real cremation or burning of ashes of the king of Edom as mentioned in the Bible (Amos 2:1) refers to a non-Jew. The burning by King

Josiah of the bones of idolatrous priests (2 Kings 23:16) was to fulfill a divine prophecy (1 Kings 13:1–3). Preuss points out several indirect references to cremation in the Talmud.[1] Ritual defilement is discussed in relation to "the ashes of burned corpses" (*Oholot* 2:2). An inheritance dispute is described in a case where the testator made the specific request "burn me" (*Jerushalmi Ketubot* 11:34). The Sadducees literally interpreted the biblical command of burning for capital offenses to mean cremation and once burned a priest's adulterous daughter (*Sanhedrin* 52b). A curse on the wicked says that even their bones should be burned (*Jerushalmi Shebiit* 8:38) or pulverized (*Genesis Rabbah* 28:3).

Recent rabbinic opinions absolutely prohibit cremation as a desecration of the dead and in total violation of Jewish law and practice.[2] Burial of the body is a religious obligation (Genesis 3:19; 1 Kings 14:13; *Sanhedrin* 46b), and nonburial is a punishment to the wicked (Jeremiah 16:4). [*See also* EMBALMING]

---

1. F. Rosner (trans.), *Julius Preuss' Biblical and Talmudic Medicine* (Northvale, NJ: Jason Aronson, 1993), pp. 521–523.
2. F. Rosner, "Embalming and Cremation," in *Modern Medicine and Jewish Ethics*, 2nd ed. (Hoboken, NJ: Ktav and Yeshiva University Press, 1991), pp. 335–350.

CRESS—White cress is used to heal a gum ailment called *chinke* (*Gittin* 69a) and for liver worms called *arketa* (*Shabbat* 109b). Pulverized cress in aged wine is a remedy for colitis (*Jerushalmi Shabbat* 14:14; *Jerushalmi Abodah Zarah* 2:40). Cress with vinegar stops bleeding (*Abodah Zarah* 28a). Garden cress has aphrodisiac properties and was, therefore, not consumed by the High Priest on the eve of the Day of Atonement (*Yoma* 2a). After eating cress, one should walk a little to avoid falling asleep (*Moed Katan* 11a).

Eating cress prior to or after bloodletting is dangerous (*Abodah Zarah* 29a; *Nedarim* 54b). A convalescing patient should not eat cress for fear of exacerbating the illness (*Berachot* 57b). He who eats cress without first washing his hands suffers fear for thirty days (*Pesachim* 111b). A woman who eats garden cress has bleary-eyed children (*Ketubot* 61a). Cress growing among flax may damage the flax (*Baba Metzia* 107a). A tasty cress dish is made from chopped cress and wine (*Yoma* 49a; *Abodah Zarah* 30b).

CUCUMBERS—The Jews in the desert yearned for the cucumbers they ate in Egypt (Numbers 11:5). The Lord provided them with whole and broken cucumbers (*Ecclesiastes Rabbah* 5:10:1). Large cucumbers are difficult to digest, whereas small ones are healthy (*Berachot* 57b). Cucumbers make the intestines expand (*Abodah Zarah* 11a). Cucumbers with holes should not be eaten in case a poisonous snake ate from them (*Chullin* 94a). The inner part of cucumbers may be bitter (*Baba Batra* 143a). Cucumbers can be grown in plant pots (*Chullin* 128a). Ordinarily, however, cucumber fields (*Baba Batra* 24b) grow from cucumber seeds (*Shabbat* 90b). Cucumber beds (*Moed Katan* 3b) or cucumber fields are guarded (*Pesachim* 6b). The Talmud describes cases of planting and gathering cucumbers by magic (*Sanhedrin* 67a and 68a). Some cucumbers are bitter (*Yebamot* 89a; *Terumot* 3:1). Cucumbers were imported from Syria, Greece, Egypt, and Remuzia (*Nedarim* 51a). Wormy cucumbers should not be consumed (*Chullin* 58a and 67b). A fibrous growth on cucumbers (*Uktzin* 2:1) may represent a fungus or other parasite.

Rabbi Judah the Prince always had cucumbers on his table (*Berachot* 57b; *Abodah Zarah* 11a). They may have been in baskets (*Shabbat* 91b and 153b). The verse "Nothing was lacking" (1 Kings 5:7) means that the king had beets in the summer and cucumbers in the winter (*Deuteronomy Rabbah* 1:5).

CUMIN—Black cumin was recommended for heart pain, although not everyone agreed (*Berachot* 40a). It was sometimes sprinkled on bread as a spice (ibid.; *Menachot* 23b). Cumin and several other ingredients boiled in wine or beer makes a therapeutic concoction for a woman with abnormal vaginal bleeding (*Shabbat* 110a–b) or with puerperal illness (*Abodah Zarah* 28a). Cumin is applied to circumcision wounds to help the healing process (*Shabbat* 133a). For this purpose, it can even be crushed on the Sabbath (ibid., 134a). Cumin is one ingredient of remedies for stomach (or heart) ailments (*Abodah Zarah* 29a) and for tertian fever (*Shabbat* 67a). Cumin and other spices are not considered life's necessities and may therefore be hoarded (*Baba Batra* 90b). Cumin can be used to heat an oven (*Terumot* 10:4). Cumin must be tithed like fruit and vegetables (*Demai* 2:1).

CUPPING—Bloodletting was performed with lancets or cupping glasses (*Gittin* 67b). Originally, horns of young cows were used. The tip of the horn was cut off, through which the cupper sucked, and the open end was placed on the patient's skin. Some cupping vessels were made of glass, bronze, or silver.[1] The cupping glass or horn is called *keren* (*Shabbat* 154b). Drinking from a cupping glass is a punishable sin (*Makkot* 16b). Two sages compared blood color in cupping horns to that of menstrual blood (*Niddah* 20a). Abba the cupper conducted his trade with sensitivity to the patient's privacy and ability (or inability) to pay (*Taanit* 21b). Rabbi Joseph never called a cupper to his house but went to the cupper's house (*Hora-*

yot 14a). Cuppers once sat under date trees and ravens, who came to suck up the blood, damaged the trees (*Baba Batra* 23a). A cupper, like other professionals, can be dismissed if his work is unsatisfactory (*Baba Metzia* 97a). The filling of one hundred cupping glasses with blood (*Shabbat* 129b) probably refers to family bleeding. [*See also* BLOODLETTING and LEECHES]

1. F. Rosner (trans.), *Julius Preuss' Biblical and Talmudic Medicine* (Northvale, NJ: Jason Aronson, 1993), p. 252.

CUSCUTA—Although cuscuta is said to have no healing properties (*Shabbat* 109a), if one swallows a snake, he should eat cuscuta with salt and run for three miles. The snake will then be excreted in strips (tapeworm?) (ibid.). Eating cuscuta out of season causes diminution of sperm (*Gittin* 70a). A nursing woman should not eat cuscuta (*Ketubot* 60b). Drinking beer containing cuscuta protects Babylonians from the illness called *raatan* (leprosy?) (*Ketubot* 77b).

Cuscuta grows in the ground (*Eruvin* 28b) and is plucked from shrubs and thorns (*Shabbat* 107b). Cuscuta growing in a vineyard may or may not (two rabbinic views) constitute a forbidden mixture of plants (*Shabbat* 139a). If an animal's lungs after ritual slaughtering resemble cuscuta (pneumonic consolidation), the animal is not fit for human consumption (*Chullin* 47b).

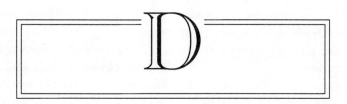

D

DANCING—Among the earliest recorded types of physical exercise are dancing and rhythmic gymnastics. The Israelites danced before the golden calf (Exodus 32:19). King David called to the people to praise God in dance (Psalms 149:3). At a circumcision, after the rabbis had eaten and drank, some recited songs or alphabetical acrostics, and some danced (*Ecclesiastes Rabbah* 7:1:8). It was common to dance before a bride (*Ketubot* 16b). The Midrash states that the righteous will one day dance before God with zest (*Song of Songs Rabbah* 1:3). Elsewhere (*Leviticus Rabbah* 12:5), the Midrash cites the eighty kinds of dances that Pharaoh's daughter danced in one night. Dancing is described in the Babylonian (*Gittin* 57a) and Jerusalem (*Betzah* 5:2) Talmuds. [*See also* EXERCISE]

DATES—Dates are a nutritious food (*Berachot* 12a). Dates are wholesome morning and evening after a meal but not in the afternoon after a rest (*Ketubot* 10b). Dates warm, satisfy, act as a laxative, and strengthen the body (ibid., *Gittin* 70a). A diced date can revive a person who faints (*Lamentations Rabbah* 1:2). Dates and figs are very important fruits (*Berachot* 41b). Black dates are good nourishment after bloodletting (*Shabbat* 129a). Black dates and marjoram heal intestinal worms (*Shabbat* 109b). Dates are helpful for melancholy, diarrhea, and hemorrhoids (*Ketubot* 10b). Persian dates were part of a folk remedy for jaundice (*Shabbat* 109b) and date stones were used to heal external inflammation (*Gittin* 69b). *Tzafdina* (stomatitis?) was treated by the local application of a compound remedy containing pulverized date stones (*Yoma* 84a).

Dates are not without side effects, however. They may intoxicate like wine; therefore, one should not teach after eating them (*Ketubot* 10b). Before meals, dates are injurious and one should not eat them on an empty stomach (*Ketubot* 10b; *Baba Metzia* 113b). Unripe dates are not healthy for nursing women (*Ketubot* 60b and 65b). Unripe dates are assimilated in the body but without benefit (*Berachot* 57b). Drinking juice made from boiling date pits may induce infertility (*Gittin* 69b).

Date honey is the sweet syrup extracted from dates (*Berachot* 38a). Dates grow on date trees (*Megillah* 28a; *Yebamot* 93a; *Baba Batra* 23a, 26a, 37a, etc.). Unripe dates blown off the trees by the wind (*Berachot* 40b) are wrapped in plaited palm branches (*Shabbat* 146a) and placed on a reed mat (*Ketubot* 50b) in the sun to dry and ripen (*Shabbat* 45b). Fresh dates are moist (*Uktzin* 2:2). Pits or stones of dates are discarded (*Shabbat* 29a). Dates are stored in sacks (*Megillah* 7b) or in storehouses (*Pesachim* 8a) and must be tithed (*Demai* 2:1). Cakes of pressed dates (*Baba Metzia* 99b) and mashes of pressed dates (*Ketubot* 80a) are ready for consumption. Date orchards (*Baba Metzia* 22a) and imported dates from Syria (inferior quality), Persia (*Shabbat* 143a), and Tabyana (*Pesachim* 53a) were sources of dates for the population in Israel. The size of a date is a legal measure or quantity for many Jewish laws (*Eruvin* 4b; *Yoma* 73b; *Sukkah* 6a; *Betzah* 7b; *Kelim* 17:12; *Tevul Yom* 3:6; *Uktzin* 1:5). A person should eat dates on Rosh Hashanah as a sign of prosperity (*Horayot* 12a).

DEAFNESS—The Bible defines a *cheresh* as a deaf person and an *illem* as a mute person (Psalms 38:14; Isaiah 56:10). In the Talmud the term *cheresh* usually refers to a deaf-mute (*Terumot* 1:2; *Menachot* 64b). Chushim, the son of Dan (Genesis 46:23), was hard-of-hearing (*Sotah* 13a). The sons of Rabbi Yochanan of Godgada were deaf (*Tosefta Terumot* 1:2; *Chagigah* 3a; *Jerushalmi Terumot* 1:1). At Mount Sinai, no Israelite was deaf (*Leviticus Rabbah* 18:4; *Song of Songs Rabbah* 4:7:1). In the world to come, all deaf people will regain their hearing (Isaiah 35:5). The causes of deafness include a divine decree (Exodus 4:11), trauma (*Baba Kamma* 85b and 91a; *Jerushalmi Terumot* 1:1; *Jerushalmi Kilayim* 8:2), old age (*Shabbat* 152a), putting one's dirty hands to the ears (ibid., 108b), and lack of modesty during cohabitation (*Nedarim* 20a). Familial and hereditary deafness was also recognized (*Jerushalmi Terumot* 1:1; *Tosefta Terumot* 1:2).

A deaf-mute is considered as a person without a mature mind (*Sanhedrin* 66a) and totally unfit for work (*Baba Kamma* 85b). He is among the most lowly and unfortunate of all people (*Sanhedrin* 85b) and exempt from biblical commandments and rabbinic decrees like a mentally retarded person (*Chagigah* 2b). Nevertheless, he must be treated with dignity and respect. It is forbidden to curse him (Leviticus 19:14) or insult him (*Baba Kamma* 86b). Even someone only hard-of-hearing is not considered intellectually perfect (*Sotah* 13a).

A number of legal regulations apply to a deaf-mute. His promises are le-

Death

gally invalid (*Arachin* 1:1). He cannot testify in a court of law (Maimonides' *Mishneh Torah, Edut* 9:11). Negotiations about sales and purchases can be effected through gestures or lip reading (*Gittin* 5:7 and 59a). Such gestures also effectuate a marriage or divorce (*Yebamot* 14:1). A guardian can be appointed for a deafmute (*Tosefta Terumot* 1:1). A deaf person should not set aside Heave Offering (*Berachot* 15a). Other legal ramifications concerning the deaf are detailed elsewhere.[1,2]

Some people stop up their ears in order not to hear (Zechariah 7:11) the cry of the poor. Such behavior is condemned (Proverbs 21:13). Occasionally, feigning deafness may be needed (Joshua 2:1; *Ruth Rabbah* 2:1). [*See also* EARS]

1. A. Steinberg, "*Cheresh*," in *Encyclopedia of Jewish Medical Ethics*, vol. 2 (Jerusalem: Schlesinger Institute at the Shaare Zedeh Medical Center, 1991), pp. 531–584 (Hebrew).
2. S.Y. Zevin (ed.), "*Cheresh*," in *Encyclopedia Talmudit*, vol. 17 (Jerusalem, 1983), pp. 495–537 (Hebrew).

DEATH—The classic definition of death in Judaism as found in the Talmud (*Yoma* 85a) and the Codes of Jewish Law (Maimonides' *Mishneh Torah, Shabbat* 2:19; Karo's *Shulchan Aruch, Orach Chayim* 329:4) is the irreversible absence of respiration in a person who appears dead (i.e., shows no movements and is unresponsive to all stimuli). Jewish writings provide considerable evidence for the thesis that the brain and the brain stem control all bodily functions including breathing and heartbeat. It therefore follows that irreversible total cessation of all brain function including that of the brain stem is equated with death. This situation is said to be the figurative equivalent of physiologic decapitation whereby the decapitated person is certainly dead even if the heart transiently continues to beat.[1,2] The other rabbinic view rejects the analogy of decapitation and requires cardiac standstill in addition to cessation of respiration before death can be pronounced.[3] Proponents of both views honestly and deeply feel the correctness of their interpretation of the classic Jewish sources.[4]

Death was ordained through Adam and Eve's sin (*Eruvin* 18b). There are nine hundred and three types of death; the worst is asphyxiation from croup, the best is death by a kiss (*Berachot* 8a). Death during childbirth was not uncommon in ancient times (Genesis 35:16–19; *Ecclesiastes Rabbah* 3:2:2; 1 Samuel 4:19–21; *Eruvin* 41b). People with dropsy or bowel diseases sometimes died suddenly (*Eruvin* 41b). Death from pestilence occurs within one day (Ezekiel 24:16–18). When Rav died, people took dust from his grave as a remedy against quotidian fever (*Sanhedrin* 47b). Death can also occur during sexual intercourse.

93

When a person is near death, the angel of death (*Berachot* 4b and 51a; *Shabbat* 89a; *Yoma* 77b; *Sukkah* 53a; *Ketubot* 77b) lets a drop of gall fall into the person's mouth and he dies (*Abodah Zarah* 20b). Dying on Sabbath eve or at the end of Yom Kippur or dying of diarrhea is a good omen because many righteous people die of diarrhea (*Ketubot* 103b).

There is no death without sin (*Shabbat* 55a; *Leviticus Rabbah* 37:2). Confession before death procures atonement for one's sins (*Yoma* 85b; *Sanhedrin* 43b). The day of death is hidden from human beings (*Pesachim* 54b; *Shabbat* 30a; *Ecclesiastes Rabbah* 11:3:1). Woe is to a man whose wife predeceases him (*Sanhedrin* 22a). Unnatural death may occur (*Taanit* 11a). When a man reaches his parents' age he should fear death (*Genesis Rabbah* 65:12). If a man dies, his brothers should fear death; if one of a company dies, the whole company should fear death (*Shabbat* 105b). Sleep is a taste of death (*Yoma* 78b). Sleep is one-sixtieth part of death (*Berachot* 57b), as if sleep is like an unripe fruit and death is the ripe fruit that falls from a tree (*Genesis Rabbah* 17:5).

When a person dies, the body orifices were stopped up to prevent air entry and to delay putrefaction (*Semachot* 1:1) because the abdomen becomes distended after death (*Shabbat* 151b). Corpses were placed on sand to preserve them prior to burial (*Jerushalmi Shabbat* 4:6). The dead were also perfumed and embalmed (see EMBALMING and PERFUMES). [*See also* BURIAL, COFFIN, CAPITAL PUNISHMENT, CORPSE, and GRAVE]

1. F. Rosner, "Definition of Death," in *Modern Medicine and Jewish Ethics*, 2nd ed. (Hoboken, NJ, and New York: Ktav and Yeshiva University Press, 1991), pp. 263–275.

2. F. Rosner and M.D. Tendler, "Definition of Death in Judaism," in *Journal of Halacha and Contemporary Society*, XVII (Spring 1989), pp. 14–31.

3. J.D. Bleich, "Establishing Criteria of Death," in *Contemporary Halakhic Problems* (New York: Ktav and Yeshiva University Press, 1977), pp. 372–393.

4. F. Rosner, "The Definition of Death in Jewish Law," in *The Definition of Death: Contemporary Controversies*, ed. R. Arnold, R. Schapiro, and S. Younger (Baltimore: Johns Hopkins University Press, 1998).

DEFECATION—The biblical verse "and closed up the place with flesh" (Genesis 2:21) is interpreted to mean that God covered man's anus with buttocks to allow him to sit in modesty during defecation (*Genesis Rabbah* 17:6). Primitive lavatories for defecation are described in the Bible (2 Kings 10:27). Defecation early in the morning is good for the body as hardening is for iron (*Berachot* 62b). He who defers his bodily functions is in violation of a biblical precept (Leviticus 11:43; *Makkot* 16b). If feces accumulate and are not excreted, dropsy develops (*Berachot* 44b). He who fails to heed the call of nature for four or five days will die (*Numbers Rabbah* 16:24). The proverbial expression is: "When your pot is boiling, empty it out (i.e., the feces)" (*Berachot* 62b). If one is unable to defecate one should repeatedly stand up and sit down on the toilet or rub the anus with a shard or concentrate hard (*Shabbat* 82a). A severe fright (*Megillah* 15a) or great fear (*Song of Songs Rabbah* 3:4) can occasionally result in defecation. A disciplinary flogging is interrupted if it induces defecation (*Makkot* 3:14). When King Eglon's abdomen was pierced with a sword, he defecated (Judges 3:21–22). Elderly people sometimes defecate before they urinate (*Leviticus Rabbah* 18:1). Straining at defecation can be painful (tenesmus?) and bring a person to tears (*Lamentations Rabbah* 2:15; *Shabbat* 151b). Massaging the abdomen helps to produce defecation (*Berachot* 62a). Normal bowel movements are a good prognostic sign in illness (*Berachot* 57b). One should behave modestly during defecation (*Berachot* 62a). Defecation in front of certain idols was part of pagan worship in antiquity (*Sanhedrin* 7:6).

After defecation little stones of varying sizes were used to clean the anus (*Shabbat* 81a). Shards (Job 2:7–8; *Yebamot* 59b) and reed skins were also used (*Shabbat* 82a) but were considered dangerous. Water from which a dog has licked should not be used to cleanse the anus (*Jerushalmi Shabbat* 8:11). One should wipe oneself with the left hand because one eats with the right hand (*Berachot* 61b). After defecation, euphemistically called "covering the feet" (Judges 3:24; 1 Samuel 24:4), it is obligatory to wash one's hands (*Yoma* 3:2). It is hygienic to cover the feces with earth after defecation and soldiers carried a special shovel for that purpose (Deuteronomy 23:10–15). Cohabitation immediately after defecation results in epileptic children (*Gittin* 70a). Children's feces were an ingredient of a remedy for scurvy (*Jerushalmi Shabbat* 14:14). Pigeon dung and white dog excrement were used for certain folk remedies (*Gittin* 69b). [*See also* HEMORRHOIDS, DIARRHEA, CONSTIPATION, INTESTINES, and ANUS]

DEFLORATION—The pain of defloration is described like the pain of venesection or "like hard bread on the palate" (*Ketubot* 39b). Defloration is a wound (*Tosefta Ketubot* 1:1) that needs to heal (*Niddah* 10:1). Defloration is also compared to a leaf falling from a tree (*Shabbat* 63b). Defloration blood may be paler and clearer than menstrual blood (*Tosefta Niddah* 9:10) although most rabbis say there is no difference (*Niddah* 65b). Defloration is not always accompanied by bleeding (*Chagigah* 14b).

A woman cannot become pregnant from the first cohabitation (defloration) (*Yebamot* 34a). Therefore, the daughters of Lot had probably deflorated themselves before their cohabitation with their father, from which they became pregnant (*Genesis Rabbah* 51:9). Some women exercised friction to destroy their hymen (*Yebamot* 34b). A woman struck by a piece of wood can lose her hymen as a result of the blow (ibid., 59a). A family in Jerusalem had women who took large steps whereby their virginity was destroyed (*Shabbat* 63b). [*See also* VIRGINITY]

DEMONS—God created demons on the sixth day of creation (*Genesis Rabbah* 7:5 and 11:9). The demons, as the angels, assist God in His work (*Numbers Rabbah* 14:3; *Song of Songs Rabbah* 1:15). In the premonotheistic period, Jews sacrificed to spirits or demons (Deuteronomy 32:17). In Egypt, magic was practiced through the agency of demons (*Sanhedrin* 87b). Incense was also offered to demons (*Keritot* 3b). Adam and Eve begat demons for one hundred and thirty years (*Genesis Rabbah* 24:6). In the time of Enosh, humans became vulnerable to demons (*Genesis Rabbah* 23:6) but the Lord protects Jews from harmful demons (*Numbers Rabbah* 11:5). Demons cannot create anything even the size of a barley corn or a camel but they move existing things from place to place by magic (*Exodus Rabbah* 10:7).

Spirits or demons play an important role in the folk medicine of the Talmud. Sick patients have to be pro-

tected from demons (*Berachot* 45b). All illness is said to be caused by a spirit or demon (*Baba Metzia* 107b). The blood demon is responsible for nosebleeds, for which several folk remedies are prescribed (*Gittin* 69a). The demon Palga is responsible for migraine (*Pesachim* 111b) and the demon Cerada for another illness (*Chullin* 105b). Only rarely is madness or insanity identified with a demon (*Rosh Hashanah* 28a), although a rabid dog is said to be possessed by a demon or evil spirit (*Yoma* 83a) that causes wanderers to go astray (*Taanit* 22b) and to violate Sabbath laws (*Eruvin* 4:1). The night demon Shabriri is responsible for certain forms of blindness (*Pesachim* 112a; *Abodah Zarah* 12b). Therapy against it consists of a folk remedy (*Gittin* 69a). Women who let their hair grow like the night demon are condemned (*Eruvin* 100b). Hands are washed upon arising in the morning to wash off the demon Shibbeta (*Yoma* 77b).

A lavatory demon exits (*Shabbat* 67a) in the form of a goat (*Berachot* 62a). A special curse is recited for demons in general and the demons of the privy in particular (*Shabbat* 67a). One should not go into a ruin because of the danger of demons (ibid., 3b). Reciting the *Shema* prayer before going to sleep keeps demons away (ibid., 5a). If one sleeps in a house alone, one may be seized by the notorious night demon Lilith (*Shabbat* 151b), who resembles a human being but has wings (*Niddah* 24b). Asmadai is the legendary king of the demons (*Gittin* 68b). Other demons identified by name include Hormin, the son of Lilith (*Baba Batra* 73a); Chamat (*Sanhedrin* 101a); Shinadon (*Genesis Rabbah* 36:3); Keter (*Lamentations Rabbah* 1: 3:29); Ben Temalion (*Meilah* 17b); Joseph, who violated the Sabbath laws with impunity (*Eruvin* 43a); and Igrat, daughter of Machalat, known as the queen of the destructive angels (i.e., demons) (*Pesachim* 112b).

Demons are more numerous than humans (*Berachot* 6a). There are three hundred kinds of demons in Sichin (*Gittin* 68a). Demons have shadows (*Yebamot* 122a; *Gittin* 66a) and change into many colors (*Yoma* 75a). They are destructive (*Numbers Rabbah* 11:7 and 12:3) and gore like an ox (*Baba Kamma* 21a). They reside in drain pipes (*Chullin* 105b). In three respects demons are like angels: They have wings, they fly, and they know the future. In three respects demons are like human beings: They eat and drink, they propagate, and they die (*Chagigah* 16a). Abaye's schoolhouse was haunted by a demon (*Kiddushin* 29b). King Solomon ruled over the demons (*Numbers Rabbah* 11:3; *Megillah* 11b; *Gittin* 68b). [*See also* ASTROLOGY, EVIL EYE, EXORCISM, MAGIC, and SORCERY]

DENTISTRY—The teeth are not counted among the 248 bones enu-merated in the Talmud (*Oholot* 1:8). Teeth are hard (*Abodah Zarah* 28a). Baby teeth are called milk teeth (*Kiddushin* 24b). Poetically, milk teeth are referred to as grinders or millers (Ecclesiastes 12:3), and the denture of the mythical Leviathan is called the "double bridle" (Job 41:13). The homiletical literature states that an ox without teeth dies (*Baba Metzia* 42b). Raba dreamed that his teeth fell out, which was interpreted to mean that his children would imminently die (*Berachot* 56a). A loud roar of a lion can make people's teeth fall out from fright (*Chullin* 59b). The Talmud states that the assertion of the *Tosefta* (*Chullin* 3:20) that animals that chew their cud have no upper teeth is incor-rect (*Chullin* 59a). A dog once barked and a pregnant woman aborted as a result (*Shabbat* 63a). A man removed the canine teeth from his she-bear so that it not harm his children (*Baba Kamma* 23b).

In his prime of life, Judah pulver-ized iron plates with his teeth (*Genesis Rabbah* 93:6). The grinders cease to work when one becomes old and there are fewer of them (Ecclesiastes 12:3). Teeth fall out as one gets older (*Niddah* 65a). Rabbi Chaggai's teeth grew back when he was eighty years old as a reward for his untiring efforts to effect the burial of Rav Huna (*Jerushalmi Kilayim* 9:32).

Broken and/or painful teeth are described in the Bible (Proverbs 25:19; Lamentations 3:16). Esau wept when he met Jacob because his teeth were loose and painful (*Genesis Rabbah* 78:9; *Targum Jonathan* on Genesis 33:4). Vinegar is harmful to the teeth, as is smoke to the eyes (Proverbs 10:26). Vinegar heals the gums, however (*Shabbat* 111a). Sour fruit juice is efficacious for toothache (ibid.). Vapors of a bathhouse are also harmful to the teeth (*Jerushalmi Abodah Zarah* 3:42). Prolonged fasting causes the teeth to blacken (*Chagigah* 22b; *Nazir* 52b). A special remedy for toothache is garlic root ground with oil and salt applied directly to the tooth (*Gittin* 69a). Rab advised his son not to have any teeth extracted (*Pesachim* 113a). Spleen is good for teeth and leeks are harmful. However, the spleen should be chewed and spit out since it is bad for digestion (*Berachot* 44b). Unripe grapes make teeth blunt (Jeremiah 31:19).

Great emphasis is placed on beautiful white teeth (*Ketubot* 111b). Lovers extol each other by describing fresh and clean teeth (Song of Songs 4:2 and 6:6). Jacob promised his son Judah "teeth whiter than milk" (Genesis 49:12). Often described is a *kisem*, which is either a toothpick or a toothbrush (*Betzah* 4:6; *Tosefta Betzah* 3:18; *Jerushalmi Demai* 3:23). It was made from fragrant wood (*Jerushalmi Shabbat* 8:11). A sharp reed should not be used to pick the teeth because it is dangerous (*Chullin* 16b). Toothpicks or wood chips were apparently constantly carried between the teeth (*Tosefta Shabbat* 5:1).

The teeth have significant legal import in Judaism. The biblical verse "a tooth for a tooth" (Exodus 21:22; Leviticus 24:19) refers to monetary compensation and is not to be taken literally. If someone knocks out the tooth of his servant, the latter goes free as a substitute for the tooth (Exodus 21:17). The tooth of a servant may be drilled if necessary (*Kiddushin* 24b). Teeth cannot be used as a ritual slaughtering instrument (*Chullin* 15b). Any part of a corpse is ritually unclean, except the teeth, hair, and nails (*Oholot* 3:3). When Rabban Gamiliel asked the Emperor how many teeth he had, the latter put his hand to his mouth and counted them (*Sanhedrin* 39a). Medications may be applied on an aching tooth even on the Sabbath (*Yoma* 8:6).

The Talmud speaks of the "drilling" of a tooth (*Baba Kamma* 26b), which the commentaries interpret as "poking and scratching around the seat of the tooth," perhaps an early form of tartar elimination. For breath improvement, one rubs the teeth with a dry powder or with ginger and cinnamon (*Shabbat* 65a). [*See also* ARTIFICIAL TEETH]

DEPILATORIES—To remove hair, known as *maavir* (*Moed Katan* 1:7), one used razors, scissors, or knives. The main depilatory used in antiquity and the Middle Ages was lime (*Shabbat* 78b; *Nazir* 3a). It was applied as a paste to the skin and then scraped off together with the skin; the process may cause pain (*Moed Katan* 1:7). Young girls in whom pubic hairs developed before menarche removed this sign of precociousness. Poor girls used lime for this purpose, rich maidens used fine flour, and royal princesses used oil of myrrh (*Pesachim* 43a; *Moed Katan* 9b; *Shabbat* 80b). This oil of myrrh is interpreted by some to represent oil of unripe olives, which causes hair to fall out and makes the body shine and the skin soft (ibid.; *Leviticus Rabbah* 5:3; *Numbers Rabbah* 10:3; *Song of Songs Rabbah* 4:8:1; *Megillah* 13a). Oil of green or unripe olives is what the prophet criticizes when the carefree Israelites anointed themselves with it (Amos 6:6). Ingested or externally applied *neshem* causes permanent depilation (*Negaim* 10:10). The identity of *neshem* is unknown.

A woman may not use lime as a depilatory during the weeks of the Passover or Tabernacle Festivals (*Moed Katan* 8b). One may not cover animals with clay, earth, or lime as a depilatory (*Betzah* 34a). [*See also* HAIR, BALDNESS, WIGS, and BEARD]

DIARRHEA—A person with diarrhea is ill in his intestines and needs to treat it before it worsens (*Sotah* 42b). Some patients also have fever and swollen abdomens (*Avot de Rabbi Nathan* 41:1). The disease may be very painful (*Shabbat* 11a) and even bring one

to tears (*Lamentations Rabbah* 2:15; *Shabbat* 151b). Because of the pain, patients with diarrhea are forgiven for their sins and do not see the face of Gehenna (*Eruvin* 41b). Thus, diarrhea may be a good omen (*Ketubot* 103b) in that righteous people die of diarrhea. Rabbi Judah the Prince suffered from diarrhea (ibid., 104a), as did King Belshazzar (*Song of Songs Rabbah* 3:4). Rabbi Jose wished diarrhea upon himself (*Shabbat* 118b). The expression *gava* for "he died" refers to diarrhea (*Genesis Rabbah* 62:2). Such people die suddenly while fully conscious (*Eruvin* 41b). King Jehoram is said to have suffered from severe dysentery so that his "bowels fell out" and he died (2 Chronicles 21:14–18).

Priests in the Temple who walked barefoot on the marble floors and ate a lot of sacrificial meat suffered from diarrhea and had a special physician to care for them (*Shekalim* 5:2). Another cause of diarrhea is a change in one's lifestyle or eating habits (*Nedarim* 37b). Eating rich foods may spoil one's Festival joy because of diarrhea (*Sanhedrin* 101a), which is called an evil affliction (Proverbs 15:15). Eating without drinking can also lead to diarrhea (*Shabbat* 42a). Thus, one should drink one cupful of water with each loaf of bread or other food (*Berachot* 40a). Also to prevent diarrhea one should eat bread immersed in vinegar or wine in both summer and winter (*Gittin* 70a). Wheatbread, fish brine, and beer can cause diarrhea (*Shabbat*

108a). So, too, coarse bread, fresh beer, and raw vegetables (*Pesachim* 42a), as well as certain types of wine (*Baba Batra* 97b). White bread, fat meat, and old wine, however, do not cause diarrhea (*Pesachim* 42a).

Remedies for diarrhea include the external rubbing of the abdomen with oil and wine (*Shabbat* 134a) or the application of heat (ibid., 40b). An Egyptian concoction of barley, safflower, and salt is a binding potion for patients with diarrhea (*Shabbat* 110a; *Pesachim* 42b). Also helpful is old apple wine (*Abodah Zarah* 40b), old grape juice (*Nedarim* 9:8), lemonade (*Leviticus Rabbah* 37:2), dates (*Ketubot* 10b), and various compounded medications (*Gittin* 69b).

Diarrhea is a favorable prognostic sign in sick patients provided it is not dysentery (*Berachot* 57b). Hydrops or leukophlegmesia is cured if the patient develops diarrhea (*Yebamot* 60b). One should not visit patients with diarrhea because of embarrassment or in order not to contract it (*Nedarim* 41a). A perfume pan was placed near patients with diarrhea (*Moed Katan* 27b). [*See also* INTESTINES, LAXATIVES, and DEFECATION]

DIETARY LAWS—Jewish dietary laws, known as *kashrut* (Esther 8:5; Ecclesiastes 10:10 and 11:6), concern themselves with which animals, birds, and fish may be eaten; the way in which they must be prepared for consumption; and the fact that meat must not be cooked or consumed with any dairy product. Many attempts have been made throughout the centuries to explain the dietary laws from hygienic, sanitary, esthetic, folkloric, ethical, or psychological viewpoints.[1] The Bible does not offer an explanation, but, in three separate passages (Exodus 22:30; Leviticus 11:44–45; Deuteronomy 14:21), the dietary laws are closely associated with the concept of holiness. The Talmud (*Yoma* 67b) states that dietary laws are divine statutes without explanation,[2] and thus serve as aids to moral conduct. Maimonides gives hygienic and sanitary reasons for the dietary laws (*Guide for the Perplexed* 3:48) and codifies the details of these laws (*Maachalot Assurot* 3:1ff.).

1. C. Roth (ed.), *Encyclopedia Judaica*, vol. 6 (Jerusalem: Keter, 1972), pp. 26–45.

2. F. Rosner (trans.), *Julius Preuss' Biblical and Talmudic Medicine* (Northvale, NJ: Jason Aronson, 1993), pp. 501–506.

DIGESTION—There are ten portions of the digestive system from mouth to gullet to stomach to small and large bowel to rectum and anus (*Ecclesiastes Rabbah* 7:19:3). The human stomach (*kevah*) grinds the food and brings on sleep (*Berachot* 61b). In old age the sound of the grinding is low (Ecclesiastes 12:4) because the stomach does not grind anymore (*Shabbat* 152a). Food should be well chewed (ibid.) and eaten slowly (*Berachot* 54b). Gourds and groats are as difficult to digest as lead (*Tamid* 27b; *Nedarim* 49b). So, too, large cucumbers (*Abodah Zarah* 11a). Spleen is harmful for digestion; it should be chewed and spit out (*Berachot* 44b). Radish dissolves food, lettuce helps digestion, and small cucumbers expand the intestines (*Abodah Zarah* 11a).

Digestion of food continues until one becomes hungry or thirsty again (*Berachot* 53b). Dogs take three days to digest their food (*Shabbat* 155b), birds and fish only one day (*Oholot* 11:7). Alteration in one's lifestyle leads to digestive disturbances (*Sanhedrin* 101a). He who travels should eat only small amounts of food in order to prevent digestive troubles (*Taanit* 10b). One should walk after eating before one lies down to prevent a bad mouth odor from undigested food (*Shabbat* 41a). [*See also* STOMACH and INTESTINES]

DISLOCATIONS—Jacob dislocated the head of his femur when he wrestled with an angel (Genesis 32:26). Legend relates that when Noah emerged from the Ark, a lion pushed him so that he limped (*Leviticus Rabbah* 20:1). Job speaks about a dislocated shoulder (Job 31:22). Mephiboshet was lame in his feet (2 Samuel 4:4), perhaps because of dislocated vertebrae sustained in a fall. Belshazzar may have had a dislocated hip (Daniel 5:6). If a person's jaw is dislocated, "the ear should be raised to its proper position" (*Abodah Zarah* 28b).

Dislocation of the jaw in an animal renders it unfit to be offered in the Temple (*Bechorot* 6:10). If most of an animal's ribs are dislocated or fractured the animal's life is in danger (*Chullin* 57a). Not so for birds (ibid.). [*See also* LAMENESS]

DOGS—Dogs eat dog biscuits (*Challah* 1:8), bones (*Shabbat* 128a), wheaten bread (*Moed Katan* 28a), and moldy bread (*Pesachim* 15b and 45b), and are fed meat from animal carcasses (*Shabbat* 30b and 155b; *Pesachim* 22a; *Betzah* 2a and 6b; *Chullin* 14a). Dogs especially like lumps of dough and pressed figs (*Bechorot* 34a; *Menachot* 56b). Sacred foods and sacrifices may not be fed to dogs (*Pesachim* 29a; *Bechorot* 15a) but they may eat semi-leaven on Passover (*Pesachim* 43a). A human being should not eat on the street or in the marketplace like a dog (*Kiddushin* 40b).

Dogs bark to protect their owners and a neighborhood or town (*Pesachim* 113b). They are very strong (Psalms 22:21; *Betzah* 25b) and hate each other (*Pesachim* 113b; *Sanhedrin* 105a). Dogs and especially wild dogs (*Kilayim* 1:6) sometimes bite humans (*Ketubot* 75a; *Numbers Rabbah* 19:23), especially if incited (*Abodah*

Zarah 18b). A mad dog who jumps up in front of a pregnant woman can cause her to abort from fright (*Shabbat* 63b). An evil spirit rests on a mad dog (*Yoma* 83b). Although dogs usually bark (*Leviticus Rabbah* 33:6), the voice of a mad dog is not heard; its mouth is open, its saliva drips, its ears flap, its tail hangs between its thighs, and it walks on the edge of the road (*Yoma* 83b) [*see also* RABIES]. A dog's tail once caught fire and was burnt (*Moed Katan* 17a).

A dog knows its owner but a cat does not (*Horayot* 13a). A shepherd's dog comes when it is called (*Bechorot* 55a). A dog urinates against the wall (*Baba Batra* 19b). Dogs are shrewd and pretend to be asleep in order to steal food (*Genesis Rabbah* 22:6). Dogs copulate in public (*Genesis Rabbah* 36:7) and are considered arrogant and brazen (*Exodus Rabbah* 42:9; *Ecclesiastes Rabbah* 1:2:1). They bear offspring after fifty days (*Genesis Rabbah* 20:4). Dogs pant even when they are not laden (*Leviticus Rabbah* 13:2). Dogs rarely devour lambs (*Ketubot* 41b; *Chullin* 53a). A dog needs three days to digest its food (*Shabbat* 155b). When dogs howl, the angel of death has come to town; when they frolic, Elijah the prophet has come to town (*Baba Kamma* 60b).

Bestiality with a dog is forbidden as an abomination (Leviticus 20:15; *Jerushalmi Sanhedrin* 6:23). A widow should not raise dogs lest she be suspected of immorality (*Abodah Zarah* 22b; *Baba Metzia* 71a). It is forbidden to castrate a dog (*Chagigah* 14b). The price of a dog or the hire of a dog (Deuteronomy 23:19) are discussed in the Talmud (*Temurah* 30a). Jacob is said to have had sixty myriads of dogs (*Genesis Rabbah* 78:11 and 96:1).

DOLPHINS—The Hebrew or Aramaic word *dolphanim* is variously translated as "dolphins, a fish about which many fables were circulated among the ancients," "a type of whale," and a "big sea fish."[1] The term probably corresponds to the Greek *delphinus*.

A most unusual passage in the Babylonian Talmud concerns the possible cohabitation of dolphins with human beings. The text in question reads as follows: "Dolphins [Heb. *Dolphanim*] are fruitful and multiple *like* human beings [Heb. *Kibnei adam*]. What are dolphins? Said Rab Judah: living beings [literally: children] of the sea" (*Bechorot* 8a). Rashi has a variant textual reading in which he states that dolphins are fruitful and multiply *from* human beings [Heb. *Mibnei adam*]; that is to say, if a human being has intercourse with a dolphin, the latter becomes pregnant therefrom. "Living beings of the sea" is explained by Rashi as follows: "There are fish in the ocean that have half the features of human beings and half the features of fish, and in Old French *syrene*." A commentator called Hametargem, who translates all the Old French

Dolphins

words in Rashi, considers *syrene* to be a mermaid (*meer vaybshen*).

Tosafot adopt the textual reading of Rashi that dolphins multiply *from* human beings. *Tosafot* further state that "dolphins are born and raised *from* human beings." Later talmudic commentators, such as Maharsha and Shitah Mekubezet (Bezalel Ashkenazi, seventeenth century), also agree with the textual variant "dolphins are fruitful and multiply from human beings." A seemingly lone dissenting viewpoint is that of Jacob Emden, who asserts that the original textual reading "dolphins are fruitful and multiply *like* human beings" is correct.

If one consults the *Tosefta* directly, one finds a discussion as to whether or not various types of animals can crossbreed with one another (*Bechorot* 1:5). The *Tosefta* then states that a human being cannot breed with them, nor they with humans. The key phrase then follows: "Dolphins reproduce and grow up *like* human beings." It is thus apparent that Rashi and all the subsequent talmudic commentators either misquoted the *Tosefta* or, more likely, possessed manuscripts of the *Tosefta* different from the printed editions of today. A single Hebrew letter makes the difference between the word *kibne* ("like") and *mibne* ("from"). Scribes in antiquity and the Middle Ages frequently made inadvertent errors in copying manuscripts. They sometimes even took the liberty of intentionally adding, deleting, or

modifying a letter, word, or phrase on their own. Be that as it may, how does one explain the entire talmudic passage and, in particular, the statement of Rashi that there are fish in the ocean that have half the features of human beings and half the features of fish?

Kohut provides one possible interpretation.[2] He points out the correct textual reading of the *Tosefta* that dolphins are fruitful and multiply like human beings. He also asserts that the intent of the Talmud is to teach us that dolphins have sexual intercourse like human beings and that the female gives birth to live offspring and suckles its young and does not lay eggs. Thus, Rashi means to say that female dolphins have breasts like humans and suckle their young like humans, yet dolphins resemble fish because they live in the sea. This interpretation seems correct in view of the fact that the talmudic text regarding dolphins is preceded by a discussion of which fish breed and which fish lay eggs (*Bechorot* 7a). The Talmud states: "Whatsoever gives birth gives suck, and whatsoever lays eggs supports its young by picking up food for it." Today we know that dolphins are mammals and thus have some features resembling human beings and others resembling fish. Kohut further asserts that dolphins are compared in the Talmud to human beings because they are extremely devoted to humans and are therefore called *philantropon zoon*

103

in Greek, meaning a philanthropic animal.

The reason Rab Judah calls dolphins "living beings of the sea," continues Kohut, is well-known from Greek writings, where the dolphin is characterized as a creature that does not live on land. In Hebrew, the expression is *ein le'dolphanim memshalah bayabashah*, meaning "dolphins have no dominion on dry land," and because they live in the sea, they are called "rulers of the sea."

One of the major commentaries on the *Tosefta*, called *Minchat Bikkurim* (Samuel Avigdor of Slonimo) raises the possibility that dolphins can be raised by suckling from human beings.

What remains difficult to explain is the original statement of Rashi that dolphins are fruitful and multiply from human beings, meaning that if a human being has intercourse with a dolphin, the latter becomes pregnant therefrom.

1. F. Rosner, "Dolphins in the Talmud," in *Medicine in the Bible and the Talmud*, 2nd ed. (Hoboken, NJ: Ktav and Yeshiva University Press, 1995), pp. 295–297.

2. A. Kohut, *Aruch Hashalem*, vol. 3 (New York: Pardes, 1955), pp. 72–73.

(Nehemiah 11:2). Open cities have fresh air, gardens, and parks. It was considered unhealthy to live in or near the city of Gerar (*Genesis Rabbah* 64:3). Concern for fresh air in one's site of residence is also expressed by Maimonides in the last chapter of his *Treatise on Asthma*.[1] A wife moves to a new residence with her husband although a new environment is sometimes detrimental and might even lead to illness (*Ketubot* 13:9). Lot refused to flee to the mountain for fear of negative consequences (Genesis 19:19) even though living on a hill is healthier than living in a valley (*Genesis Rabbah* 50:11). The high altitude of Sepphoris and its fresh air is praised over that of Bet Shean in the valley (*Ketubot* 104a).

On the other hand, one can avert misfortune by changing one's place of residence (*Genesis Rabbah* 44:12). Abraham did so at God's command (Genesis 12:1). A scholar should not live in a city without a physician (*Sanhedrin* 17b). A beautiful dwelling enlarges a man's spirit (*Berachot* 57b).

1. F. Rosner, *Moses Maimonides' Treatise on Asthma* (Haifa: Maimonides Research Institute, 1994).

DOMICILE—It is healthier to live in an open city rather than in a fortified city (*Ketubot* 110b). Special thanks were given to people who offered to live in the fortified city of Jerusalem

DOVES—The nation of Israel is often compared to a dove (Song of Songs 5:2; Psalms 68:14; *Gittin* 45a) because the dove is innocent, graceful, distinguished, chaste, faithful, etc.

(*Song of Songs Rabbah* 1:15:2). The dove is the symbol of chastity (*Eruvin* 100b). Noah sent forth a dove from the Ark (Genesis 8:8ff.). On top of the golden scepter was a dove (*Numbers Rabbah* 12:17). Doves flutter in and out of their nests (*Betzah* 11a) and hover over their young without touching them (*Chagigah* 15a). They hop about (*Betzah* 10b) and beat their wings (*Sanhedrin* 95a). They can also fly (*Nazir* 12a) over considerable distances (*Baba Kamma* 83a). When a dove tires, it draws in and rests one of its wings and flies on with the other (*Genesis Rabbah* 39:8).

The Talmud discusses white doves and black doves (*Betzah* 10b), golden doves (*Berachot* 53b), Hardisian doves (*Shabbat* 155b), Herodian doves (*Betzah* 24a; *Chullin* 138b), and Zuzimian doves (*Chullin* 62b). Also described are nets to trap doves (*Baba Kamma* 83a) and dove nests or dovecotes (*Eruvin* 34a; *Pesachim* 55b; *Betzah* 9a; *Baba Metzia* 102a; *Baba Batra* 11a; *Chullin* 139b). He who sells a dovecote has also sold the doves (*Baba Batra* 78b). Wild doves of the dovecote as well as doves of a loft are subject to the law of sending the dam away (Deuteronomy 22:6; *Baba Metzia* 102a).

A woman after childbirth brought two turtle doves or young pigeons as offerings (Leviticus 12:1–8). Elisha was called the man of wings because he once opened his hands to find the wings of a dove (*Shabbat* 49a and 130a).

When Titus died, his skull was opened and something like a dove was found (brain tumor?) (*Genesis Rabbah* 10:7; *Gittin* 56b). The figure of a dove was worshiped by the Cutheans (*Chullin* 6a). [*See also* BIRDS, CHICKENS, GEESE, and PIGEONS]

DREAMS—In the Bible, dreams are divine communications (Genesis 20:3–6 and 31:10–11) or a variety of prophecy (*Genesis Rabbah* 17:5). Dreams are regarded as omens (*Baba Kamma* 55a). Joseph's dreams (Genesis 37:5ff.) and those of Pharaoh (ibid., 41:1–5) and his butler and baker (ibid. 40:1ff.) are symbolic.[1] In the Talmud, some sages posit that dreams are of no consequence, neither help nor harm (*Horayot* 13b; *Gittin* 52a), and have no importance for good or evil (*Sanhedrin* 30a). Dreams speak falsehood (Zechariah 10:2). Other sages state that dreams foreshadow the future (*Baba Batra* 10a; *Yoma* 87b). A good dream is a blessing from God (Isaiah 38:16; *Berachot* 55a). Dreaming is a good prognostic sign for sick patients (*Berachot* 57b). No dream, good or bad, is ever wholly fulfilled (ibid., 55a) because every dream has some nonsense in it (ibid.; *Nedarim* 8b). One should wait up to twenty-two years for the fulfillment of a good dream (ibid.). Going to sleep in good spirits promotes happy dreams (*Pesachim* 117a).

One may have frightening dreams (*Yoma* 22b) or even nightmares (*San-*

hedrin 103a). Job's sleep was disturbed by terrifying dreams (Job 7:14). A bad dream is worse than flogging (*Berachot* 55a). A man once saw white casks full of ashes in a dream (ibid., 28a). Unchaste dreams may result in nocturnal pollution (*Moed Katan* 25a; *Niddah* 43a; *Mikvaot* 8:3). Ahasuerus had a bad dream that Haman seized a sword to kill him (*Esther Rabbah* 10:1). If one dreams one is under a ban, ten people are needed to lift the ban (*Nedarim* 8a). Fasting counteracts an evil dream (*Genesis Rabbah* 44:12; *Shabbat* 11a; *Taanit* 12b). A bad dream is nullified by prayer, charity, and repentance (*Ecclesiastes Rabbah* 5:5:1) and by the lapse of time (*Genesis Rabbah* 64:5). A special prayer concerning dreams is recited on festivals during the priestly benediction (*Berachot* 55b). This prayer saves one from bad dreams (*Song of Songs Rabbah* 3:7:1).

In talmudic times, there were twenty-four professional dream interpreters (*Berachot* 55b). Balaam was originally an interpreter of dreams (*Numbers Rabbah* 20:7). Joseph was both a dreamer (Genesis 37:5) and a dream interpreter (Genesis 41:12–15). A dream that is not interpreted is like a letter that is not read (*Berachot* 55a). No dream is without its interpretation (*Genesis Rabbah* 68:12). All dreams depend on their interpretation except for dreams about wine (ibid., 89:8).

1. C. Roth (ed.), *Encyclopedia Judaica*, vol. 6 (Jerusalem: Keter, 1972), pp. 208–211.

DRINKING WATER—Water is a proper nutritional substance (*Eruvin* 30a), although one should not drink it in public (*Bechorot* 44b). Water is cheap and wine is expensive, yet the world can exist without wine but not without water (*Jerushalmi Horayot* 3:48). One should drink lots of water after meals to avoid intestinal problems (*Berachot* 40a). River water has healing powers (2 Kings 5:14; Ezekiel 47:9; *Exodus Rabbah* 15:21). During baths, one drinks water to compensate for perspiration losses (*Shabbat* 40b).

If one drinks contaminated water one may develop *chatatin*, a type of skin rash (*Jerushalmi Terumot* 8:45). Drinking water from a channel that flows through a cemetery is harmful to one's mind (*Horayot* 13b). One should not drink directly from rivers or pools lest one swallow a leech (*Abodah Zarah* 12b) nor drink from them at night because of the night demon Shabriri (*Pesachim* 112a). Various remedies against this demon are described (*Gittin* 69b). It is forbidden to drink from water left uncovered overnight lest a snake deposited poison there. If one drinks some by oversight, one should quickly drink a cup of strong wine (*Gittin* 69b). Such uncovered water should not be poured out on the floor lest venom therein harm someone who walks barefoot (*Baba Kamma* 115b), nor should it be given to animals to drink, nor should one wash one's hands and face therewith (*Abodah Zarah* 30b). If the water is boiled or heated, it is safe to drink, especially if spice roots are added (*Chullin* 84b; *Jerushalmi Terumot* 8:45). The waters of the Siloa well outside Jerusalem allowed meat to be digested like normal food (*Avot de Rabbi Nathan* 35:5), perhaps an early use of mineral water with medicinal intent. [*See also* WATER SUPPLY and BEVERAGES]

DROPSY—Dropsy or *hydrakon* (hydrops) is a divine punishment for immoral sexual behavior (*Yebamot* 60b) and other sins such as the golden calf (*Yoma* 66b). Dropsy also occurs as a result of withholding one's bowels (*Berachot* 62b; *Tamid* 27b); therefore, the maxim: "Much feces, much dropsy; much wine, much anemia" (*Bechorot* 44b). Dropsy is said to be caused by an abnormal mixing of water and blood in the body (*Leviticus Rabbah* 15:2). The sages describe three types of dropsy: the thick one is punishment for sin, the swollen one is caused by hunger (hypoproteinemia or nephrotic syndrome?), and the thin one is caused by magic (*Shabbat* 33a). Several famous talmudic sages suffered from it (*Shabbat* 33a), probably due to hunger. A person afflicted with dropsy may die suddenly (*Eruvin* 41b). It is not clear whether the abdominal swelling of a suspected adulteress after she drank the bitter waters represents dropsy [*see* SOTAH].

DROWNING—Moses was saved from drowning by Pharaoh's daughter (Exodus 2:5). If one sees one's fellow man drowning, one is obligated to try to save him (*Sanhedrin* 73a). If a man drowns in a large lake, his wife is forbidden to remarry (*Yebamot* 115a) unless his leg and knee is found, in which case he is presumed dead and his widow can remarry (ibid., 120b). People who drown at sea have no burial (*Ecclesiastes Rabbah* 3:2:2). Four hundred captured children who were being transported by boat for immoral purposes jumped into the sea and drowned (*Gittin* 57b). Abdan was punished for his sins in that his two sons drowned (*Yebamot* 105b). He who in former times would be sentenced to strangulation may drown in the river as divine punishment (*Sanhedrin* 37b).

DRUNKENNESS—Wine gladdens the heart (Psalms 104:15). Therefore bitter souls and poor people drink to drown their sorrow (Proverbs 31:6–7). However, the side effects of alcohol are significant. Adam drank wine that Eve gave him and the world was cursed on his account (*Numbers Rabbah* 10:4). The face of intoxicated people shines (*Ecclesiastes Rabbah* 8:1:4). Woe to the man and woman who drink wine, become intoxicated, and commit sins (*Numbers Rabbah* 10:1). Women who drink behave immorally (*Ketubot* 65a). Judges who drink prevent justice (ibid., 10:4). An intoxicated person behaves like a madman (*Megillah* 12b) and has red eyes (Proverbs 24:29–30; Genesis 49:12). Drunk people totally expose themselves (*Habakkuk* 2:15) as did Noah when he was drunk (Genesis 9:21). A drunkard sells all his possessions to buy wine (*Leviticus Rabbah* 12:1) and becomes poor (Proverbs 23:21). A person is recognized by the amount of alcohol he drinks (*Eruvin* 65a–b). A drunkard drinks his entire glass in one gulp (*Betzah* 25b), sees strange things (hallucinations?), speaks confused words (Proverbs 23:33), has wounds on his skin (ibid., 23:29), and may fly into a drunken rage (*Exodus Rabbah* 30:11). Drunkards fall by themselves (*Shabbat* 32a). The Lord hates Torah scholars who frequent wine shops (*Niddah* 16b) and loves those who do not become intoxicated (*Pesachim* 113b).

The amount of alcohol one can tolerate varies. Some people drink only a little and feel it from head to toes (*Shabbat* 14a). One rabbi suffered from headaches for seven weeks after the four cups of wine on Passover night (*Ecclesiastes Rabbah* 8:1; *Nedarim* 49b). Mar Samuel became dizzy solely from the aroma of wine (*Eruvin* 65a). A walk or a little sleep counteract the effects of a little wine but not if one is drunk (*Sanhedrin* 22b; Leviticus 37:3). The sleep of an intoxicated man benefits himself and the world is spared of his wickedness while he sleeps (*Sanhedrin* 72a). The prayer of a drunkard is an abomination (*Eruvin* 64a).

A king should not drink lest he pervert justice (Proverbs 31:4–5). The sons of Aaron died because they were drunk when they performed the priestly service (*Leviticus Rabbah* 12:3). Lot became drunk from the wine his daughters gave to him (Genesis 19:32–35). He should have avoided wine the second time (*Nazir* 23a). The talmudic expression is "drunk as Lot" (*Eruvin* 65a). Wine is especially dangerous for women; if they drink four cups of wine, they solicit even an ass and are not ashamed (*Ketubot* 65a). [*See also* WINE, BEER, and *KORDIAKOS*]

DUNG—Animal dung was recommended as a plaster to cure a foot problem (*Song of Songs Rabbah* 2:3). Meat roasted over cattle dung, followed by wine, was used to treat weakness of the heart (*Eruvin* 29b). Cow dung was also used in bandaging material (*Abodah Zarah* 28a). One of many remedies for abnormal vaginal bleeding contains dung from a white mule (*Shabbat* 110b). Trees with missing bark can be treated by applying dung there (*Abodah Zarah* 50b).

Dung must be stored at least three handbreadths from a neighbor's wall (*Baba Batra* 17b). Dung heaps (*Baba Metzia* 24a) were present near houses, on the street (*Chullin* 12a), and in courtyards (*Baba Batra* 11b). Some dung heaps are cleared away and the dung taken out to dunghills (*Pesachim* 55b). Dung heaps sometimes hid important vessels and articles (*Baba Batra* 19a). A starving child was once found on a dung heap (*Sanhedrin* 63b). Because of the unpleasant odor (*Berachot* 25a), dung heaps were forbidden in Jerusalem (*Tosefta Negaim* 6:2). Jerusalem's Dung Gate (Nehemiah 2:13; *Eduyot* 1:3) is probably the gate through which dung was removed from the city (*Shabbat* 15a).

DWARFISM—Nebuchadnezzar, king of Babylon, is said to have been a midget or dwarf (*Genesis Rabbah* 16:4). A male dwarf should not marry a female dwarf, lest their offspring be a dwarf of the smallest size (*Bechorot* 45b). According to the commentaries of Ibn Ezra and Targum Jonathan, the biblical term *dak* (Leviticus 21:20) refers to a midget or dwarf.

A dwarf is described in the Talmud in relation to violation of Sabbath laws (*Shabbat* 5a). Bald-headed people, dwarfs, and the bleary-eyed are unfit for the priesthood because "they are not like the seed of Aaron" (*Bechorot* 43b). The suggestion that Abba Saul was a dwarf is rejected in the Talmud (*Niddah* 24b).

A woman whose son was a dwarf saw him in her imagination as "tall and swift" (*Genesis Rabbah* 65:11) but everyone else saw him only as a puny dwarf (*Song of Songs Rabbah* 2:15:12).

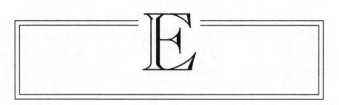

EARS—In the Bible, the word *ozen* refers to equilibrium (Ecclesiastes 12:9) or the organ of hearing or hearkening (Exodus 15:26; Psalms 135:17). Although earrings (Genesis 35:4; Exodus 32:2) or rings (Ezekiel 16:2; *Shabbat* 11b and 57a) were placed in ears, the latter's main function was for hearing (Deuteronomy 29:3; Ezekiel 12:2). The ear tip or cartilage is called *tenuch ozen* (Exodus 29:20; Leviticus 8:23) or *bedal ozen* (Amos 3:12). In the Talmud the earlobe is called *alyah* (*Ketubot* 5:2), *meylat* (*Bechorot* 37b), or *milta* (*Kiddushin* 20b). The ear cartilage is called *tenuch* (*Bechorot* 6:1) and the rest of the auricle is called *or ha' ozen*, or "skin of the ear" (*Bechorot* 37a).

Convulsing animals twitch their ears (*Chullin* 38a). A rabid dog flaps its ears (*Yoma* 83b). A mule's ancestors determine the size of its ears (*Chullin* 79a). Scratching in one's ear is dangerous since it can lead to deafness (*Shabbat* 108b). Aural secretions are beneficial when in small amounts (*Numbers Rabbah* 18:2) but harmful when present in large quantity (*Baba Metzia* 107b). Pain in the ear and remedies for it are frequently described in the Talmud (*Abodah Zarah* 28b; *Shabbat* 67a). Wet ear sores are treated with dry powders but dry ear sores require liquid ear drops (ibid.). Placing a grasshopper in one's ear to treat an earache is rabbinically forbidden (*Shabbat* 6:10 and 67a). Absorbent cotton can be inserted into the ear for an earache, even on the Sabbath (*Shabbat* 64b).

Many Jewish laws relate to the ear. For certain ritual purifications (e.g., of a leper), oil is sprinkled on the tip of the right ear (Leviticus 14:14 and 17; *Negaim* 14:9). Aaron the High Priest and his sons placed ram's blood on the tips of their right ears at the consecration of the Tabernacle (Exodus 29:20). Tips of the ears do not contract ritual impurity on account of quickflesh (*michyah*) (*Negaim* 6:7). A Hebrew manservant's ear is bored if he wishes to remain with his master after six years of servitude (Exodus 21:6). If a master strikes his servant's ear and renders him deaf, he obtains his freedom as a result (*Baba Kamma* 98a).

If one harms another person's ear, one must pay for damages, pain, and medical expenses.

A variety of ear blemishes in humans and animals may disqualify a priest from Temple service or an animal from being offered as a sacrifice (*Bechorot* 37a). These include nicks or perforations in the ear cartilage, dryness or duplication of the earlobe, excessively large or small ears, or unequal sizes of the two ears (*Bechorot* 44a; *Tosefta Bechorot* 4:15). Other legal ramifications of ear abnormalities are discussed elsewhere.[1,2] The ear is also mentioned in a variety of proverbs such as "The walls have ears" (*Ecclesiastes Rabbah* 10:20) and others (*Genesis Rabbah* 45:7 and 74:2). [*See also* DEAFNESS]

---

1. F. Rosner (trans.), *Julius Preuss' Biblical and Talmudic Medicine* (Northvale, NJ: Jason Aronson, 1993), pp. 289–291.
2. A. Steinberg, *"Ozen,"* in *Encyclopedia of Jewish Medical Ethics,* vol. 1 (Jerusalem: Schlesinger Institute at the Shaare Zedek Medical Center, 1988), pp. 24–30 (Hebrew).

EATING HABITS—General rules of nutrition include eating in moderation. More people die of overeating than of undereating (*Shabbat* 33a). One should not eat excessively (*Gittin* 70a). One should also eat simple foods. A man once ate fine bread and fat meat and drank old wine and suffered harm while his friend who ate coarse bread and vegetables escaped harm (*Ecclesiastes Rabbah* 1:18). Eat cress rather than fat tails (*Pesachim* 114a). One should eat slowly and chew the food well (*Shabbat* 152a). Drawing out a meal prolongs one's life (*Berachot* 54b). One should eat regularly since altering one's schedule leads to indigestion (*Sanhedrin* 101a). It is preferable to eat during the day when one can see well rather than at night (Ecclesiastes 6:9). For this reason, too, the blind eat but are not satiated (*Yoma* 74b).

A person should consume more solid food than liquid (*Megillah* 12a) although one should drink abundantly (*Berachot* 40a), one cupful of water per loaf of bread or other food (ibid.). Eating without drinking destroys one's vitality (*Shabbat* 41a). One should eat only one main meal per day, at an appropriate hour (*Shabbat* 10a; *Sukkah* 27a). One should not sit on food lest it be crushed and wasted, but one may sit on a basket of legumes (*Kallah Rabbati* 2:52) or on a cake of pressed figs because these are not spoiled by sitting on them (*Soferim* 3:14). One should not eat while standing nor lick one's fingers (*Derech Eretz Zutah* 5:1). One should eat porridge with a spoon and not with one's fingers (*Nedarim* 49b). One should wash one's hands before eating (*Chullin* 106a). One should not eat in the marketplace or on the street (*Kiddushin* 40b).

Terminally ill patients may eat whatever they desire (*Exodus Rabbah* 30:

22; *Ecclesiastes Rabbah* 5:6). Such patients may ask for delicacies (*Song of Songs Rabbah* 2:5) such as fragrant apples (*Soferim* 16:4). Fresh eggs and fish are healthy for sick patients (*Sanhedrin* 64a and 98a). *Arsan*, a barley food cooked like beef (*Nedarim* 41b and 49a), is good for ill people. Corn flour mixed with honey (*shatita*) is a remedy for sick patients (*Berachot* 38a), especially for those with fever (*Gittin* 70a). The following foods are good for convalescing patients: cabbage; mangold; chamomile; the maw, womb, and large lobe of the liver; and small fish (*Berachot* 57b). Physicians prescribe special diets for injured people (*Baba Kamma* 85a).

Nourishment relating to bloodletting, eye disorders, pregnancy, lactation, and the teeth is discussed in those respective sections [*see* BLOODLETTING, EYES, REMEDIES, PREGNANCY, LACTATION, and DENTISTRY]. See also specific foods and vegetables.

EGGS—The Talmud states that an egg is superior in food value to the same quantity of any other food (*Berachot* 44b). A lightly cooked or roasted egg is superior to six measures of fine flour; a hard boiled egg is better than four (ibid.). A boiled egg is better than the same quantity of any other boiled food except meat (ibid.). Eggs were eaten either very soft so that they were sucked out, or hard-boiled, requiring the peel to be removed (*Uktzin* 2:6). Eggs were also fried by being placed in hot sand or dust or cracked on a hot cloth and allowed to roast in the sun (*Shabbat* 3:3). Eggs were also roasted by rolling them in hot ashes (*Numbers Rabbah* 9:10) or placing them on the side of boilers (*Shabbat* 38b). Roasted eggs were sometimes beaten into a hash (*Shabbat* 109a). It is not clear whether eggs were also eaten raw (*Tosefta Sotah* 1:2).

Foods made from fine flour and eggs soften the stool but stimulate the sexual drive (*Yoma* 18a). Addled eggs upon which a hen brooded may be eaten by those who are not squeamish. If a blood spot is found on the egg it may not be eaten, unless the blood spot is on the white, in which case only the blood spot is forbidden (*Chullin* 64b). A very-hard-boiled egg when swallowed whole and excreted through the bowels helps the physician prescribe therapy for an internal ulcer (*Nedarim* 50b). Shrunken eggs that are boiled or roasted down to a very small size are delicious but forbidden on the Sabbath (*Shabbat* 58a).

The Talmud relates that the mother of Abaye told him that eggs with *kutach* make children strong (*Yoma* 78b). A soft-boiled egg without salt is said to be able to restore one's forgotten learning (*Horayot* 13b). On the other hand, eating peeled eggs that were kept overnight without their peels can be dangerous (*Niddah* 17a). Eggs and chicken are easy-to-digest food for ill people (*Jerushalmi Baba Kamma* 8:6). Fresh eggs are particularly therapeutic for sick patients (*Sanhedrin* 64a). Eggs are not recommended after bloodletting (*Abodah Zarah* 29a). He who eats eggs has children with big eyes (*Ketubot* 61a). Eggwhite is an ingredient in healing ointments (*Shabbat* 77b). A cook once offered to teach someone how to prepare one hundred dishes made from eggs (*Ecclesiastes Rabbah* 1:8:2).

Eggs that are arched and rounded with one end broad and the other end narrow are derived from clean (i.e., kosher) birds (*Chullin* 64a). If the yolk and the white are mixed together, it is a reptile's egg (ibid.). Locust eggs were worn around the neck as a prophylactic against earache (*Shabbat* 67a). Turtle doves have light (i.e., small) eggs (*Shabbat* 80b). An egg laid on the Sabbath or on a Festival may not be consumed until after the Sabbath or the Festival (*Shabbat* 43a). Egg shells could be pierced, filled with oil, and placed over the mouth of an oil lamp to provide a continuous source of oil (*Shabbat* 29b).

EMACIATION—Rabbi Zadok fasted for forty years to ward off the downfall of Jerusalem and he became extremely emaciated (*Gittin* 56a). Puberty can be delayed because of emaciation (*Yebamot* 97a). If a man has intercourse immediately after blood-letting, he will have feeble children (*Niddah* 17a). [*See also* FASTING]

EMBALMING—Jewish practices and procedures after death, including the washing and ritual purification of the body, the use of coffins, different types of graves, the funeral, and the like are discussed in detail elsewhere.[1,2] Embalming of bodies was an Egyptian and not a Jewish custom although the Bible describes embalmers (Genesis 52:2) and mentions embalming with reference to Jacob and Joseph, who both died in Egypt (Genesis 50:2–3 and 50:26). The embalming of Jacob is explained differently by the biblical commentators. Rashi and others say that embalming means to use aromatic spices to perfume the body. Hertz and others claim that Joseph's aim in "embalming" his father Jacob was to preserve it from dissolution before it reached Israel for burial. Ralbag states that the embalming of Jacob did not involve any desecration of the body. The embalming of Joseph (Genesis 50:26) is also variously interpreted by the commentaries.

King Herod is said to have "embalmed" his beloved by preserving the body in honey for seven years (*Baba Batra* 3b). Most current rabbinic decisors prohibit embalming as a desecration of the body.[3] [*See also* CREMATION]

---

1. F. Rosner (trans.), *Julius Preuss' Biblical and Talmudic Medicine* (North-

vale, NJ: Jason Aronson, 1993), pp. 511–521.

2. I. Jakobovits, *Jewish Medical Ethics* (New York: Bloch, 1975), pp. 116–152.

3. F. Rosner, "Embalming and Cremation," in *Modern Medicine and Jewish Ethics*, 2nd ed. (Hoboken, NJ: Ktav and Yeshiva University Press, 1991), pp. 335–350.

EMETIC—One may not induce vomiting on the street, out of decency (*Shabbat* 12a). One should not induce vomiting after a meal so as to be able to eat more, because it is a waste of food (ibid., 147b). One should not induce vomiting on the Sabbath with an emetic drug but may do so by hand (ibid., 147a). Newborns were induced to vomit to cleanse their mouths of mucus (*Shabbat* 123a). *Afiktazon* is an emetic (ibid., 147b). Cultured plants were used as emetics (*Sukkah* 40b). Wheat cakes streaked with honey followed by strong wine is an emetic (*Gittin* 69b). A person can become nauseous and vomit when discussing obscene matters (*Sanhedrin* 55a). After eating a certain chicken stew, one can prevent nausea and vomiting by drinking old wine (*Shabbat* 145b).

EPILEPSY—The biblical term "fallen down" probably refers to epilepsy. Hence, Balaam (Numbers 24:16) and King Saul (1 Samuel 19:24) are said to have suffered from epilepsy (Mai-

monides' *Mishnah Commentary, Gittin* 7:5). Body humors and gases play a role in the causation of epilepsy (ibid., *Gittin* 7:1). Demons may also play a role (*Gittin* 70a; *Rosh Hashanah* 28a; *Leviticus Rabbah* 26:5). Hereditary factors were also recognized in that a person should not take a wife from a family of epileptics (*Yebamot* 64a). Immoral sexual behavior is strongly discouraged in Judaism and may be the basis for several talmudic statements about epilepsy: A woman who copulates in a mill will have epileptic children (*Ketubot* 60b). He who copulates immediately after defecation (*Gittin* 70a) or by the light of a lamp will have epileptic children (*Pesachim* 112b). He who stands naked in front of a lamp or who cohabits in a bed in which a baby is sleeping will become epileptic (*Pesachim* 112b). Cohabitation after bloodletting may also lead to the birth of epileptic children (*Leviticus Rabbah* 16:1). Some post-talmudic rabbinic decisors consider epilepsy to be an infectious disease but most agree with modern medical knowledge that it is not.[1] The talmudic sages knew that certain epileptics had seizures at specified times (*Ketubot* 77a).

The diagnosis and treatment of epilepsy was carried out by competent physicians, not by priests or exorcists (*Leviticus Rabbah* 26:5). Amulets were used both to prevent and to treat epilepsy (*Shabbat* 61a; *Tosefta Shabbat* 4:9). One also recited incantations

(*Shabbat* 67a). The condition known as *kordiakos* (*Gittin* 7:1) is interpreted to refer to withdrawal seizures in the course of delirium tremens, secondary to alcoholic intoxication.[2] Some rabbis rule that a single convulsive episode defines a person as an epileptic, whereas other rabbis require three episodes. Controversy exists as to whether or not epilepsy is a life-threatening illness.[1]

Legally, an epileptic is unfit to serve as a priest in the Temple even if he only had a single seizure (*Bechorot* 7:5). An epileptic may serve as a cantor in the synagogue if his epilepsy is dormant or controlled (Responsa *Chatam Sofer*, *Yoreh Deah* #7). Similarly he may serve as a ritual slaughterer (ibid.). Undisclosed epilepsy may be grounds for divorce.[1] An epileptic can testify in a legal proceeding while he is well, provided his mind is clear (*Ketubot* 20a; Maimonides' *Mishneh Torah*, *Edut* 9:9).

---

1. A. Steinberg, *Encyclopedia of Jewish Medical Ethics*, vol. 4 (Jerusalem: Schlesinger Institute of the Shaare Zedek Medical Center, 1994), pp. 210ff. (Hebrew).

2. F. Rosner, "Kordiakos," in *Medicine in the Bible and the Talmud*, 2nd ed. (Hoboken, NJ: Ktav and Yeshiva University Press, 1995), pp. 60–64.

EPISPASM—Circumcision is the sign of the covenant between God and Abraham and the people of Israel (Genesis 17:13). According to the Talmud (*Avot* 3:11), anyone who abrogates this covenant has no share in the world to come. It is alleged that during Hellenistic times some Jews who wanted to participate nude in the Greek games in the gymnasia attempted to make their circumcisions unrecognizable by methodically pulling the foreskin to the front. These epispastics (Greek meaning "to draw in"), according to Josephus (*Antiquities* Book 12, chapter 5:1), covered the circumcision of their penis, so that even when they were naked, they could not be distinguished from the Greeks. Some authors believe these Jews "underwent painful operations to obliterate the signs of circumcision [epispasm]."

The Talmud (*Yebamot* 72a) rules that a circumcised male whose prepuce has been drawn forward to cover up the corona must be recircumcised. A similar rule is found in the extratalmudic collection of rabbinic sayings known as *Tosefta* (*Shabbat* 16:6). In the course of the persecutions that preceded the Judean revolt led by Bar Koziba against Rome in 132 C.E., many Jews became epispastics by forcibly drawing their prepuces forward. After the liberation, many were recircumcised without any harm occurring to their health or procreative ability, thus contradicting the assertion of Rabbi Judah in the Talmud that to recircumcise an epispastic is dangerous (*Yebamot* 72a). Elsewhere (*Sanhedrin* 44a), the Talmud states that Achan was an epispastic, based on the biblical passage in Joshua 7:11. The rabbinic exegetical work entitled *Midrash Tanhuma*, in its commentary on the book of Genesis, implied that Esau was also an epispastic. Preuss cites several additional references to epispastics in ancient Hebrew writings.[1] [*See also* CIRCUMCISION]

---

1. F. Rosner (trans.), *Julius Preuss' Biblical and Talmudic Medicine* (Northvale, NJ: Jason Aronson, 1993), pp. 246–247.

ESOPHAGUS—The foodpipe or esophagus (*veshet* in Hebrew) is known as the "place of swallowing" (*beth habeliyah*) (*Ketubot* 30b; *Niddah* 42a; *Zavim* 5:19). The esophagus has an outer muscular and an inner mucous membrane (*Chullin* 43a). The muscular layer causes the esophagus to retract when it is cut, as during the ritual slaughtering of an animal (*Chullin* 43b). The ritual slaughtering of animals requires the severance of both trachea and esophagus (*Chullin* 27a). Perforation of both membranes or layers of the esophagus is a life-threatening situation in an animal (*Chullin* 43a). If the lower jawbone of an animal is gone, one can keep the animal alive by putting food directly into its gullet (*Chullin* 55b).

One should not speak while eating (*Taanit* 5b) nor recline on the right side while eating, lest the food go into the windpipe instead of the esophagus (*Pesachim* 108a). The esophagus is one of the ten digestive organs (*Ecclesiastes Rabbah* 7:3). Injuries to the esophagus in humans are dangerous. These include a needle or a small hook stuck in the esophagus (*Jerushalmi Sanhedrin* 9:27). Esophageal atresia (literally: closed or obliterated esophagus) in a newborn is fatal (*Niddah* 23b). If one chokes on a piece of meat that is stuck in the throat, one should try to wash it down with water (*Berachot* 45a). Magical incantations were also recited for someone with an object stuck in the throat (*Shabbat* 67a). [*See also* THROAT, STOMACH, and NECK]

EUNUCH—A congenital eunuch is called a *saris chama* (sun castrate) as opposed to acquired sterility due to an illness or injury (*Yebamot* 80a). The signs of a eunuch are that he has no beard, his hair is soft, his skin is smooth, his urine has a weak stream and does not bubble or ferment, his semen is like water, and his voice is soft (*Yebamot* 80b). A eunuch can marry (*Tosefta Yebamot* 2:5–6) but may not be able to cohabit with his wife (*Tosefta Bechorot* 5:4) and cannot beget children (*Jerushalmi Yebamot* 9b). He is like a dry tree (Isaiah 56:3) but may retain his libido (*Sirach* 20:2). To embrace him is like embracing a statue (*Exodus Rabbah* 43:7). Some men have a few bristles as their beard and can be mistaken for eunuchs (*Yebamot* 80b).

God blesses the Jews by saying there will be no eunuchs or women incapable of procreation (Deuteronomy 7:14). Yet some exist. Men were castrated in ancient times (Isaiah 39:7) to serve as harem watchers (2 Kings 9:32 and 24:12). Eunuchs also served as military supervisors (2 Kings 25:19; Daniel 1:3), brewmasters (*Kiddushin* 52b; *Baba Metzia* 42b), or servants of the courts (*Megillah* 28a; *Kiddushin* 33a). A eunuch priest is unfit to serve in the Temple (*Tosefta Bechorot* 5:2). A eunuch is not appointed to the Sanhedrin (*Sanhedrin* 36b) and cannot judge criminal cases (*Tosefta Sanhedrin* 7:5). Eunuchs are consoled by God for their misfortune (Isaiah 56:4). A palace eunuch, reproached for his useless existence, committed suicide (*Ecclesiastes Rabbah* 10:7:1; *Shabbat* 152a). [*See also AYLONIT*, CASTRATION, CHILDLESSNESS, and STERILITY]

EUTHANASIA—Jewish teaching in regard to mercy killing is based on the principle of the infinite value of human life (*Yoma* 85b). One is prohibited from doing anything that hastens death (*Semachot* 1:1ff.). He who closes the eyes of a dying person even as the soul is departing and thereby shortens life by a few seconds is considered a murderer (*Shabbat* 151b). Probably the first recorded instance of euthanasia is the merciful death of King Saul

at the hands of an Amalekite (2 Samuel 1:5–10) after Saul's unsuccessful attempt at suicide (1 Samuel 31:1–6). The death of Rabbi Chanina ben Teradion by fire at the hands of the Romans is an illustrative case involving euthanasia (*Abodah Zarah* 18a).

On the other hand, thirteenth-century Rabbi Judah the Pious sanctions the removal of an impediment to death (*Sefer Chasidim* #723). So do Rabbi Moshe Isserles (*Rama, Shulchan Aruch, Yorah Deah* 339:1) and many others. Based on these and other sources, rabbinic decisors[1,2,3,4,5] conclude that any form of active euthanasia is strictly prohibited and condemned as plain murder. At the same time Jewish law sanctions the withdrawal of any factor that may artificially delay the patient's death in the final phase. Some rabbinic views do not allow any relaxation of efforts, however artificial and ultimately hopeless they are, to prolong life. Others, however, do not require the physician to resort to "heroic" methods, but sanction the omission of machines and artificial life-support systems that serve only to draw out the patient's agony, provided, however, that basic care (such as food and good nursing) is provided.

1. F. Rosner, *Modern Medicine and Jewish Ethics*, 2nd ed. (Hoboken, NJ, and New York: Ktav and Yeshiva University Press, 1991), pp. 197–246.
2. I. Jakobovits, *Jewish Medical Ethics* (New York: Bloch, 1975), pp. 119–125.

3. J.D. Bleich, *Judaism and Healing* (New York: Ktav, 1981), pp. 134–145.

4. A.S. Abraham, *Comprehensive Guide to Medical Halachah* (Jerusalem and New York: Feldheim, 1990), pp. 174–180.

5. B.F. Herring, *Jewish Ethics and Halakhah for Our Time: Sources and Commentary* (New York: Ktav and Yeshiva University Press, 1984), pp. 67–90.

EVIL EYE—A widespread belief among nearly all people in antiquity and also in more recent times is the belief that the evil eye, or *ayin hara*, can be the cause of illness. The Talmud states that the evil eye, the evil inclination, and hatred of one's fellow man can remove a person from the world (*Avot* 2:11). A person should not have a grudging nature that is equivalent to an evil eye (*Avot* 2:9 and 5:13). A person with an evil eye is considered wicked (*Avot* 5:19). Rab and Chiya are of the opinion that ninety-nine percent of all people die through the evil eye, and only one percent die of natural causes. Both lived in Babylonia, "where the evil eye was extremely prevalent" (*Jerushalmi Shabbat* 14:14). Even this belief, therefore, originated in Babylonia. When Scripture states "And the Lord will take away from thee all sickness" (Deuteronomy 7:15), it refers to the evil eye (*Baba Metzia* 107b), from which the Israelites would be immune. One is protected from the evil eye by placing the right thumb in the left hand, and the left thumb in the right hand (*Berachot* 55b). The evil eye has no power over the descendants of Joseph (*Berachot* 20a; *Baba Metzia* 84a). A fox's tail was suspended between a horse's eyes to ward off the evil eye (*Shabbat* 53a). Hair ribbons were worn by women for the same reason (ibid., 57b). Market traders are exposed to the public gaze and hence to the evil eye (*Pesachim* 50b). Some people sell their property with an evil eye (*Baba Batra* 64b). A person should always be on guard against an evil eye (ibid., 118a). The birth of a daughter is a good sign because the evil eye has no influence over her siblings (ibid., 141a). A woman with menstrual bleeding on the night of her ritual bath is afflicted by the evil eye and has no cure (*Niddah* 66a). [*See also* DEMONS, EXORCISM, MAGIC, SORCERY, INCANTATIONS, and ASTROLOGY]

EXERCISE—Jacob, the ostensibly sedentary dweller in tents (Genesis 25:27), wrestled with an angel and prevailed (Genesis 32:26). He also rolled two large stones from the mouth of the well and watered the flock of Laban (Genesis 29:13). Lifting or moving a huge stone was later recognized as a test of one's strength (Zechariah 12:3).

After the conquest of Canaan, the Jews of ancient times were farmers who tilled the soil and raised and bred cattle and other livestock. Physical activity was recognized as a good soporific, as stated: "The sleep of a laboring man is sweet" (Ecclesiastes 5:11).

The strength of the heroes and mighty men of Judaism such as Joshua, Samson, Gideon, David, and others was praised as the "glory of young men in their strength" (Proverbs 20:29). Even God is characterized as "strong and mighty" (Psalms 24:8). Jewish youth served in the armed forces, beginning at twenty years of age (Numbers 1:4) and, among other things, were taught archery (2 Samuel 1:18). They became equally adept at shooting arrows using both the right and left hand (1 Chronicles 12:2). Some also became experts at slinging stones at a hairsbreadth and not missing (Judges 23:16). They shot arrows and great stones from towers (2 Chronicles 23:15), proving their great strength. Shooting arrows at a specific target is described (1 Samuel 20:20), as is the bending of the bow (Lam. 3:12). Thrusting one's enemy through with a sword (2 Samuel 2:15) and scaling a wall (Psalms 18:30) also required considerable strength and some practice.

In talmudic times, it was recommended to the Jews by the Sages that physical perfection engenders spiritual fulfillment. Thus, the Talmud says (*Shabbat* 92a; *Nedarim* 33a): "The Divine Presence rests only on a wise man, a strong man, a healthy man, and a tall man." Furthermore, God takes pride in men of high stature (*Bechorot* 45b).

The Midrash states (*Numbers Rabbah* 20:24) that a man should be fierce as a leopard, swift as an eagle, fleet as a hart, and strong as a lion in the performance of God's will. The same recommendation is found in the Talmud (*Avot* 5:23). The talmudic rabbis advised the people regarding appropriate exercise regimens and their legal decisions reflect the prevalence of exercise practices. Rabbi Yochanan said, "Do not sit too long, for long sitting provokes hemorrhoids; do not stand too long because long standing is injurious to the heart; do not walk too much because excessive walking is harmful to the eyes. Rather, spend one-third of your time in sitting, one-third in standing and one-third in walking" (*Ketubot* 111a).

Apparently, oil rubs or embrocations were commonly employed in bathhouses. After the embrocation, the person did physical exercise to tire himself (*Kallah Rabbati* 9:54d); in some cases, the oil rubbing routine itself caused considerable exertion (*Jerushalmi Sheviit* 38b). Scales were present in the bathhouse to note changes in body weight due to perspiration, a clinical problem encountered by the bather drinking hot water (*Genesis Rabbah* 4:4).

The Talmud (*Shabbat* 147a) states that one may oil and lightly massage the body on the Sabbath but not massage it strongly or scrape it to invigorate or stimulate the circulation because that constitutes healing on the Sabbath, a prohibited act unless essential to preserve life or limb. Rabbenu Chananel explains this talmudic passage as follows: "One bent and stretched the arms forwards and backwards as well as the legs on the haunches so that one became warm and perspired," apparently describing deep knee bends.

Rabbi Joseph used to cure the shivers by working at the mill, Rabbi Sheshet by carrying heavy beams. He said, "Work is a splendid thing to make one warm" (*Gittin* 67b). Discussions and rulings on exercise are also found in the codes of Jewish law of Maimonides (*Mishneh Torah*), Karo (*Shulchan Aruch*), and others.[1] [*See also* RUNNING, WALKING, DANCING, BALLPLAYING, and SWIMMING]

---

1. F. Rosner, "Exercise and Judaism," in *Medicine in the Bible and the Talmud*, 2nd ed. (Hoboken, NJ: Ktav and Yeshiva University Press, 1995), pp. 140–149.

EXORCISM—The placenta of a black cat was once used for a demonic exorcism (*Berachot* 6a). A man possessed by the demon of madness is treated by making smoke with roots and then sprinkling water to chase the demon away (*Numbers Rabbah* 19:8). A demon was once driven away with smoke made from fish heart and fish liver (*Tobit* 8:2). An extensive procedure to exorcise the "demon" causing a burning fever is depicted in the Talmud (*Shabbat* 7a). [*See also* ASTROLOGY, DEMONS, EVIL EYE, INCANTATIONS, and MENTAL ILLNESS]

EYES, ANATOMY—The eye sits in its socket in the skull (*Niddah* 23a and 23b). The pupil is known as the black of the eye (*Niddah* 31a; *Bechorot* 40a) or the apple of the eye (Deuteronomy 32:10; Psalms 17:8; Proverbs 7:2; Lamentations 2:18; Zechariah 2:12), a term denoting love and affection. The pupil is round (*Niddah* 23a). The white of the eye is considered as fat (*Bechorot* 38b). In man the white is predominant, whereas in animals it is the black (*Jerushalmi Niddah* 3:50). The *galgal* or globe is round in humans and oblong in animals (ibid.). Only the snake has a round pupil (*Niddah* 23a). The eyeball lies in a hollow. The eyes of the prosperous stand out with fatness (Psalms 73:7), whereas poor people suffering from hunger have sunken eyes (Midrash Psalms 73:7). The iris is called *sira* (*Bechorot* 38a).

The eyebrows above the eyes are called *gabinim* (Leviticus 14:9; *Baba Kamma* 117a). The biblical term *afapayim* refers both to the eyebrows and the eyelids (Psalms 11:4; Proverbs 6:4; Job 16:16), whereas the Talmud interprets this word to refer only to eyebrows (*Shabbat* 109a). The Aramaic word *timora* means "protectors" (*Shabbat* 77b). The talmudic term *ris* refers mostly to the eyebrows (*Tosefta Negaim* 8:5; *Sanhedrin* 104b) but sometimes also to eyelids (*Bechorot*

38a; *Kiddushin* 31a). Eyebrows can become very bushy and overgrown in old age (*Baba Kamma* 117a). According to legend, the white (i.e., cornea) of the eye is derived from the father, the black (i.e., pupil) from the mother, and vision is a gift from God (*Niddah* 31a). In man the eyes are in front of the face whereas in some animals and birds they are on the side (*Niddah* 23a).

EYES, BLEMISHES—Numerous eye blemishes or defects that have legal consequences are discussed in the Bible and Talmud, such as disqualifying a priest from Temple service, nullification of a marriage for nondisclosure, or disqualifying an animal from being sacrificed.[1] Rav studied with a shepherd for eighteen months to become expert in animal blemishes (*Sanhedrin* 5b). Eye defects in humans include *gibben* (Leviticus 21:20), which refers to a person without eyebrows or with only one eyebrow (*Bechorot* 43b) or a person with overhanging eyebrows or thick eyebrows (ibid., 44a). *Dak* (Leviticus 21:20) refers to clouding of the cornea (cataract?) or covering of the eye by a thin membrane (*Bechorot* 38b).

A *tebalul* (Leviticus 21:20) is a person whose white of the eye mixes with the black. *Bilbul* means "confusion" and, therefore, *tebalul* refers to coloboma (*Bechorot* 38a and 44a). *Yabelet* (Leviticus 22:22) is a wart or verruca in the eye (Rashi, Leviticus 22:22) and can be filled with hair (*Bechorot* 40b). *Charutz* (Leviticus 22: 22) refers to a hole or slit in the eyebrows (*Bechorot* 41a). *Chalazon* or *nachash* refers to an extra membrane on the cornea that reaches the pupil (*Bechorot* 38b), probably a pterygium or a chalazion. The talmudic commentaries (Rashi, Rabbenu Gershom) say it is called *Chalazon* because it resembles a worm or a snake. *Enab* is a berry-like excrescence (*Abodah Zarah* 28a). *Petzilah* is strabismus, where one sees several simultaneous images (*Bechorot* 43b–44a).

Chawarwar, meaning "white," refers to another type of corneal clouding, perhaps punctate keratitis. *Mayim*, or water in the eye, may refer to a cataract with a lot of tears. *Zavir* (*Bechorot* 44a) refers to a person with protruding eyes (exophthalmos?) or one with receded eyes or whose eyes are constantly shaking (nystagmus?) (*Bechorot* 44a). *Lufyan* is a person with thick and long eyebrows (ibid.). *Tamir* is a person whose eyebrows fell out (ibid.). *Zagdan* is a person with unequal eyes, such as if one eye is larger or of a different color than the other (*Bechorot* 44b). Other abnormalities include a large eye (*Bechorot* 40b), a small eye (ibid.), and a single eye (*Tosefta Bechorot* 4:4).

---

1. F. Rosner (trans.), *Julius Preuss' Biblical and Talmudic Medicine* (Northvale, NJ: Jason Aronson, 1993), pp. 259–265.

EYES, COSMETICS—Painting of the eyes is frowned upon in the Bible. It was only practiced by immoral women such as Jezebel (2 Kings 9:30) and others (Ezekiel 23:40) and was strongly condemned by the prophets (Jeremiah 4:30). The Talmud, however, recognized—although somewhat disapprovingly—that it was a generally accepted custom (*Tosefta Sotah* 3:3). Some rabbis even allow a woman to paint her eyes on the Sabbath (*Tosefta Shabbat* 10:13; *Shabbat* 95a). It is considered a necessary adornment of a woman even on Festivals (*Moed Katan* 1:7). For a man to use eye makeup is biblically prohibited (Deuteronomy 22:5).

Eye painting and other eye makeup was omitted during periods of mourning (*Ketubot* 4b) and during a woman's menstrual period (*Shabbat* 64b). If not veiled, both eyes were painted (*Shabbat* 80a). Mothers also painted the eyes of their newborn children (*Kiddushin* 73b). The expression "to paint the eyes" is commonly found in the Talmud (*Berachot* 58a; *Yoma* 69b).

For eyebrow painting, women used *puch* or stibium, which is an antimony powder (2 Kings 9:30; Isaiah 54:11; 1 Chronicles 29:2). *Puch* is an eye remedy and increases eyebrow hair (*Shabbat* 109a). *Cuchla* is a light blue powder containing antimony and is applied to the eye with a metal spoon called *makchol* (*Tosefta Kelim* 3:4) or a wooden spoon called *mekuchla* (*Shabbat* 151b) or *makchali* (*Gittin* 69a). The act of painting or anointing the eyes for cosmetic or therapeutic purposes is called *kachal* (Ezekiel 23:40). Turks, Persians, and Arabs to this day call an eye doctor *kochol*.[1] The eye makeup was applied by the cosmetic-impregnated crayon or stick horizontally between the closed eyelids. This cosmetic stick, also called *makchol*, was rounded at one end and pointy at the other (*Kelim* 13:2). The spoon described above was probably used to remove the makeup from the holder (Rashi, *Gittin* 69a). The spoon could even be made of silver (*Baba Kamma* 117a). The cosmetic stick in its holder, called *shefoferet*, was kept in a case by the woman (*Kelim* 16:18).

---

1. F. Rosner (trans.), *Julius Preuss' Biblical and Talmudic Medicine* (Northvale, NJ: Jason Aronson, 1993), pp. 280–282.

EYES, DISEASES—The rabbinic Sages describe various stages of eye inflammation (*Betzah* 22a; *Abodah Zarah* 28b; *Bechorot* 44a). *Techila uchla* is the first sign of eye inflammation. *Rira* is a discharge of pus (conjunctivitis). *Ditza* refers to shooting or sharp pain in the eyes. *Dama* refers to bloodshot eyes. *Dimata* means excessive tearing. *Kadachta* means local inflammation.[1] *Meridah* is said to be protrusion of the eye (Rashi, *Abodah Zarah* 28b) or the flow of infectious pus from the eye (Rashi, *Negaim* 6:8). *Sof uchla* is the final stage of eye inflammation. When the infectious secretion dries on the eyebrows, it becomes like a membrane called *lifluf* (*Mikvaot* 9:2; *Niddah* 67a). *Zabalgan* (*Megillah* 26b) is one from whose eyes tears flow (Rashi, *Megillah* 24b).

The eyes of a man afflicted with a *raatan* (*Ketubot* 77b) tear because of inflammation and his vision is defective as a result. Also, beware of contagion from flies near him (ibid.). A *tziran* (*Bechorot* 44a) is said to be a person with tearing eyes (Maimonides' *Mishneh Torah, Biyat Mikdash* 8:6) or with round eyes. Eyes that are *terutot* (*Shabbat* 31a; *Taanit* 24a; *Sotah* 47a; *Sanhedrin* 107b; *Bechorot* 44a) are round (Rashi, *Shabbat* 31a) and the eyelids are only partially open (Maimonides, *Biyat Mikdash* 8:5). *Simuka* (*Jerushalmi Shabbat* 14:4) is a person with redness of the eyes as a sign of a dangerous eye ailment. *Pekiat ayin* (*Abodah Zarah* 28b) refers to perforation of the eye as the final stage of a serious infection. *Barkit* or *barka* (*Bechorot* 38b; *Baba Metzia* 78b; *Shabbat* 78a) is a white tissue that protrudes from the eye and is compatible with a corneal inflammation (keratitis). *Atzev* or *einav* (*Bechorot* 38a) is a protrusion of part of the uveal layer secondary to corneal inflammation (Maimonides' *Mishnah Commentary, Bechorot* 6:2). This condition may be the same as *barkit*.

Chavarvar (*Bechorot* 38b) refers to sudden blindness from nerve weakness (Maimonides, *Bechorot* 6:3) or blindness (*Mishneh Torah, Issurei Mizbeah* 2:7) or cataract (*Aruch*, s.v. *eever*). Some authors consider it to refer to white spots on the eye and therefore a condition resembling *barkit*. The rabbis distinguish between permanent and temporary or transient *chavarvar* by repetitive examinations of the eye during an eighty-day period (*Bechorot* 38b). Water in the eye (ibid.) refers either to constant tearing (Rashi, *Bechorot* 38b) or the flow of water within the eye (Maimonides, *Bechorot* 6:3) which, according to some authors, refers to the development of a cataract.

Causes of eye ailments and diseases are extensively discussed in the Talmud. A woman who eats cress has bleary-eyed children; if she eats small fish she has children with small or blinking eyes; if she eats eggs, her children have large eyes (*Ketubot* 60b–61a). Drinking water from rivers or pools at night is dangerous and may lead to blindness (*Pesachim* 112a). Drinking water in a pot is harmful and may cause *barkit* (*Pesachim* 11b; *Gittin* 89a). Living in a dark house causes one's eyes to blink (*Berachot* 59a). Prolonged weeping causes the eyelashes to fall out (Genesis 29:17; *Baba Batra* 123a). People who live in sandy places have eyes that are *terutot* (*Shabbat* 31a).

Causes of blindness are described in the section BLINDNESS.

1. F. Rosner (trans.), *Julius Preuss'
Biblical and Talmudic Medicine* (Northvale, NJ: Jason Aronson, 1993), pp. 267–
270.

EYES, REMEDIES—Therapeutic
remedies cited in the Talmud for eye
disorders include liquids, salves, and
nonmedical measures. Coriander
leaves, applied to the eyes, cool them
and alleviate inflammation (*Shabbat*
109a). Compresses of other green
leaves can also be used (ibid.). Garden cress, the biblical *orot* (2 Kings
4:39), placed on the eyes, soothes and
heals eye ailments and improves vision
(*Shabbat* 109a; *Yoma* 18b). Metallic
objects, such as bowls or utensils,
placed on the eye cool it (ibid.). A
metal ring to minimize swelling can
also be placed on the eye (*Sanhedrin*
101a).

Among liquids, water is used to
wash out the eyes (*Shabbat* 78a and
108b). Wine or water from the Dead
Sea can also be applied locally to the
eye (*Shabbat* 108b). The spittle of a
firstborn son applied to his father's
eyes has healing properties (*Baba
Batra* 126b). Saliva after an overnight
fast is also efficacious (*Shabbat* 108b).
The most widely used eye remedy in
talmudic times was the paste called
collyrium rubbed on the eyes as an
ointment. The ingredients are mixed
and applied to the eyes (*Jerushalmi
Betzah* 4:4). The paste is applied with

water (*Shabbat* 8:1), wine (*Niddah*
19), human milk (*Tosefta Shabbat* 8:8),
dew (*Jerushalmi Shabbat* 8:11), or eggwhite (*Shabbat* 77b). The most famous
of all is the collyrium of Mar Samuel
(*Shabbat* 108b), which cured the eye
ailment of Rabbi Judah the Prince
(*Baba Metzia* 85b). These collyria
healed without producing a crust on
the eye.

An artificial eye made of gold is
described in the Talmud (*Jerushalmi
Nedarim* 9:8). Eyeglasses are not mentioned in the Talmud, although some
authors interpret *okselit* (*Tosefta Kilayim* 5:26) to represent eyeglasses. A
telescope used for distance vision, however, is mentioned (*Eruvin* 43b).

A variety of dietary recommendations for the prevention and treatment
of eye ailments and disorders are discussed. Well-cooked mangold or beets
are good for the eyes (*Berachot* 39a).
Figs are a delight to the eyes (*Ecclesiastes Rabbah* 5:10:1). Wine prepared
from cole sprouts is a good eye remedy (*Berachot* 51a). Honey consumed
after meals has a propitious effect on
the eyes (*Yoma* 83b). White bread, fat
meat, and old wine give light to the
eyes (*Pesachim* 42a). The lung of a
goose "brightens the eyes" (*Chullin*
49a). Mar Samuel said that a drop of
cold water in the eye in the morning
. . . is better than all the collyria in the
world (*Shabbat* 108b).

Babylonian *kutach* bread, because
of the Sodomite salt therein, is harm-

ful to the eyes. Excessive walking or taking big strides destroys a little of one's vision (*Ketubot* 111a). Fish consumption is harmful to the eyes (*Nedarim* 54b). Smoke is damaging to the eyes (Proverbs 10:26). The eye atrophies in the dark; daylight or sunlight nourishes the eye (*Oholot* 13:4). Patients with fever and eye ailments should not go to the bathhouse, and bloodletting is dangerous for someone with painful eyes (*Abodah Zarah* 20b–29a). Talking is also harmful for such patients (*Nedarim* 41a).

---

1. F. Rosner (trans.), *Julius Preuss' Biblical and Talmudic Medicine* (Northvale, NJ: Jason Aronson, 1993), pp. 276–284.

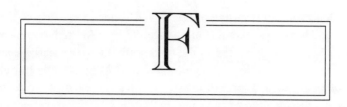

FACE—Adam is said to have had a double face and Eve was created from one of these faces, not from one of his ribs (*Berachot* 61a). The Lord creates all people with different faces so that people do not appropriate the wife or property of another person (*Jerushalmi Sanhedrin* 4:22). The prophet Ezekiel's vision included human faces on angelic beings (Ezekiel 1:1ff.). A corpse cannot be identified with certainty unless the face including the nose is clearly recognizable (*Yebamot* 16:3). Disfigurement of the face is described in the Talmud (*Niddah* 24a). Fasting results in pallor of the face and blackened teeth (*Nazir* 52b). Perspiration from anywhere on the body except the sweat from the face is said to be harmful (*Jerushalmi Terumot* 8:45).

Faces, even of idolatrous images, were engraved on signet rings (*Tosefta Abodah Zarah* 5:2) or embroidered into fabrics (*Tosefta Shekelim* 3:14). Fountains were adorned with faces on statues (*Tosefta Abodah Zarah* 6:6). In Judaism one is prohibited from making graven images or likenesses of human faces (*Rosh Hashanah* 24b), although pictures of the planets, animals, and nature scenes are permissible (*Abodah Zarah* 42b). "To turn one's face" means to be angry at someone. The Lord turns his face from those who sin against Him (*Chagigah* 5b). Facial makeup is discussed in the section entitled COSMETICS. [*See also* FOREHEAD, NOSE, MOUTH, and LIPS]

FAINTING—Weak people faint during profuse perspiration and need time to recuperate (*Shabbat* 9b). A man fainted when he saw that his father was about to be killed (*Chullin* 56b). After bloodletting, a poor man fainted from lack of food when he ate garlic (*Taanit* 25a). A dried date or fig may be sufficient to revive a person who faints (*Lamentations Rabbah* 1:2). Faint people are revived by honey (1 Samuel 14:27).

FAMINE—Famine, hunger, and starvation are punishments for wrongdoing (Deuteronomy 38:48; Ezekiel 7:15). God Himself proclaims famine (*Berachot* 55a). Famine occurs for the crime of robbery (*Shabbat* 32b) and the sin of giving all one's priestly gifts to a single priest (*Eruvin* 63a). When famine becomes severe, people eat even their own flesh (*Taanit* 5a), as foretold by the prophet (Isaiah 9:19) and as happened during the destruction of the Temple (*Lamentations Rabbah* 1:16:45). Famine visits the world ten times: in the days of Adam, Lemech, Abraham, Isaac, Jacob, the Judges, Elijah, and Elisha; one that travels about the world; and one in the Messianic future (*Genesis Rabbah* 25:3). Other famines such as in the time of David are described in the Bible (2 Samuel 21:1), which has 101 references to famine.[1]

During the famine in Egypt, Joseph's brothers came to buy bread (Genesis 47:18–19). During droughts with fear of famine, fast days were decreed and the warm baths were closed (*Taanit* 1:5 and 24b; *Genesis Rabbah* 33:3). Famine is worse than war (*Yebamot* 114b). Famine produces black skin features, withered and shriveled skin, and loss of hair (*Lamentations Rabbah* 4:10). Dried figs are distributed to the poor during times of famine (*Jerushalmi Eruvin* 4:22). Deaths from starvation are described in the Talmud (*Baba Batra* 91b). In Jerusalem, a child faint with hunger was once found lying upon a dungheap (*Sanhedrin* 63b).

In times of famine, cohabitation should be restricted to preserve body strength (Genesis 41:50; *Genesis Rabbah* 31:12 and 34:7). Only childless couples are exempt from this rule (*Taanit* 11a). However, hunger may weaken such couples and not allow them to engage in procreative activities (*Ketubot* 10b). One should flee from a place of famine or pestilence (*Baba Kamma* 60b). [*See also* FASTING and HUNGER]

---

1. A. Even-Shoshan, *A New Concordance of the Bible* (Jerusalem: Kiryat Sefer, 1981), pp. 1083–1084.

FASTING—An entire talmudic tractate (*Taanit*) is devoted to fasting and fast days and the laws pertaining thereto. Fasting is biblically required on Yom Kippur (Leviticus 16:29 and 23:27). The sages also decree fast days in times of calamity such as pestilence or drought (Joel 1:14; *Taanit* 14 and 21b). A person may not fast privately lest he damage his health (*Tosefta Taanit* 2:12). He who fasts for the sake of self-affliction is termed a sinner (*Taanit* 11a). Fasting weakens one's strength (*Lamentations Rabbah* 1:14:43), yet several talmudic sages fasted for long periods of time (*Baba Metzia* 33a). Rabbi Yochanan ben Zakkai lived only on figs for forty years to try to ward off the destruction of Jerusalem and the Temple. He nearly died of starvation (*Gittin* 56b). In the Temple, some Levites fasted on Mondays for the safety of sea travelers and on Tuesdays for the safety of wayfarers. On Wednesdays they fasted so that children would not be afflicted with *askara* (diphtheritic croup) and die, and on Thursdays they fasted so that pregnant women would not miscarry and nursing mothers would have adequate milk (*Lamentations Rabbah* 1:16:51; *Taanit* 27b).

Fasting for various purposes is detailed by the prophet (Isaiah 50:3ff.). One fasts for a sick person, praying for their recovery (*Taanit* 10b), as did King David for Bathsheba's child (2 Samuel 12:22). Lengthy fasting produces a bad mouth odor (*Genesis Rabbah* 42:1; *Avot de Rabbi Nathan* 6:3) and black teeth (*Nazir* 62b; *Jerushalmi Shabbat* 5:7). Eating following a prolonged fast may lead to pollution (*Avot de Rabbi Nathan* 8:8). The spittle of a fasting person is efficacious for treating eye ailments (*Shabbat* 108b). [*See also* FAMINE and HUNGER]

FENUGREEK—Fenugreek is a leguminous plant allied to clover. Its fruit and stalk taste alike (*Kilayim* 2:5). It is most edible when it is tender (*Maaser Sheni* 2:3). It is an ingredient in compound remedies for mouth abscesses (*Gittin* 69a) and for vaginal bleeding (*Shabbat* 110b). If one eats fenugreek on an empty stomach and then drinks water, intestinal worms may develop (*Shabbat* 109b). One should eat fenugreek regularly, especially on Rosh Hashanah since it grows in profusion and is symbolic of prosperity and fertility (*Horayot* 12a). Fenugreek is bought and sold by the bundle (*Orlah* 3:5; *Betzah* 13a; *Yebamot* 81b; *Zevachim* 72a). Fenugreek is liable to tithes (*Maaserot* 1:3) from the time when it grows (*Rosh Hashanah* 12b). So, too, for its shoots and berries (*Maaserot* 4:6). One can test the blue thread of fringes (*tzitzit*) with a liquid mixture containing fenugreek (*Menachot* 42b). Blood may occasionally be the same color as fenugreek juice (*Niddah* 19a).

FETUS—The fetus is known as the "fruit" (Lamentations 2:20; *Chullin* 114b; *Shabbat* 135b) or the "fruit of the womb" (Genesis 30:2). A woman's womb is wide below and narrow above so it may contain the fetus (*Eruvin* 18b). Forty days before the embryo is formed, a heavenly voice announces: So-and-so is to be the wife of so-and-so (*Moed Katan* 18b; *Sanhedrin* 22a). God insures that an embryo does not fall out of the mother's womb as money falls out of a bag whose opening is downward (*Leviticus Rabbah* 14:2–3). When the embryo is in its mother's womb, God causes a light to shine for it wherewith it can see from one end of the world to the other (ibid.). Job compares the generation of a fetus with coagulation (Job 10:10). It is also thought of as congelation of the sperm (*Leviticus Rabbah* 14:9). The body is shaped into flesh in the mother's womb (Wisdom of Solomon 7:12). First, there develops an amorphous mass (Psalms 139:16). The fetus begins to take shape after forty days from conception (*Genesis Rabbah* 32:5, *Bechorot* 21b; *Niddah* 25b). Queen Cleopatra of Alexandria cut open her pregnant slaves and found the male fetus to be completely formed at forty days and the female fetus at eighty days of gestation (*Tosefta Niddah* 4:17). An early human embryo has two eyes, two nostrils, and two ears that resemble two fly droppings; its two arms are like two threads of crimson silk; its mouth is like a barley grain; its trunk is like a lentil . . . (*Niddah* 30b). Three partners are involved in the formation of an embryo: God, the father, and the mother. Each contributes specific components to the fetus (*Niddah* 31a; *Ecclesiastes Rabbah* 5:10:2).

Fetal development begins either from the head or from the navel, from which its roots spread in all directions (*Sotah* 45b; *Yoma* 85a). The embryo lives only from its navel (*Song of Songs Rabbah* 7:3:1). Antoninus asked Rabbi Judah the Prince whether the soul and the evil inclination enter the body at the time of conception or the time of birth (*Sanhedrin* 91b). The embryo in a woman's womb is compared to a nut floating in a bowl of water (*Niddah* 31a). An embryo in its mother's womb

also resembles folded writing tablets. Its hands rest on its temples, its elbows on its legs, and its heels against its buttocks. Its head lies between its knees, its mouth is closed, and its navel is open . . . (*Niddah* 30b). An embryo is externally recognizable at three months of pregnancy (*Yebamot* 37a; *Niddah* 8b). The sex of a fetus can be determined by a "splinter test" (*Niddah* 25b) although its sex is already decided at the moment of cohabitation [*see* SEX DETERMINATION]. Mar Samuel says that fetal sex can only be decided with certainty if it has hair (*Niddah* 25a). During the first three months of pregnancy the fetus occupies the lowest chamber, during the middle months it occupies the middle chamber, and during the last months it occupies the uppermost chamber. When its time to emerge arrives it turns over, and this is the cause of the mother's pains of childbirth. The pains of a female birth are more intense than those of a male birth (*Niddah* 31a). Conception in an eleven-year-old girl may be dangerous for both mother and fetus (*Yebamot* 12b). Legally, the fetus may be considered to be merely an appendage of its mother (*Yebamot* 78a; *Baba Kamma* 78b; *Sanhedrin* 8b; *Chullin* 58a; *Temurah* 19a and 30b) or as an independent entity in regard to inheritance, eating Heave Offering (*Yebamot* 67a), or acquiring possessions (*Baba Batra* 141b). A fetus exempts its mother from levirate marriage (*Yebamot* 87a). Payment is required for the accidental killing of a human fetus, based on Exodus 21:22 (*Baba Kamma* 42a, 49a, 53b, and 87a). Miscarriage by a woman requires the process of ritual purification as if she gave birth to a baby (*Abodah Zarah* 42a).

Animal embryos are also discussed in the Talmud, including reptile and bird embryos in their eggs (*Chullin* 64a), animal embryos with two backs and two spinal columns (*Niddah* 24b), animal cesarean sections to extract fetuses (*Bechorot* 47b; *Temurah* 17a) and breech delivery of an animal fetus (*Chullin* 32a). An embryo in a cow increases its market value (*Baba Kamma* 47a). Financial compensation is required for the loss of a cow's embryo from goring by an ox (*Baba Batra* 93a). Animal embryos in their mother's wombs are tithed together with their mothers (*Bechorot* 56a). It is not clear whether or not an animal embryo is holy and can be offered in the Temple if it was dedicated by its owner for that purpose (*Temurah* 10a and 17a). Embryos from animals and birds are included in the prohibition against consuming or cooking milk and meat products together (*Chullin* 116a).

Embryotomy is only allowed to save the mother's life (*Oholot* 7:6) [*see also* ABORTION]. Postmortem cesarean section in an attempt to save the fetus was performed in talmudic times (*Arachin* 7a). Women buried their dead fetuses in earth mounds (*Tosefta Oholot* 16:1) or in cisterns (ibid.,

16:13). Genitalia of a fetus within the mother's womb can be torn off (*Jerushalmi Yebamot* 8:9d), probably secondary to a pelvic presentation and difficult birth. Psychic maternal influences on the fetus are well known and extensively discussed by Preuss.[1] [*See also* PREGNANCY and CHILDBIRTH]

---

1. F. Rosner (trans.), *Julius Preuss' Biblical and Talmudic Medicine* (Northvale, NJ: Jason Aronson, 1993), pp. 391–392.

FEVER—*Kadachat* (Leviticus 26:16), *daleket*, and *charchur* (Deuteronomy 28:22) are all types of fever. A fever in the winter is severer than in the summer (*Yoma* 29a). A furuncle called *simta* sometimes causes fever (*Abodah Zarah* 28b). For a bee sting or eye ailment associated with fever, bathing is dangerous (ibid.). One should visit a sick patient only after the fever subsides (*Nedarim* 41a). Circumcision is postponed in a baby with fever (*Yebamot* 70a). Patients with fever often go for days without eating; hence the hypothesis that "fever nourishes" (*Sanhedrin* 108b). If fever is not life-threatening it is salutary to the body, but one sage said: "I want neither the fever nor the theriac" (*Nedarim* 41a).

Numerous folk remedies are discussed for fever (*Shabbat* 67a; *Gittin* 67b). Radishes are good for a patient with fever (*Abodah Zarah* 28b). A fever present for two days is an indication for bloodletting (*Gittin* 67b). The nail from the gallows of an executed person is efficacious against the febrile illness *ababita* (*Jerushalmi Shabbat* 6:8). One sage with fever was cured by an incantation (*Song of Songs Rabbah* 2:16). When Rav died, people took dirt from his grave as a remedy for quotidian fever (*Sanhedrin* 47b). Rav Assi died of pyemia with high fever (*Nedarim* 36b). Burning fevers are considered life-threatening (*Abodah Zarah* 28a). Fig juice was rubbed on one such patient (*Pesachim* 25b). Another was treated with exorcism (*Shabbat* 67a). Other types of fever, including *achilu*, are detailed elsewhere.[1]

---

1. F. Rosner (trans.), *Julius Preuss' Biblical and Talmudic Medicine* (Northvale, NJ: Jason Aronson, 1993), pp. 160–164.

FIGS—The tree of knowledge in the Garden of Eden is said to have been a fig tree (*Genesis Rabbah* 15:7; *Sanhedrin* 70b). Adam and Eve ate figs, which are good to eat, fair to behold, and increase wisdom (*Ecclesiastes Rabbah* 5:10:1). Figs are nutritious and are eaten as dessert after meals (*Berachot* 41b; *Shevuot* 12b). Noah took fig cakes into the Ark as a nutritional substance for humans and animals (*Genesis Rabbah* 31:14). Fig cakes, made from dried and pressed summer figs, are highly nutritional (1 Samuel 30:12; *Kelim* 8:10). Fig trees were cultivated in ancient Israel (Numbers 13:23) and

fig honey was plentiful (*Ketubot* 111b). Dried figs were distributed to the poor (*Peah* 8:5), especially during times of famine (*Jerushalmi Eruvin* 4:22). Rabbi Zaddok lived only on figs for forty years (*Gittin* 56a).

Medically, fig cakes were used as cataplasms to heal wounds (2 King 20:7; *Sheviit* 8:1) and boils (Isaiah 38: 21). Fig juice was used to treat a burning fever (*Pesachim* 25b) and was imbibed as a beverage (*Pesachim* 107a). Figs were also used to treat bulimia (*Yoma* 83b) and were prescribed for sick patients (*Menachot* 64a). Fig gruel is difficult to digest (*Nedarim* 49b). The first ripe figs are of better quality than the late figs (*Genesis Rabbah* 22:5). Figs on the eastern side of fig trees are the sweetest (*Yoma* 83b). Figs from Beth Hini never fully ripen (*Pesachim* 53a) and figs from Keilah (1 Samuel 23:1, *Yoma* 76a; *Shevuot* 23a) are intoxicating (*Bechorot* 45b; *Keritot* 13b).

Figs grow on regular fig trees (*Eruvin* 32a) or on wild fig trees (*Demai* 1:1; *Rosh Hashanah* 15b). They can shrivel up on the tree (*Chullin* 127b). Goats graze under fig trees (*Ketubot* 111b). Most fig trees are worm-free (*Zevachim* 58a) although some figs are wormy (*Baba Batra* 93b). Black figs and white figs (*Terumot* 4:8; *Chullin* 136b) are cut off the trees with special fig-cutting knives (*Sheviit* 8:6). The figs may have remnant stalks on them (*Uktzin* 1:6; *Sanhedrin* 40a and 81b). Figs are dried on the roof (*Shab-*

bat 45a; *Betzah* 26b). While drying, they may be covered with straw to protect them from the rain (*Moed Katan* 13b). Fresh or dried figs (*Terumot* 2:4; *Demai* 5:5) are stored in jars (*Terumot* 4:10; *Baba Batra* 19b), casks (*Betzah* 33b), or barrels (*Oholot* 6:2) in storerooms (*Baba Batra* 20b). Fresh figs are also stored on the roof to keep them fresh (*Machshirin* 6:2). Figs can be pressed into fig cakes (*Terumot* 2:1; *Yebamot* 81a) and consumed by all people (*Genesis Rabbah* 31:14). The fig cakes can be round or square (*Terumot* 4:8–9; *Baba Metzia* 21b) and some are very juicy (*Shabbat* 7b and 99b). Dried figs are sold by measure and fig cakes by weight (*Ketubot* 64b). Baskets of figs (*Numbers Rabbah* 3:2; *Baba Batra* 143a) or baskets of fig cakes (*Shabbat* 120a) are sold in the market (*Berachot* 62b). The size of a dried fig is a quantity or measure for a variety of halachic or legal matters (*Shabbat* 70b, 76a–b, 78b, 80a, and 91a; *Eruvin* 4a and 80b; *Kelim* 17:7).

FINGER—Fingers are composed of roots, or *ikarim* (*Nazir* 50b), which are the connections to the metacarpals; the knuckle or joint, known as *perek*; and the fingertips, or *rashim* (*Negaim* 6:7). The thumb, or *bohen*, is used in the consecration of priests (Exodus 29:20). The Israelites intentionally crushed their thumbs to avoid playing music for the wicked king Nebuchadnezzar (Midrash Psalms 137:

5). A folk remedy for toothache was to tie a stalk of garlic to the thumbnail and place it on the aching tooth (*Gittin* 69a). The right thumb was placed in the left hand and the left thumb in the right hand to recite a magical incantation against the evil eye (*Berachot* 55) or to exorcise demons (*Pesachim* 110a). Hagrus the Levite (*Yoma* 3:11) had great musical talent. He produced musical sounds by placing his thumb in his mouth (*Jerushalmi Shekalim* 5:48) and a finger between his teeth (*Yoma* 38b). Alternatively, he placed both thumbs in his mouth, thus producing beautiful melodies (*Song of Songs Rabbah* 3:5:6).

The index finger is called *etzba* (Exodus 8:15). The middle finger is called *amma* or *etzba tzeredah*, meaning "snapping finger." To keep the High Priest awake on the night of Yom Kippur, the young priests snapped with this finger (*Yoma* 1:7) against the thumb of the right hand (*Tosefta Yom Hakkipurim* 1:9). Another view is that this finger was struck against the mouth (*Jerushalmi Yoma* 39b). The ring finger is called *kemitza* and the little finger *zeret* or *etzba ketanah*. It is forbidden to gaze even at the little finger of a woman lest it arouse lewd thoughts (*Shabbat* 64b). "My little finger is thicker than my father's loins" (1 Kings 12:10) is an expression of firmness. Putting one's fingers between the teeth (*Ketubot* 52a, 59b, and 71a) refers to the commission of an error. "The work of God's fingers" refers to His creations (Psalms 8:4) and "His finger" (Exodus 8:15) refers to His might. If one hears something unpleasant one plugs one's ears with one's fingers (*Ketubot* 5b). Refined people do not lick their fingers after eating (*Derech Eretz Zuta* 5:1).

A cubit is the distance from the elbow to the tip of the middle finger (*Ketubot* 5b). A span is the distance from the little finger to the thumb of a spread hand (ibid.). The ring finger is used for taking a fistful of the meal offering (Leviticus 2:2). The index finger is used for priestly services (ibid., 4:6). The thumb has its own function (ibid., 8:23–24; ibid., 14:14ff.; *Menachot* 11a). Every finger has a nail or *tziporen* (*Niddah* 6:2). Long nails were cut short but not discarded; rather, nails were buried or burned (*Niddah* 17a). A person in mourning does not cut his fingernails (*Moed Katan* 18a). A woman captured in war lets her nails grow (Deuteronomy 21:12). The psychotic King Nebuchadnezzar's nails grew like birds' claws, long and curved (Daniel 4:30). In old age, Rabbi Chiya's nails were lustrous and rosy like those of a child (*Chullin* 17b). To test whether a ritual slaughtering knife is completely notch free, it must first be examined with one's fingernail (*Chullin* 17b).

Webbed fingers (*Niddah* 23b) and extra fingers (polydactyly) are described in the Talmud (*Bechorot* 45b) and in the Bible (2 Samuel 21:20). Injury to or severance of fingers makes

people unable to spin flax or silk (*Song of Songs Rabbah* 8:11). The king of Bezek had his thumbs cut off (Judges 1:6). An injured finger is treated by an application of remedies (*Eruvin* 103b; *Shabbat* 50a). [*See also* HAND]

FISH—Fish live in the sea (*Sanhedrin* 108a) and are extremely fertile (*Baba Batra* 74b). The fish were blessed by God on the fifth day of creation (Genesis 1:22; *Ketubot* 5a). The fish of the sea said "And the truth of the Lord endureth forever" (*Pesachim* 118b). Everything is blessed by rain, including fish who feel it (*Genesis Rabbah* 13:16; *Deuteronomy Rabbah* 7:6). Fish are caught out of the water by their mouths (*Genesis Rabbah* 97:3). The Jews' complaint about not having fish in the desert (Numbers 11:5) is discussed at length in the Talmud (*Yoma* 75a). In the wilderness, the well brought up for the Jews various kinds of exceedingly rich fish (*Genesis Rabbah* 66:3). There are about seven hundred species of fish (Lamentations, *Proem* 34; *Chullin* 63b) including white fish and black fish (*Abodah Zarah* 39b), Egyptian fish, and Spanish tunny (*Machshirin* 6:3). Fish ponds (*Eruvin* 47b; *Yebamot* 121a; *Moed Katan* 4a; *Ketubot* 79a), fish pantries (*Pesachim* 8a), fishing boats (*Baba Batra* 73a and 78b), fishing nets (*Baba Batra* 21b; *Yebamot* 121a), and fishermen (*Moed Katan* 13b) are all described in the Talmud. A fish, a serpent, and a swine become stronger as they become older (*Shabbat* 77b; *Abodah Zarah* 30b). All copulate face-to-back except three who copulate face-to-face: humans, serpents, and fish (*Genesis Rabbah* 20:3).

Fish are clean (kosher) and fit for consumption if they have fins and scales (Leviticus 11:9; *Chullin* 59a and 66b). All fish that have scales have fins but some species have fins but no scales (*Niddah* 51b). Certain fish that shed their fins and scales when drawn out of the water are permitted for human consumption (*Abodah Zarah* 39a; *Chullin* 66a). Various types of clean and unclean fish are described in the Talmud, including mud fish and eels (*Abodah Zarah* 39a). The head and backbone help identify the species of fish (ibid., 40a). An unclean fish breeds, whereas clean fish lay eggs and hatch them (*Bechorot* 7b; *Abodah Zarah* 40a). If an unclean fish swallows a clean fish, it is permitted to be eaten but if a clean fish swallows an unclean fish, the latter is forbidden (*Bechorot* 7b). Fish do not require ritual slaughter (*Genesis Rabbah* 7:2; *Leviticus Rabbah* 22:10; *Numbers Rabbah* 19:3; *Ecclesiastes Rabbah* 7:23:3; *Chullin* 27b) and their blood is permitted (*Keritot* 21a) except if it is collected in a container (*Keritot* 21b).

Fish is considered as an independent food (*Pesachim* 114b). Salted fish are used as hors d'oeuvres at banquets (*Baba Batra* 60b). Fish is eaten salted, roasted, cooked, or seethed (*Nedarim*

20b); roasted on coals (*Kallah Rabbati* 1 fol. 52a); or boiled or broiled (*Moed Katan* 11a). Fish were strung together with ropes (*Baba Metzia* 21a and 23b) and pickled (*Shabbat* 39a and 145b) like herring (*Abodah Zarah* 40a) or made into a pie (*Shabbat* 37b). Fish innards were dissolved to make lighting oil (*Shabbat* 21a) and fish skin was used to polish the surface of wooden utensils (*Sanhedrin* 20b). Fish roe or eggs (*Chullin* 63b; *Abodah Zarah* 40a) are a delicacy but should be bought only by a reliable person to ensure that they are from a kosher fish (*Abodah Zarah* 40a). Fish are roasted with their skin over the fire and eaten with two loaves of bread (*Sanhedrin* 100b).

Medically, people who regularly eat small fish do not suffer from intestinal disorders. Fish strengthen the whole body (*Berachot* 20a) and serve as an aphrodisiac (*Berachot* 40a). Eating fish helps patients recover from illness (*Berachot* 57b; *Sanhedrin* 98a). Salted fish is tastier than unsalted fish (*Baba Batra* 74b). It was recommended that fish be pressed in salt sixty times before being eaten (*Moed Katan* 11a). Adda the fisherman said that one should broil fish with salt, plunge it in water, eat it with its sauce, and drink water after it (*Moed Katan* 11a). Also, after eating fish, cress, and milk, one should walk a little before lying down (ibid.). Fish heart and liver contain substances to fumigate people possessed with an evil spirit (*Tobit* 6:8 and 8:2). The evil eye is said to have no power over fish (*Genesis Rabbah* 97:3; *Berachot* 20a).

On the other hand, one should abstain from eating fish before bloodletting (*Abodah Zarah* 29a) and fish may be detrimental to the eyes (*Nedarim* 54b). Small salted fish can be deadly if imperfectly roasted (*Berachot* 44b). Fish soup ingestion may lead to uterine bleeding (*Tosefta Zavim* 2:5). Hemorrhoids may be caused by eating fish bones or salted fish (*Berachot* 55a; *Shabbat* 81a). The milk of a nursing woman who eats small fish may decrease in amount or turn turbid (*Ketubot* 60b). Fish consumption is said to have caused leprosy (*Pesachim* 112b) among the Israelites who complained about their sustenance in the wilderness (Numbers 11:5).

Honoring the Sabbath includes sending workers home early on Friday to allow them to broil their fish (*Genesis Rabbah* 72:4). Fish are given to poor people for their Sabbath meals (*Tosefta Peah* 4:8). A man named Joseph honored the Sabbath by buying fish at any price (*Genesis Rabbah* 11:4; *Shabbat* 118b). Fishermen catch fish privately for their Sabbath and Festival requirements (*Moed Katan* 13b). Fish may not be caught on the Sabbath or Festival (*Shabbat* 106b–107a).

Fish are hunted like beasts and birds (*Pesachim* 23a). Birds and fish digest their food in a few hours (*Oholot* 11:7). Fish are not susceptible to ritual uncleanness when they are alive (*Uktzin* 3:8). If fish and fowl are salted to-gether, the fish are forbidden because the blood exuded from the fowl is absorbed by the fish (*Chullin* 112b).

FISH BRINE—Muries is a kind of pickle, containing fish hash and wine with salt and water (*Shabbat* 108b). It is measured in a special cup (*Pesachim* 109a). Muries and fish brine are stored in casks or barrels (*Abodah Zarah* 31b) or in earthenware bottles (*Abodah Zarah* 33a). If these containers are left uncovered overnight the fish brine is not prohibited from use (*Chullin* 49b). Pickled herring is stored and served in brine (*Abodah Zarah* 39b). One species of fish (*kabbit*) only breeds in brine (*Abodah Zarah* 35b).

Medicinally, fish brine has a purgative effect on the intestines (*Shabbat* 108a). Sciatica can be treated by rubbing fish brine sixty times on each hip (*Gittin* 69b). Fish brine is also aphrodisiac in its effect (*Tosefta Zavim* 2:5) and, therefore, the High Priest is not fed fish brine for a week before the Day of Atonement lest he experience a semen flow and be rendered ritually unclean (*Yoma* 18a). Small fish in brine are recommended after fasting (*Abodah Zarah* 29a). The sharpness of vinegar and fish brine aid in cooking stews (*Maaserot* 1:7). Some rabbis bought fish brine with second tithe money (*Eruvin* 27a).

On the other hand, fish brine is not considered to be a fit beverage (*Yoma* 81a). Putting pressed or dried figs in fish brine spoils them (*Terumot* 11:1). Spices should not be put into brine because they might boil and spoil from the sharpness of the brine (*Shabbat* 42b; *Pesachim* 40b). A pregnant woman who consumes fish brine will have children with blinking eyes (*Ketubot* 60b).

Fish may be squeezed for their brine even on the Sabbath (*Shabbat* 145b), but one may not prepare pickling brine on the Sabbath (*Shabbat* 108a). Fish brine of Gentiles was forbidden since wine was often mixed in (*Abodah Zarah* 29b). If it was prepared by an expert, it is permitted since no wine would have been added (*Abodah Zarah* 34b). Fish brine that falls into a ritual bath renders it invalid (*Mikvaot* 7:2).

FISH HASH—Fish hash is prepared in honor of the Sabbath (*Pesachim* 112a) and may have a pungent odor (*Eruvin* 65a). Fish pie is prepared with fish hash and flour (*Abodah Zarah* 38a). Fish hash is better fresh than old (*Baba Batra* 916). Joab (1 Chronicles 11:8) only tasted his fish broth and fish hash and gave the rest to the poor (*Sanhedrin* 49a). A pot of fish hash was once part of an inheritance (*Baba Batra* 144a).

On the other hand, fish hash is harmful for pregnant women (*Ketubot* 60b). Residue of fish hash is related to the development of leprosy (*Pesachim* 112b). Scurvy or bleeding gums is caused by eating overnight remnants of a pie of fish hash and flour (*Yoma* 84a; *Abodah Zarah* 28a).

FLIES—Flies are carriers of disease (*Baba Kamma* 80b). They swarm all over patients suffering from *raatan* (*Ketubot* 77b). Beware of those flies (ibid.; *Leviticus Rabbah* 16:1). God's plans on earth can be carried out even by the most superfluous of creations such as flies, fleas, and gnats (*Genesis Rabbah* 10:7). The eyes and nostrils of an embryo are like two fly droppings (*Niddah* 25a).

FLOGGING—The Talmud enumerates many offenses for which the Bible prescribes disciplinary flogging (*Makkot* 13a, 17a, and 20a). The maximum is forty stripes save one (Deuteronomy 25:2–3; *Makkot* 22a). If one cannot tolerate that many, he receives less (*Makkot* 22b). Flogging is incidental to offenses punishable by heavenly death. In fact, flogging is considered a substitute for death (*Sanhedrin* 10a). The methodology of administering flogging is described in graphic detail (*Makkot* 22b–23a). Stripes are administered with the lash or whip (*Sanhedrin* 7b) made of calf hide (*Makkot* 23a). The lash is short so that it not reach the heart when being applied to the back (ibid.). A flogging in progress is stopped if the culprit urinates or defecates because of the humiliation (*Makkot* 23a). Judicial flogging is imposed for a variety of prohibited sexual activities, as well as for eating eels, ants, or hornets (*Eruvin* 28a); taking a false oath (*Sukkah* 53a); planting diverse seeds (*Moed Katan* 2b); ploughing in the sabbatical year (ibid., 3a); falsely accusing others of immorality (*Gittin* 57a); and a variety of other offenses.

In addition to judicial flogging ordained by biblical law (Deuteronomy 25:2–3) and imposed by a court of three judges (*Sanhedrin* 10a), the rabbinic sages imposed disciplinary flagellation for disobedience (*Shabbat* 40b; *Sanhedrin* 46a; *Chullin* 132b). An entire tractate of Talmud (*Makkot*) is devoted to flogging and flagellation.

FLOUR—Various kinds of flour are life's necessities (2 Samuel 17:28; *Baba Batra* 90b). Foods made from fine flour and eggs have both laxative and aphrodisiac properties (*Yoma* 18a). Wheat and wine are mentioned as food for children (*Nedarim* 8:7). Barley bread is preferable to wheat bread (*Shabbat* 140b). A wife must be provided with wheat and other food staples for her sustenance if her husband does not live with her (*Ketubot* 5:8). In the desert, the manna tasted like flour mixed with honey (*Exodus Rabbah* 5:9). Fine flour was used for meal offerings in the Temple (Leviticus 2:1). Flour is used in the tanning of hides (*Pesachim* 45b).

Therapeutically, flour paste (*Eduyot* 5:2) is used as a plaster on wounds

(*Tosefta Pesachim* 2:3; *Tosefta Demai* 1:25). Fine flour is part of a remedy for abnormal vaginal bleeding (*Shabbat* 110b). On the other hand, fine flour can become worm-eaten (*Shekalim* 4:9). Barley flour may contain *kukyane* worms (*Berachot* 36a), which can be destroyed with specific remedies (*Shabbat* 109b). Moldy flour can weaken the body (*Pesachim* 42a). Fish hash and flour may produce gum disease (*Abodah Zarah* 28a). [*See also* BREAD]

FOLK MEDICINE—Many of the medical therapies in the Talmud belong to folk medicine. Even laymen recommend home remedies (*Song of Songs Rabbah* 2:3). Some laymen are "knowledgeable in healing remedies" (*Yoma* 49a). For toothache, a folk remedy is to bind garlic on the thumbnail and place it on the aching tooth (*Gittin* 69a). To be able to sleep, one should wear a fox's tooth (*Shabbat* 67a). Exorcism (ibid.) and amulets are said to be efficacious for a variety of illnesses [*see* AMULETS and EXORCISM].

Numerous folk remedies are suggested for fever (*Gittin* 67b; *Shabbat* 67a), for splenic maladies (*Gittin* 69b), for vaginal bleeding (*Shabbat* 110a–b), and for eye ailments [*see* EYES, REMEDIES]. Folk remedies are prescribed for weakness of the heart (*Eruvin* 29b), pain in the heart (*Berachot* 40a), heaviness of the heart (*Gittin*

69b; *Shabbat* 140a) and palpitations of the heart (*Gittin* 69b). A person bitten by a snake either sits on the fetus of a white ass (*Shabbat* 109b) or applies squashed gnats to the site of the bite (ibid., 77b). Folk remedies for a scorpion bite include the gall of a white stork (*Ketubot* 50a), ointment from a black and white lizard (*Shabbat* 77b), or forty-day-old urine (ibid., 109b). Very unusual folk remedies are described for bladder stones (*Gittin* 69b). Patients with sciatica rub their hips sixty times with fish brine to obtain relief (ibid.). [*See* specific illnesses, specific body organs, and specific plants and vegetables]

FOREHEAD—The upper part of the face is the forehead (*metzach*). An obstinate person has a copper forehead (Isaiah 48:4), and a defiant person has a hard forehead (Ezekiel 3:7). To have "the forehead of a whore" (Jeremiah 3:3) is a designation of shamelessness and insolence. The temples or thin parts of the skull are located on both sides of the forehead (Judges 4:21). The talmudic term for forehead is *tzida*, meaning "side" (*Shabbat* 8:4). The "corner of the head" that may not be sheared (Leviticus 19:27) refers to the temples (*Makkot* 20b). The forehead becomes darkened in old age (*Shabbat* 151b). A priest with a receding or markedly protruding forehead (*makban*) is unfit to serve in the Temple (*Bechorot* 43b). Leprosy of the head

can affect the forehead (*Negaim* 10:10). Gourds placed on the forehead serve as a remedy for patients with fever (*Yoma* 78a). The high priest wore the golden front plate or *tzitz* (Exodus 28:36–38) on his forehead (*Sanhedrin* 12b). [*See also* FACE]

FORENSIC MEDICINE—The Talmud describes seven substances that, when properly applied to a garment, can distinguish a blood stain from dye (*Niddah* 63a and ff.). These are tasteless spittle, the liquid of crushed beans, urine, *natron, borit, kimonia,* and *eshlag.*

These seven substances are mentioned elsewhere in the Talmud (*Sanhedrin* 49b; *Zevachim* 95a), and all but the first two are discussed in *Shabbat* 90a. The efficacy of these substances in being able to distinguish a blood stain from a dye stain is undisputed in the Talmud. In fact, the matter is stated as fact in both the code of Maimonides (*Issurei Biah* 9:36–38; *Mishkav Umoshav* 4:13) and the code of Joseph Karo (*Shulchan Aruch, Yoreh Deah* 190:31). Karo adds, however, that today (he lived from 1488 to 1575) "We are not knowledgeable in some of these names." Apparently Karo wished to put a stain to the test to ascertain whether it was blood or dye but was unable to do so because he was not sure of the exact identity of the seven substances.[1]

Regular soap apparently washes out both blood and dye stains from a garment and would be perfectly suitable to cleanse the stain from the garment no matter what it is. However, regular soap would not resolve the question of ritual impurity that applies to a blood stain. The question to which the seven substances address themselves is the problem of blood versus dye. The seven substances apparently do not distinguish between different types of blood (i.e., animal versus human blood), since they wash out all types of blood stains. It is not clear whether this forensic pathology can be reliably used nowadays. [*See also* MENSTRUATION]

1. F. Rosner, "'Forensic Medicine' in the Talmud," in *Medicine in the Bible and the Talmud*, 2nd ed. (Hoboken, NJ: Ktav and Yeshiva University Press, 1995), pp. 269–272.

FRIGHT—Fear suspends menstruation (*Niddah* 9a) but sudden fright can bring on menses (*Niddah* 71a; *Megillah* 15a; *Sotah* 20b). Fright can cause a person to become pale (*yerakon*) (*Ketubot* 103b; *Abodah Zarah* 20b). A patient on the verge of death may be frightened, open his mouth, and turn green like gall (*Abodah Zarah* 20b). One can die from sudden fright (*Jerushalmi Terumot* 8:46). A man once lost his hair from fright after stepping on a snake (*Exodus Rabbah* 24:4). A pregnant woman once aborted when a dog jumped in front of her (*Shabbat* 63b). Fear of war can cause

impotence in soldiers (*Zevachim* 116b) and even involuntary loss of urine (*Sotah* 44b). Severe fright can also induce defecation or diarrhea (*Megillah* 15a). Therapeutically, one frightens patients with *avit* to stop shaking or trembling (*Tosefta Shabbat* 7:21).

FRUIT—Apples are considered a special delicacy (Song of Songs 2:5). Cherries do not provide the body with any benefit (*Berachot* 57b). Nuts are considered harmful to patients convalescing from illness (ibid.), particularly hazelnuts. The most important fruits are dates and figs. Dates constitute a full course at a meal and figs are served for dessert (ibid., 41b). Dates (ibid., 12a) and other fruits are nutritious (*Eruvin* 30a). Figs and dates are described in detail elsewhere in this Encyclopedia.

God created the fruit trees (Genesis 1:11). Adam is said to have eaten from the fig tree in the Garden of Eden (*Ecclesiastes Rabbah* 5:15). "The fruit of the land" (Joshua 5:12) probably refers to both fruits and vegetables. Some fruits, such as figs, grapes, quinces, and peaches, are spread out to dry (*Shabbat* 45a), often on the roof (*Abodah Zarah* 70b). Unripe fruit is put into straw to ripen (*Eruvin* 77a). It is also stored on the roof to keep it free from maggots (*Chullin* 13a; *Machshirin* 6:1). Worm-eaten grapes (*Nazir* 34b), decayed fruit (*Sanhedrin* 14b), and insects in fruits (*Chullin* 67b) are cited in the Talmud. Fruit suspected of being wormy must be carefully examined (Leviticus 11:41). Fruit is stored in vessels, in heaps (*Baba Metzia* 24b), in sacks, or in jars (*Machshirin* 3:1–2). Fruit purchased from fruit vendors (*Moed Katan* 13b) is packed in large bags (*Baba Batra* 86b).

Fruits are beneficial to the eyesight (*Sanhedrin* 18a). One sage received a basket of fruit every Sabbath eve from his tenant (*Yebamot* 93a). The poor eat fruit fallen from trees (*Pesachim* 56a). Peddlers who came to private homes to sell their wares also sold fruit (*Maaserot* 2:3). Hand washing was practiced for hygiene before fruit consumption (*Chullin* 106a).

Fruit juices including wine are popular beverages (*Berachot* 38a). Sour fruit juice is efficacious for a toothache and does not harm healthy teeth (*Shabbat* 111a). [*See also* APPLES, DATES, FIGS, and other specific fruits]

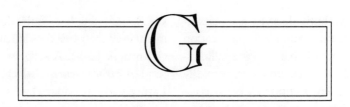

GALLBLADDER—The Hebrew word *marah*, meaning "bitter," is used in the Talmud to denote both bile and the gallbladder. Bitterness, poison (*Terumot* 8:5), and gall are all derived from this term. *Maror* refers to the Passover bitter herbs (*Pesachim* 39a) but also is the root for the Hebrew word for "embittered" (Exodus 1:14). Zophar says to his friend Job that man's ill-gotten gains turn to gall and do not endure (Job 20:14). The angel of death has a drop of gall hanging from his sword (*Abodah Zarah* 20b). The word *machalah*, meaning "sickness" (Exodus 23:25 and Deuteronomy 7:15), refers to diseases of the gall (*Baba Metzia* 107b). Such illnesses can be counteracted by partaking in the morning of bread dipped in salt followed by a jugful of water (ibid.; *Baba Kamma* 92b). Water of palm trees is also recommended for dysfunction of the gall because such water is sharp and pierces the gall (*Shabbat* 110a; *Jerushalmi Shabbat* 14:3). The illness of Rabbi Yochanan (*Berachot* 5b) is said to have been gallstones (*Song of Songs Rabbah* 2:16:2).

The gallbladder was thought to be the organ of jealousy (*Leviticus Rabbah* 4:4), probably based on the ancient concept of gall meaning "anger" or "bitterness." In his *Aruch Hashulchan* (*Yoreh Deah* 42:1), Yechiel Michael Epstein explains that the function of the gallbladder is to assuage the heat of the liver and its anger. Therefore, if the gallbladder is pierced and the bile lost, the heat of the liver cannot be tolerated. For this reason, a pierced gallbladder renders an animal *terefah*, or nonviable (*Chullin* 3:1 and 42b). Job speaks of a sword or arrow piercing the gallbladder (Job 20:25) and that God "pours out my gall on the ground" (Job 16:13). Another biblical account of a pierced gallbladder (2 Samuel 2:23) is discussed in the Talmud (*Sanhedrin* 49a).

In their respective codes of Jewish law, Maimonides (*Mishneh Torah, Shechitah* 6:6) and Karo (*Shulchan Aruch, Yoreh Deah* 42:1) both rule that if the gallbladder is pierced but the perforation is completely sealed by the liver, the animal is permitted for human consumption. Also discussed by the rabbinic decisors are cases of absence, duplication, ectopic location of, and foreign objects in the gallbladder.[1] These discussions are primarily of Jewish legal importance to determine whether an animal with such a defect is capable of living or whether a fatal outcome can be expected. In the latter case, the animal is *terefah* and unfit for human consumption.

---

1. F. Rosner, "The Gallbladder," in *Medicine in the Bible and the Talmud*, 2nd ed. (Hoboken, NJ: Ktav and Yeshiva University Press, 1995), pp. 107–112.

GARGLING—The illness known as *askara* (diphtheria) is a form of mouth disorder (*Shabbat* 33a), affects primarily children (*Taanit* 27b), and kills by asphyxiation (*Leviticus Rabbah* 18:4). A variety of liquid medications can be prepared and used as gargles.[1] Gargling is known as *irer* (*Tosefta Shabbat* 12:10) or *gargir* (*Berachot* 36a) in Hebrew. He who gulps down fluids is known as a *gargeran* (*Pesachim* 86b). Olive oil was used as a gargle for pain in the throat (*Berachot* 36a). Mangold broth served as a vehicle for using oil in gargling (*Jerushalmi Eruvin* 6:23). [*See also* THROAT]

---

1. F. Rosner (trans.), *Julius Preuss' Biblical and Talmud Medicine* (Northvale, NJ: Jason Aronson, 1993), pp. 157–158.

GARLIC—The Jews in the desert remembered the garlic they ate in Egypt (Numbers 11:5). A serpent is very fond of garlic (*Genesis Rabbah* 54:1). Eating garlic produces bad-smelling breath (*Shabbat* 31b; *Sanhedrin* 11a). Garlic root is a wholesome vegetable, whereas garlic leaves may be unhealthy (*Eruvin* 56a). Eating peeled garlic may be dangerous to one's health (*Niddah* 17a). Garlic is often spread out to dry (*Sanhedrin* 109b; *Abodah Zarah* 28b) and ground with a mortar and pestle (*Shabbat* 123a–124a). It is sometimes mixed with mustard or with beans and grits for consumption (*Shabbat* 140a). Garlic consumed on an empty stomach may cause faintness (*Taanit* 25a). Garlic was customarily eaten on Fridays (*Nedarim* 31a and 63b), as ordained by Ezra (*Baba Kamma* 82a), for its aphrodisiac effect. Garlic satiates, keeps the body warm, brightens the face, increases semen, and kills parasites in the bowels (ibid.). Some say that it fosters love and removes jealousy (ibid.). Garlic is used as an ingredient in stew (*Nazir* 36a). For toothache, a folk remedy is to place a stalk of garlic over the tooth (*Gittin* 69a). The consumption of garlic may induce menstrual bleeding in some women (*Niddah* 63b). Garlic and onion peels, placed on a wound, help it to heel (*Tosefta Shabbat* 5:3–4). One should eat garlic starting from the upper end, not from the bulb outwardly (*Betzah* 25b).

In Jewish law, garlic roots can both contract and impart ritual uncleanness (*Uktzin* 1:3). Of all vegetables, only garlic and onions are subject to the law of the corner (*Chullin* 137a; *Niddah* 50a). Garlic stalks tied in bundles do not come under the law of the forgotten sheaf (*Peah* 6:10) or the law of "if water be put" (*Machshirin* 6:2). Such bundles of garlic are not delivered in sacks (*Baba Batra* 86a). Garlic and small wild garlic do not constitute mingled seeds or *kilayim* (*Kilayim* 1:3). Crushed garlic (*Eduyot* 2:6) from which juice exudes on the Sabbath may be consumed on the Sabbath provided it was crushed on Friday (*Shabbat* 19a). If one carries a measure of garlic into a public domain on the Sabbath, one is liable for transgressing Sabbath laws (ibid., 76a).

GEESE—The goose is a clean bird and fit for human consumption after ritual slaughtering (*Chullin* 4a). Goose fat was smeared with a goose quill in the mouth to treat gum bleeding (*Abodah Zarah* 28a). Goose lung is said to "brighten the eyes" and is more expensive than the rest of the goose (*Chullin* 49a). Goose meat is cheaper than beef (*Chullin* 84a). One should not eat geese excessively lest one develop a greedy appetite for them (*Pesachim* 114a).

Geese live in orchards (*Betzah* 25a) and are caught in nets (*Betzah* 24a).

Geese can be used to thresh corn (*Sanhedrin* 59b). Very fat geese lose their feathers (*Baba Batra* 73b). A heathen once behaved immorally with a goose, strangled it, roasted it, and ate it (*Abodah Zarah* 22b). "White geese" is a metaphor for "old men" (*Ketubot* 85a). [*See also* BIRDS, CHICKENS, DOVES, and PIGEONS]

GENITALIA, FEMALE—The biblical word *ervah*, meaning "nakedness" (Leviticus 18:6ff.; Ezekiel 16:36), refers to the female genitalia. Rarely, the term *kovah* is used (Numbers 25:8). The uterus is called *beten* (Genesis 25:23; Deuteronomy 7:13; Job 1:21; Micah 6:7) or *rechem* (Genesis 29:31). The Talmud compares the female genitalia figuratively to the parts of a house: the *cheder* or inner chamber is the uterus, the *prosdor* or vestibule is the vagina, and the *aliyah* or upper chamber is the bladder (*Niddah* 2:5). The *lul* is probably the vaginal (or cervical) orifice (*Niddah* 71b). The terms are interpreted somewhat differently by Maimonides in his *Mishnah Commentary* (*Niddah* 2:5) and his legal code (*Mishneh Torah, Issurei Biyah* 5:3–4). Other talmudic expressions for the female genitalia include "that place" and "the site of shame" (*Niddah* 20a; *Nedarim* 20a; *Chullin* 9:2). The vagina is also called the *bet hachitzon*, or "outer house" (*Niddah* 5:1). The terms *sefayot*, meaning "lips"

(*Jerushalmi Yebamot* 6:7), and *erva* (*Bechorot* 6:5) portray the labia majora and minora.

Vaginal specula were used for internal examinations for blood (*Niddah* 66a). All women are subject to ritual uncleanness if blood is found in the vagina (ibid., 40a) since it is assumed to be of uterine origin. If the blood is from a cervical or vaginal wound, the woman remains clean (ibid., 17b). Physicians are called to diagnose and treat vaginal bleeding (*Niddah* 22b). A variety of folk remedies are described (*Shabbat* 110a–b). [*See also* UTERUS, BREASTS, VIRGINITY, PUBERTY, and MENSTRUATION]

GIGANTISM—Giants existed in biblical times (Genesis 6:4; *Genesis Rabbah* 31:12). The spies whom Moses sent to explore the promised land claimed they saw giants (Numbers 13:33). Og, king of Bashan, was the only giant remaining in his kingdom (Deuteronomy 3:11). His bed was nine cubits long and four cubits wide and his thigh bone was more than three parasangs long (*Niddah* 24b). Josephus describes giants in Hebron (*Antiquities*, Book 5, Chapter 2:3). The Philistine Goliath was a giant (1 Samuel 17:4) and his exploits are described in the Talmud (*Sotah* 42b). Whether or not any of these giants were acromegalics cannot be established with any degree of certainty.

The biblical term *sarua* (Leviticus 21:18) is interpreted to refer to excessive growth and size of one limb, which disqualifies a priest from serving in the Temple (*Bechorot* 3b). Ben Batiach is said to have had an unusually large hand or fist (*Kelim* 17:12). A certain Rabbi Ishmael is also said to have had huge hands and was able to grasp four *kabs* in one hand (*Yoma* 47a). Tall stature (gigantism?) was thought to be hereditary in that the offspring of a tall man who marries a tall woman are tall children (*Bechorot* 45b). The terms *kippuach* (*Tosefta Berachot* 7:3; *Jerushalmi Berachot* 9:13) and *kippeach* (*Bechorot* 7:6; *Berachot* 58b) refer to a very tall person or a giant (*Bechorot* 45b). A series of very tall rabbis is enumerated in the Talmud (*Niddah* 24b).

GINGER—Ginger placed in the mouth makes the breath pleasant (*Shabbat* 65a). Skin boils were treated by the application of a ginger-containing salve (*Gittin* 86a). Most ginger is beneficial to the whole body (*Pesachim* 42b). Preserved ginger is considered a food (*Yoma* 81a). A rabbi once sent his colleague a sackful of ginger as a gift (*Megillah* 7b).

GOATS—The goat is a kosher (i.e., edible) animal (Deuteronomy 14:5) and is classified among small cattle

(*Betzah* 25b). These include forest goats and goats from Lebanon (*Chullin* 80a). Goats have horns and beards (*Shabbat* 52a). Their udders are tied to prevent milk from dripping (*Shabbat* 52b) and to protect the udders from thorns (ibid., 53b). Goat's hair is washed and spun directly on the goats (ibid., 74b). Their flesh is of high quality (*Pesachim* 57b) and is tender when roasted (ibid., 84a).

Goat fat is used to treat internal rectal slits (fissures?) (*Abodah Zarah* 28b). The spleen of a she-goat is used to cure splenic ailments (*Gittin* 69b). Juice from a goat's kidney is recommended to treat earache (*Abodah Zarah* 28b). Goat's milk is not only a delicacy (Proverbs 27:27) but is effective in treating the illness called *barsam* (*Gittin* 69a). A sick person with heart disease can suck goat's milk directly from the udder (*Baba Kamma* 80a). Fat meat from a goat that has not yet sired young decreases bowel movements, straightens the stature, and gives light to the eyes (*Pesachim* 42a–b). Pregnant wild goats bitten in their genitals by a *darkon* (snake?) deliver their offspring easily (*Baba Batra* 16b). An ewe can give birth to a species of goat and vice versa (*Bechorot* 5b and 6b).

Goats are considered despicable animals (*Song of Songs Rabbah* 6:5:1). They can do considerable damage and even kill bears (*Taanit* 25a; *Baba Metzia* 6a). The goats of Job killed wolves (*Baba Batra* 15b). Goats can break utensils (*Baba Kamma* 21b), eat up dough (ibid., 48a) or barley of other people (*Baba Batra* 36a). The wild goat is heartless toward her young (ibid., 16a–b). On the other hand, they can pull wagons (*Sanhedrin* 59b) and graze peacefully under fig trees (*Ketubot* 111b). Goatskins are made into water containers (*Baba Batra* 58a). A goat with a shrunken kidney the size of a bean (chronic renal disease?) is not viable (*Chullin* 55a–b). [*See also* ASSES, MULES, and HORSES]

GONORRHEA—A male with flux from his genitalia (Leviticus 15:2ff.) is called a *zav* (Leviticus 15:1–18) and a woman with intermenstrual flux is called a *zava* (ibid., 15:25–28). After the first emission, the man is called a *baal keri* and is ritually unclean for the day. After the second emission, he is unclean and has to count seven days, wash his garments, immerse in a ritual bath, and wait for sunset. After the third emission, he also has to bring sacrifices on the eighth day (*Nedarim* 43b). If a woman observes a flux after her menses, she is unclean until evening. From then on, she is "on the wait" and if there is a flux on the second day, she becomes unclean for seven days. A third day certifies her as gonorrheic and she must then bring a sacrifice after ritual purification (*Zavim* 2:3).

Excessive eating and drinking was thought to be a cause of gonorrhea (*Yoma* 18a; *Kiddushin* 2b). A sufferer from gonorrhea who has a seminal emission requires ritual ablution (*Berachot* 26a). He or she may take the bath during the day (*Yoma* 6b), even in swiftly running waters (ibid., 78a) and even on Yom Kippur (ibid., 88a). A man with gonorrhea causes defilement by touching or carrying (*Baba Kamma* 25a). He cannot eat the paschal lamb (*Bechorot* 33a). His spittle is the direct cause of levitical impurity (Leviticus 15:18; *Bechorot* 38a). He must examine himself to determine the number of emissions he has had (*Niddah* 13a). A woman can have gonorrhea before or after she gives birth (*Keritot* 9b).

When Israel stood at Mount Sinai, there were none among them with gonorrhea or leprosy (*Leviticus Rabbah* 18:4). In the desert, however, people with gonorrhea were sent out of the camp (Numbers 5:2). Gonorrheal flux and sperm emission differ in that the former resembles incubated egg whites and is pale, whereas sperm is "bound" and resembles the white of eggs (*Tosefta Zavim* 2:4). Sperm issues from an erect penis whereas flux issues from a flabby penis. The talmudic discussion about confirming the diagnosis of gonorrhea and a variety of laws pertaining to such patients are detailed by Preuss.[1]

___
1. F. Rosner (trans.), *Julius Preuss' Biblical and Talmudic Medicine* (Northvale, NJ: Jason Aronson, 1993), pp. 354–357.

GOURDS—Gourds and pumpkins are food for humans as well as animals (*Shabbat* 156b; *Betzah* 2a, 6b, and 27b; *Chullin* 14a). Chewing pumpkins produces very thick spittle (*Tamid* 27b). The Talmud discusses gourd seeds (*Shabbat* 90b), gourd stalks (*Uktzin* 1:6), gourd beds (*Moed Katan* 3b), and gourd blossoms (*Betzah* 13b). Gourds float on water (*Sanhedrin* 108a) and come from Greece (*Betzah* 3b; *Yebamot* 81b; *Orlah* 3:7), Egypt (*Kilayim* 1:5), and Ammon (*Sanhedrin* 106a). The Greek ones have long leaves (*Kilayim* 2:11). Pumpkin seeds are planted (*Shabbat* 103a) in pumpkin fields (*Baba Batra* 24b). Pumpkins can shrivel on the stem during growth (*Chullin* 127b). Pumpkins shells, when dried and hollowed, can be used to draw water from wells (*Shabbat* 125a; *Kelim* 3:5; *Parah* 5:3). They can be roasted prior to consumption (*Sanhedrin* 33b).

Therapeutically, pumpkin peels were used to close skull defects (*Tosefta Oholot* 2:6). Ripe and unripe gourds were placed on the foreheads of patients with fever (*Yoma* 78a). However, gourds are harmful for some patients (*Nedarim* 49a). Gourds and pumpkins are unhealthy for nursing women since they injure the milk (*Ketubot* 60b). A gourd or pumpkin with a hole should not be consumed lest a poisonous snake ate from it (*Chullin* 94a; *Terumot* 8:6). Pumpkins and gourds are difficult to digest (*Nedarim* 49b; *Tamid* 27b). Nevertheless, one should eat pumpkins on Rosh Hashanah as a sign of prosperity and fertility (*Horayot* 12a; *Keritot* 6a). Seeing a pumpkin in a dream is auspicious (*Berachot* 52b).

The popular saying "Better one grain of pungent pepper than a basketful of pumpkins (*Chagigah* 10a; *Megillah* 7a; *Yoma* 85b) means that a sharp mind is better than mere learning. Other proverbs include the following: "Every pumpkin can be told by its stalk" (*Berachot* 47b); "A young pumpkin in hand is better than a full-grown one in the field" (*Sukkah* 56b; *Ketubot* 83b); and "He with large pumpkins and his wife with small pumpkins" (*Megillah* 12a–b).

GOUT—King Asa of Judah (915–875 B.C.E.) reigned for over forty years. In his old age he suffered from a disease in his feet considered to be gout (I Kings 15:23). The Talmud (*Sanhedrin* 48b; *Sotah* 10a) describes King Asa's illness as *podagra*, which feels "like a needle in the raw flesh." Rabbi Nachman also suffered from it. Rashi (*Sanhedrin* 48b) states that the name of this illness, *podagra*, "is the same even in our language," i.e., French, Rashi's native tongue. The expression "like a needle in the raw flesh" is used elsewhere in the Talmud

(*Berachot* 18b; *Shabbat* 13b and 152a). Further mention of King Asa's illness is found in 2 Chronicles 16:12.[1]

Another pertinent reference to gout is the Mishnah, which describes a foot ailment called *tzinit* (*Shabbat* 6:6). The Jerusalem Talmud interprets this word to mean *podagra* or gout (*Shabbat* 6:8). The Babylonian Talmud, however, considers *tzinit* to refer to a corn or a bunion (*Shabbat* 65a).

1. F. Rosner, "Gout," in *Medicine in the Bible and the Talmud*, 2nd ed. (Hoboken, NJ: Ktav and Yeshiva University Press, 1995), pp. 58–59.

GRAPES—Grapes are an essential part of human nutrition (*Sirach* 39:26), although a Nazirite is prohibited from drinking wine or eating grapes (Numbers 6:3: *Nazir* 34a–b). Grapes are harvested and trodden in wine presses (*Abodah Zarah* 55a) or kneading troughs (*Sheviit* 8:6) to extract the wine or they are eaten as grapes (*Terumot* 1:9 and 8:3). They are cut off the vine with a sharp flint (*Oholot* 18:1), gathered in baskets (*Demai* 2:5; *Oholot* 18:1), and put into the wine press (*Tohorot* 10:4; *Shabbat* 15a and 17a; *Pesachim* 3b). The grapes are first weighed on the scales of a balance (*Machshirin* 5:11) as whole clusters (*Betzah* 35a; *Ketubot* 112a) and eventually pressed out to make wine (*Baba Batra* 97b). Sometimes grapes are spread out to dry (*Shabbat* 45a) to make them into raisins (*Betzah* 26b).

The Talmud cites undeveloped grapes that are less than a third grown (*Orlah* 1:8), late grapes (*Demai* 1:1, *Pesachim* 6b), fully ripe grapes (*Kilayim* 7:7), white grapes, black grapes (*Keritot* 19a), wild grapes (*Baba Metzia* 105a), and even worm-eaten grapes (*Nazir* 34b). Ripe grapes, if not gathered, deteriorate (*Sanhedrin* 15a). Bitter wine is made from unripe grapes and sweet wine results from grapes sweetened by the heat of the sun (*Abodah Zarah* 30a). Wine is said to be the red blood of grapes (Genesis 49:11). Also discussed are grape stones and husks as well as grape skins (*Orlah* 1:8; *Shabbat* 47b; *Taanit* 26b; *Abodah Zarah* 29b and 34a; *Nazir* 3b and 34b).

Medically, grapes from a vine trailed on a palm tree in water are used (*Gittin* 69b). A dough made from unripe grapes was applied to the head of newborns to ward off insects (*Genesis Rabbah* 34:15). Homiletically, grapes in the world to come will contain enormous amounts of wine (*Ketubot* 111b). [*See also* WINE and DRUNKENNESS]

GRASSHOPPERS—Certain grasshoppers or locusts are fit for human consumption (i.e., kosher) (Leviticus 11:22; *Shabbat* 90b). These have four legs, four wings, leaping legs, and wings covering the greater part of the body (*Chullin* 59a and 65a). Other grasshoppers are "unclean" (i.e., not kosher) (*Eduyot* 7:2). The antennas of a grasshopper are soft so that it does not go blind when they hit a hard object (*Shabbat* 77b). "Locusts' horns" may refer to the antennas (*Pesachim* 48b). The soul of a person resembles a winged grasshopper (Midrash Psalms 11:6).

Invasion of locusts is divine punishment for the crime of robbery (*Shabbat* 32b). They may come in swarms (*Shabbat* 106b). They can be found in shopkeepers' baskets (*Abodah Zarah* 39b), in warehouses, or on ships (ibid., 40b). Grasshoppers can eat up a whole crop (*Baba Metzia* 106a; *Menachot* 71b). The alarm is sounded and fasting is decreed for the calamity of grasshoppers or locusts (*Taanit* 19a–b). For diseases caused by locusts, prayers are recited and repentance is solicited (*Baba Kamma* 80b). Grasshopper eggs were used to prepare remedies for ear afflictions (*Shabbat* 67a). One of the remedies for jaundice is to rub the patient with juice of locusts in a warm bathhouse (*Shabbat* 109b–110a).

GRAVE—Burial is effected in caves or in the ground. Abraham bought a cave as a family burial plot (Genesis 23:9ff.). The Hittites offered Abraham sepulchers (Genesis 23:11). Such sepulchers were hewn out of rock even during one's lifetime (Isaiah 22:16). Graves in the ground (as opposed to caves) are not mentioned in the Bible. Absalom was buried under a heap of rocks (2 Samuel 18:17) as was Achan (Joshua 7:25). Sepulchers were sealed with a large stone (*Chullin* 72a; *Oholot* 2:4; *Sanhedrin* 47b) or a beam or barrel (*Oholot* 15:8–9). The number of vaults (i.e., graves) in a sepulcher varied with the character of the rock (*Baba Batra* 6:8). Some tombs were built above ground (*Moed Katan* 8b). There existed a separate sepulcher of the pious and of judges (*Moed Katan* 17a). A field of burial crypts (*kuchin*) is described within which a family burial site was lost (*Tosefta Oholot* 17:11). Plowing a field may unearth such crypts and break bones. Such a field is called *bet haperas*, meaning an area or house of pieces (*Oholot* 17:1). One might accidentally fall into a burial vault by ploughing above it (*Niddah* 24b).

He who touches a grave becomes ritually unclean (Numbers 19:18). Therefore, before the three pilgrimage Festivals (Exodus 23:17), burial sites were identified or marked (*Shekalim* 1:1; *Niddah* 56b) with white lime reminiscent of the color of bones (*Baba Batra* 69a). People can hide in a grave (*Sanhedrin* 29b). Women and lepers buried their abortuses and leprous limbs, respectively, in "earth mounds" near cities (*Tosefta Oholot* 16:1). Graves must be kept fifty cubits from a town because of the bad smell (*Baba Batra* 25a). Grave robbers (*Baba Batra* 58a) and grave diggers (*Yebamot* 65b; *Sanhedrin* 26b; *Niddah* 24b) are also described.

Homiletically, decay of the corpse in the earth was believed to be painful to the body (*Berachot* 18b; *Sanhedrin* 47b). The lips of Torah scholars move gently in the grave when their teachings are quoted in their names (*Yebamot* 97a; *Bechorot* 31b). Smoke

arose from Acher's grave, indicating that he was burning in hell (*Chagigah* 15b). The grave (*kever*) receives and gives forth (*Berachot* 15b; *Sanhedrin* 92a). Thus, the Hebrew word *kever* for grave is also used to denote the uterus (*Niddah* 21a; *Shabbat* 129a), perhaps because the fetus is enclosed in the uterus like a corpse in the grave.

Entering a cemetery ritually defiles a person (*Eruvin* 47a). Imbeciles sleep in the cemetery (*Chagigah* 3b). Spending a night in a graveyard causes one to forfeit one's life (*Niddah* 17a). Executed people were buried in separate graveyards (*Yebamot* 47b; *Sanhedrin* 47a). Wine merchants once left their merchandise in a cemetery (*Leviticus Rabbah* 12:1). If one ploughs over a graveyard, one may unearth corpses and crush skeletal remains (*Niddah* 57a). [*See also* BURIAL, COFFIN, and CORPSE]

GUMS—For an abscess of the gums, pyrethrum and other ingredients placed in the mouth is beneficial (*Gittin* 69a). An illness of the gums or teeth called *tzafdina*, associated with gum bleeding (scurvy or stomatitis?), is discussed in the Midrash (*Genesis Rabbah* 33:2 and 96:2) and Talmud (*Yoma* 84a; *Baba Metzia* 85a; *Abodah Zarah* 28a) and a variety of remedies for it are prescribed [*see* SCURVY]. Eating hard bread causes the gums to bleed (*Keritot* 21b). Vinegar heals diseased gums and teeth (*Shabbat* 111a).

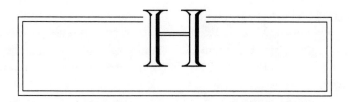

H

HAIR—The full unsheared hair on the head is called *pera* (Numbers 6:5). Tufts or locks of hair are described on Samson (Judges 16:13) and Ezekiel (Ezekiel 8:3) and on a biblical lover (Song of Songs 5:2 and 7:6). Nebuchadnezzar let his hair grow wild (Daniel 4:29ff.). Semites normally have black hair (Leviticus 13:31). Some red-haired people such as Esau (Genesis 25:25) are bloodthirsty, whereas others such as David (1 Samuel 16:12) kill only with court sanction or divine approval (*Genesis Rabbah* 63:8). A hair can sometimes have a black root and a red tip (*Parah* 2:5). Axillary hair has a shorter lifespan than hair on the head. In elderly, obese men, it gradually falls out (*Nazir* 59a). In old age, hair becomes white. Rabbi Eleazar ben Azariah's hair miraculously turned white overnight when he was eighteen years old and appointed head of the talmudical academy (*Berachot* 28a). Hair can turn white from leprosy as well (Leviticus 13:3).

In homiletics, each hair has its own groove (*Baba Batra* 16a). In fact, two hairs may grow from a single follicle in both humans (*Niddah* 52a) and animals (*Parah* 2:5). Each hair follicle also has its own source of nutrients (*Tanchuma, Tazria* on Job 38:25). Hairs grow out from their roots (*Nazir* 39a). Eunuchs have soft hair and no beards just like women (*Yebamot* 80b).

People with a full head of thick, long hair include Esau, who was born "like a hairy garment" (Genesis 25:25) and was later still called a hairy man (hypertrichosis?) (Genesis 27:11). The prophet Elijah had wavy hair and was ridiculed by being called a hairy man (2 Kings 1:8). Allowing one's hair to grow into long locks is designated in Judaism as a heathen practice (*Tosefta Shabbat* 6:1) or idolatrous custom (*Deuteronomy Rabbah* 2:18). These are called "people with polled hair" (Jeremiah 9:25). The sons of David who were raised with heathen war captives let their locks grow (*Sanhedrin* 21a), as did the Israelites in Egypt to imitate the Egyptians (*Leviticus Rabbah* 23:2).

Hair styles in men were frowned upon. A man who curled his hair was ridiculed (*Megillah* 18a). Petuel is so called because he used to curl his hair like a young woman (Midrash Psalms 80:1). Polling one's hair is discussed in relation to priests (Ezekiel 44:20). Special coiffures are described (*Shabbat* 9b), which required considerable time and expertise (*Shabbat* 9b) and were very expensive (*Nedarim* 51a).

For women, beautiful hair is an adornment. God Himself braided Eve's hair, adorning her like a bride (*Genesis Rabbah* 18:1) before He brought her to Adam (*Berachot* 61a). A famous rabbi's wife sold her hair braids so that her husband could study Torah undisturbed (*Jerushalmi Sotah* 9:24). Well-to-do women hired permanent coiffeuses to skillfully weave and braid their hair (*Shabbat* 94b and 104b; *Kiddushin* 49a).

It is prohibited for men to pray in the presence of women whose hair is uncovered (*Berachot* 24a) since it is proper for Jewish women to cover their hair (*Tosefta Ketubot* 7:6). A woman who was meticulous in her observance of the law merited to have seven sons, all of whom became high priests in succession (*Yoma* 47a). Part of the ceremony in the case of a suspected adulteress is to uncover her hair (Numbers 5:18). A woman standing in a doorway with uncovered hair should be avoided (*Sanhedrin* 110a). Financial compensation must be paid to a woman by someone who intentionally uncovers her hair in public (*Baba Kamma* 8:6). Only unmarried women do not cover their hair (*Ketubot* 2:1).

Traditionally in Judaism, the father, mother, and God are partners in the creation of a human being. The mother contributes the skin, the blood, hair, and the black of the eye (*Niddah* 31a). After a bath, one either combed one's hair (*Shabbat* 41a) or had a barber (*sappar*) (*Esther Rabbah* 10:4) or hairdresser (*chappan*) (*Tosefta Baba Metzia* 9:14) do so. Hair loosening is part of the isolation procedure for a leper (Leviticus 13:45–46).

Pubic hairs are a sign of maturity (*Niddah* 52a). A hairy mole in a child can be mistaken for pubic hair (*Niddah* 46a). A eunuch has no pubic hair (*Tosefta Yebamot* 10:5). An infertile woman may also lack pubic hair (*Yebamot* 80b). Pubic hair may interfere with intercourse, occasionally leading to divorce (*Gittin* 6b). Jewish women who removed their pubic and axillary hair were considered beautiful (*Sanhedrin* 21a; Ezekiel 16:14). [*See also* BEARD, BALDNESS, DEPILATORIES, WIGS, HAIRCUTTING, HAIRCUTTING INSTRUMENTS, and HAIR GROOMING AND WASHING]

HAIR GROOMING AND WASHING

ING—A comb or *masrek* was used to arrange one's hair (*Berachot* 18b). Special head combs were available (*Kelim* 13:7). In antiquity, combs were made of box-tree or ivory and used by hairdressers (*Nazir* 42a). They resembled curry combs used to comb horses (*Moed*

Katan 10b). Combing was part of the grooming of both men and women (*Leviticus Rabbah* 6:8; *Berachot* 18b). To wash or cleanse the head, one used soda (*neter*), soapwort (*ahala*), or earth (*adama*) (*Niddah* 66b). Soda or carbonate of soda loosens the hair, whereas soapwort makes it stick together. One should use only warm water to cleanse the hair because cold water makes the hairs stick together (ibid.). Earth has the same effect (*Nazir* 6:3). The combination of soda and sand may result in hair falling out (*Shabbat* 50a). Such cleansing of the head was customary even among men such as Hillel (*Shabbat* 31a). A Nazarite may cleanse or shampoo his hair and part it, but must not comb it (*Shabbat* 50b; *Nazir* 42a). He may not poll his hair (*Nazir* 5a) or thin it (*Nazir* 4a). Combing and cleansing are two separate acts (*Nazir* 42a).

For women, hair washing and cleansing is specifically required before their ritual bath at the end of their menstrual period (*Niddah* 66b), as decreed by Ezra (*Baba Kamma* 82b).

Hairs that are stuck together from perspiration or dust anywhere on the body (*Mikvaot* 9:2–3) can be separated with the fingers (*Nazir* 6:6). In healthy people, they may be so firm as to be thereby torn out (*Nazir* 42a). Because of extreme poverty, Rabbi Akiba and his wife slept on straw on the floor even in the winter. In the morning, he removed the stubble from her hair (*Nedarim* 50a). It was forbidden for men to pluck out white hairs from among their black hairs in order to look more youthful (*Shabbat* 94b) because this was considered to be a womanly custom (Deuteronomy 22:5). [*See also* HAIR, BEARD, BALDNESS, WIGS, DEPILATORIES, and HAIRCUTTING]

HAIR WHITENING—The spontaneous development of localized poliosis (whitening of the hair) has several common causes, including radiation therapy, alopecia areata, severe dermatitis, and vitiligo. Two additional possibilities are described in ancient Hebrew writings. The Babylonian Talmud (*Berachot* 27b–28a) relates that when the wise and sagacious Eleazar ben Azariah was asked whether or not he would consent to become head of the rabbinical academy, his wife said to him, "You have no white hair." He was eighteen years old on that day, and a miracle was wrought for him as eighteen rows of hair on his beard turned white. That is why he said, "Behold, I am like seventy years old," and did not simply say "seventy years old."

Rashi states that Rabbi Eleazar ben Azariah looked like an old man although he was really not old. Hoariness came on him suddenly on the day that Rabban Gamliel was deposed from his leadership role and Rabbi Eleazar ben Azariah was appointed in his stead.

In his talmudic commentary, Maimonides asserts that Rabbi Eleazar ben

Azariah studied so industriously and pored over his learning day and night with such fervor that his strength waned and he became hoary like an old man, even though he was chronologically much younger.

Other commentators agree with Rashi that the poliosis occurred overnight as a miraculous event. In the parallel tractate in the Jerusalem Talmud, the statement is made that Rabbi Eleazar ben Azariah was really an old man and said "like seventy years" because he was sixty-eight or sixty-nine years old. From the foregoing, two additional causes of acquired poliosis are evident: divine intervention and extreme industriousness in pursuing one's studies.[1]

---

1. F. Rosner, "Can hair turn white overnight?" in *Medicine in the Bible and the Talmud*, 2nd ed. (Hoboken, NJ: Ktav and Yeshiva University Press, 1995), p. 304.

HAIRCUTTING—Joseph had a haircut before he appeared before Pharaoh (Genesis 41:14) to show respect to royalty (*Genesis Rabbah* 89:9). Dreaming that one is having a haircut is a good omen (*Berachot* 57a). One cuts one's hair in preparation for the Sabbath or a Festival (*Shabbat* 1:2), including Passover eve (*Tosefta Pesachim* 2:18). An apron or sheet is placed by the barber on the knees before the hair-

cut (*Shabbat* 9b). During the haircut one looks into a mirror (*Abodah Zarah* 29a). Hand mirrors are used to cut off loose-hanging hair (*Shabbat* 149a).

The King had his hair cut daily because "Thine eyes shall see the king in his beauty" (Isaiah 33:17); the High Priest only on Fridays because the Temple watches were changed on that day; and ordinary priests only every thirty days (*Taanit* 17a). Those people assigned to the priestly watches could not leave their positions to obtain a haircut except on Thursdays, in honor of the Sabbath (ibid.). One may not gaze at the King while his hair is being cut (*Sanhedrin* 2:5) because he is to be revered (*Sanhedrin* 22a). The same applies to the High Priest (*Tosefta Sanhedrin* 4:1).

It is forbidden to cut off the hair from the "corners of the head" (Leviticus 19:27) or the "end of the head" (*Makkot* 20b). Cutting one's hair on the Sabbath or on Holy Days is prohibited in Judaism. It is permitted on the intermediate days of Passover and Tabernacles for those who were not able to do so prior to the Festival (*Moed Katan* 3:1; *Tosefta Pesachim* 2:18). A child's first haircut may also be done on the intermediate Festival days (*Moed Katan* 14b). A Nazarite is prohibited from cutting his hair (Numbers 6:5). A lifetime Nazarite may do so once a year to "lighten his hair" (*Nazir* 46). A person who is very anxious may omit cutting his hair (*Jerushalmi Rosh*

Hashanah 1:57). A seriously ill patient should not cut his hair lest he suffer a relapse (*Berachot* 57b).

Mourners are also forbidden to cut their hair (*Moed Katan* 14b). An exception is the High Priest, who is specifically forbidden to let his hair grow even during his period of mourning for a close relative (Leviticus 21:10). The same prohibition applied to the sons of Aaron when their brothers died (ibid., 10:6). There was a time in antiquity, however, when the opposite was true. Job cut his hair when he heard of the death of his children (Job 1:20). *Komi* is a special type of hairstyle or coiffure in which the corners of the head are shaven but a line of hair is left at the back of the head. It is prohibited (*Deuteronomy Rabbah* 2:18) except for Jewish officials who have to deal with foreign governments (*Baba Kamma* 83a; *Meilah* 17a). When not in mourning, the High Priest had a special haircut called *lulyanit* (*Shabbat* 9b). One should wash one's hands after a haircut (*Pesachim* 112a).

Hair on the chest was called "a hairy heart" in antiquity when it referred to exceedingly strong and intelligent people, such as Aristomenes and Leonidas.[1] In Jewish homiletics, Judah, son of the Patriarch Jacob, became enraged so that the hair of his heart would protrude through his clothes (*Genesis Rabbah* 93:6). [*See also* HAIR, BEARD, BALDNESS, DEPILATORIES, and HAIR GROOMING AND WASHING]

1. F. Rosner (trans.), *Julius Preuss' Biblical and Talmudic Medicine* (Northvale, NJ: Jason Aronson, 1993), p. 104.

HAIRCUTTING INSTRUMENTS—

The Bible and Talmud describe a variety of haircutting instruments including *mora* (Judges 13:5, 1 Samuel 1:11) and *taar* (Numbers 6:5 and 8:7; Isaiah 7:20), both of which refer to a razor. Scissors are called *zug shel misparayim*, meaning "pair of cutters" (*Kelim* 13:1) or the abbreviated version *zug* (*Shabbat* 94b) or *zuga* (*Megillah* 16a). Sometimes, only one blade of the scissors is used for cutting to "make the hair lighter" (Rashi, *Taanit* 13a; *Jerushalmi Moed Katan* 3:82). The *zug* removes hair (*Niddah* 6:12) or pinches off hair (*Negaim* 4:4). Cutting scissors, hair shears, and razors were stored in an instrument case (*Kelim* 16:8) or a large leather box (*Kelim* 24:5).

A *shachor* is a small hair shear that can be dismantled (*Kelim* 13:1). A *rehitani* is a small folding hair-removing instrument (*Tosefta Makkot* 4:10). The same term is used for a carpenter's axe (*Baba Kamma* 119a; *Shabbat* 97a). *Malkat* or *malketet* refers to forceps with which to pull hair out (*Makkot* 3:5). Two broken teeth from a carding comb can also be used for this purpose (*Kelim* 13:8). *Melkachayim* are forceps used as candle snuffers for the candelabra in the Temple (Exodus 25:38 and 37:23). *Negustre* or *genustre*

157

represents a nail-cutting knife (*Tosefta Kelim* 3:12). [*See also* HAIR, HAIRCUTTING, BEARD, BALDNESS, DEPILATORIES, and HAIR GROOMING AND WASHING]

HAND—The word *yad* for hand, or a variant thereof, occurs 1617 times in the Bible.[1] An entire tractate of Talmud, entitled *Yadayim* (hands), deals mainly with the ritual uncleanness of the hands and the rules governing their cleansing. Man is master over his mouth, his hands, and his feet (*Genesis Rabbah* 68:3). The hand of God contains soul and justice; His right hand contains the Torah and righteousness (*Leviticus Rabbah* 4:1). The Lord writes with His hand in the Heavenly Book of Records (*Avot* 2:1 and 3:16; *Malachi* 3:13; Exodus 32:32; Daniel 7:10). The hands of a newborn are clenched, but when one dies the hands are spread open (*Ecclesiastes Rabbah* 5:14).

One lifts up one's hand to take an oath (Genesis 14:22). Hand clapping is a sign of grief and mourning (*Moed Katan* 28b), of joy and happiness (2 Kings 11:12), or of ridicule and gloating (*Nahum* 3:19). Rivers (Psalms 98:8) and trees (Isaiah 55:12) also clap their hands as they pay homage to the Lord. Thrusting the hand is a symbol of befriending someone (*Sotah* 47a). To lift one's hands against a neighbor means to assault him (*Baba Kamma* 90a; *Sanhedrin* 58b). Strik-

ing hands (Proverbs 17:18 and 22:26) makes one a security for another person. It is a superstition to believe in a "lucky hand" (*Tosefta Shabbat* 6:12). Laying of hands on the head of an animal (Leviticus 1:4 and 3:2) is part of the ritual of offering sacrifices in the Temple (*Shabbat* 15a; *Pesachim* 89a; *Yoma* 5a, etc.). A woman lays her hands on the spindle and her hands hold the distaff (Proverbs 31:19). She stretches out her hands to the poor and the needy (ibid., 31:20). The chief butler placed the Pharaoh's goblet of wine in his hand (Genesis 40:21).

A physician visiting a patient takes his hand to feel the pulse (Midrash Psalms 73:1) and a visitor grasps the patient's hand to raise him in the bed (*Berachot* 5b). During prayer, a person raises his hands toward God (Exodus 9:29; 1 Kings 9:3; Psalms 44:21). Raising the hands is part of the priestly benediction (*Megillah* 4:7). Only the skull, feet, and hands of Jezebel were found for burial (2 Kings 9:35). The king saw his hand in silhouette on the wall (Daniel 5:5). A drop of cold water in the morning and bathing one's hands and feet in hot water in the evening is better than all the eye salves in the world (*Shabbat* 108b). Unwashed hands that touch the eye can cause blindness (*Shabbat* 109a). The evil spirit rests on one's hands during the night; hence, one must wash one's hands upon arising in the morning (ibid.). Solomon also decreed handwashing before eating (*Shabbat* 109a).

Handwashing is mandatory before (*Yoma* 30a) and after meals (*Numbers Rabbah* 20:21), the latter to remove salt and grease from one's hands (*Chullin* 105a). One sanctifies one's hands by washing them (Exodus 30:19; *Yoma* 22a and 45a). Unclean hands convey ritual impurity (*Tohorot* 1:7 and 4:7; *Tevul Yom* 2:2). One must travel great distances, if necessary, to obtain water for handwashing (*Chullin* 122b).

The hand ailments of Eleazar (2 Samuel 23:10) and Jeroboam (1 Kings 13:14) and the hand condition of the Benjaminites (Judges 20:16) are not clear. Hand amputation secondary to leprosy or injury (*Jerushalmi Nazir* 9:58) and a hand squashed in a moving cylinder (*Jerushalmi Makkot* 2:31) are described. The hands and feet of the murderers of Ishboshet were cut off after they were dead (2 Samuel 4:12). Someone who cuts off his neighbor's hand is punished appropriately (*Baba Kamma* 85a). The legal status of a handless person is detailed by Preuss.[2]

Handfuls of meal were burnt on the altar (Leviticus 2:2) in association with certain offerings (*Menachot* 72b). From a handful of grain, a person can support his family. One fistful of Moses contained eight handfuls (*Genesis Rabbah* 5:7). Handmills to grind flour and corn are described (*Pesachim* 11a; *Ketubot* 69a; *Gittin* 61a; *Baba Batra* 21b, 57a, and 66b; *Niddah* 60b; *Tohorot* 7:4; *Zavim* 3:2). A handbreadth is a legal measure. A notch of that size on the Temple altar renders it unfit (*Chul-*

lin 18a). A garment is defined as a minimum of three handbreadths square (*Shabbat* 26 and 29a). A wall has to be a certain number of handbreadths wide (*Sanhedrin* 4a). The Ark measured ten handbreadths in height (*Sanhedrin* 7a). A placenta is ten or more handbreadths wide (*Niddah* 26a).

The clenched fist is called *egrof*. A man called Ben Batiach had an unusually large fist (*Kelim* 17:12). The wicked smite with the fist of wickedness (Isaiah 59:4). If one strikes another with one's fist (Exodus 21:18), one is liable (*Sanhedrin* 78a). "The fist of flattery" is an expression of bias (*Sotah* 41b). In the Temple, the priest took fistfuls of incense (Leviticus 16:12; *Yoma* 49b). A fistful of meal offering accompanied some sacrifices (*Zevachim* 11a, 13b, 25a, and 30a). It was eaten by male priests (ibid., 63a). [*See also* ARM and FINGERS]

1. A. Even-Shoshan, *A New Concordance of the Bible* (Jerusalem: Kiryat Sefer, 1981), pp. 422–430.
2. F. Rosner (trans.), *Julius Preuss' Biblical and Talmudic Medicine* (Northvale, NJ: Jason Aronson, 1993), pp. 234–235.

HEAD—The head is called the king of limbs (*Avot de Rabbi Nathan* 31:3). There are nine bones in the head (*Oholot* 1:8). The crown (*kodkod*) is the point of intersection of the coronal and sagittal sutures and corresponds to the anterior fontanel of infants (*Menachot* 37a). The crown of the head is cited several times in the Bible (Deuteronomy 28:35; 2 Samuel 14:25; Job 2:7). Sometimes the term *kodkod* is used for the head (Genesis 49:26). The phylacteries are placed on this area of the head (*Eruvin* 95b). The fontanel is the place where the "brain of a child is soft" (*Menachot* 37a) or "pulsating" (*Jerushalmi Eruvin* 10:26). The term *kodkod* is sometimes translated as "summit" or "high point" (Isaiah 3:17; Jeremiah 2:16 and 48:45). *Kodkod sear* refers to the scalp or hairy part of the head (Psalms 68:22).

Old people have hoary heads (*Kiddushin* 33a). Such people are seventy or more years of age (*Avot* 5:21). In talmudic times, people wore turbans (*Berachot* 24a) or *sudarim*, which are pieces of cloth used as head coverings (*Kiddushin* 29b; *Moed Katan* 24a). Scholars had distinctive headgear (*Kiddushin* 8a), although Rav Kahana wore only a scarf on his head. One should not walk four cubits bareheaded because God is above one's head (*Kiddushin* 31a), although the head is unveiled as a sign of mourning (*Moed Katan* 24a). Married women do not uncover their heads in public (*Ketubot* 16a and 72a). If a man intentionally uncovers a woman's head, he must pay her a fine for her shame (ibid., 66a).

A headplate of pure gold with God's name on it (Exodus 28:36–38) was placed on the forehead of Aaron the High Priest as he officiated, and it propitiated certain sacrifices (*Shabbat* 12a; *Pesachim* 16b, 34b, and 77a; *Sanhedrin* 49b; *Zevachim* 22b and 82a). Various malformations of the head disqualify a priest from serving in the Temple [see BLEMISHES]. Leprosy on the head or beard (Leviticus 13:29) is discussed in detail in the Talmud (*Negaim* 10:1; *Tosefta Bechorot* 5:3; *Megillah* 24b), as are the purification rites (*Negaim* 14:8). Injuries to the head are described in several incidents. Jael hammered a nail into Sisera's head (Judges 4:21). The story is depicted again more clearly (ibid., 5:26–27). A certain woman threw a millstone on Abimelech's head and broke his skull (Judges 9:53). David stunned Goliath by smiting him on the forehead with a stone from his slingshot (1 Samuel 17:49).

Rounding of the corners of the head is biblically prohibited (Leviticus 19:27), except for a leper or a Nazarite (*Nazir* 57b; *Yebamot* 5a). To remove the hair from the sideburns is to make the temples as bald as the skin behind the ears and on the forehead (*Makkot* 20b).

Metaphorically, it is said that it is "better to be a tail to lions than a head to foxes" in regard to sitting at the head of the table (*Sanhedrin* 37a; *Avot* 4:15). The head teacher means just that (*Baba Batra* 21a).

HEADACHE—The famous talmudic sage Rab said that he could tolerate any pain except headache (*Shabbat* 11a). Another famous rabbi suffered from headaches for seven weeks following the imbibition of the four prescribed cups of wine on the first night of Passover (*Ecclesiastes Rabbah* 8:1; *Nedarim* 49b). Yet another talmudic sage was unable to wear the head phylactery during the summer because his head was heavy from the heat (*Jerushalmi Berachot* 2:4). The final illness of Titus, in which a gnat flew into his nose, ascended into his head, and gave him incessant headaches, is vividly depicted in the Talmud (*Gittin* 56b). An eminent rabbi cried out that the generation of the deluge brought headaches upon mankind (*Genesis Rabbah* 34:11). A king once reminded his son about the place where the latter had a headache (*Numbers Rabbah* 23:3).

One cause of headache is the blowing away of the froth or foam of beverages such as beer or mead (*Chullin* 105b). Divinely induced headaches require repentance and the performance of good deeds (*Shabbat* 32a). When Jabez prayed to the Lord to keep evil away from him (1 Chronicles 4:10), he was referring to headache (*Temurah* 16a). Another remedy for headache is to study Torah (*Eruvin* 54a) because the words of Torah are an ornament of grace on one's head (Proverbs 1:9). The standard medical therapy for headache was to rub the head with wine, vinegar, or oil (*Tosefta Shabbat* 12:11; *Jerushalmi Maaser Sheni* 2:53). A person with a headache should imagine that he is being put in irons (*Shabbat* 32a).

Someone with a headache is exempt from living in a *sukkah* (booth) on the Festival of Sukkot (*Sukkah* 26a). One should not visit patients with headache because speech is said to be harmful to them (*Nedarim* 41a). Perhaps they prefer to lie quietly without speaking. The name of King Ahasuerus associated with the holiday of Purim is interpreted to mean "headache-inducer" (Hebrew: *chash berosh*) (*Esther Rabbah* 1:3; *Megillah* 11a). Numerous discussions about the causes and treatment of headache are found in the writing of Moses Maimonides.[1]

Plethora, or an excess of blood, is the cause of many illnesses (*Baba Batra* 58b) of the ancients, including migraine or hemicrania.[2] People or animals with congestion or plethora were placed in cold water to cool off (*Shabbat* 53b). Once such an animal cools off, its flesh is not harmful for human consumption (*Tosefta Chullin* 3:19). A variety of folk remedies are detailed in the Talmud to treat blood rushing to the head and migraine (*Gittin* 68b). Animals with plethora were also treated with phlebotomies (*Tosefta Bechorot* 3:17). Leprosy is said to be caused by plethora (*Leviticus Rabbah* 15:2; *Bechorot* 44b).

---

1. F. Rosner, "Headache in the Writings of Moses Maimonides and Other Hebrew Sages," *Headache*, vol. 33 (1993), pp. 315–319.

2. F. Rosner (trans.), *Julius Preuss'
Biblical and Talmudic Medicine* (Northvale, NJ: Jason Aronson, 1993), pp. 305–
306.

HEART—The Hebrew word for heart
is *lev*. In the Bible, this term is used
mostly in a figurative sense. For example, the Bible speaks of "circumcis-
ing the foreskin of the heart" (i.e.,
opening the heart) (Deuteronomy 10:
16; Jeremiah 4:4), the "heart of the
ocean" (Exodus 15:8; Ezekiel 27:25–
27; Proverbs 23:34 and 30:19; Psalms
46:3), the "heart of heaven" (Deuteronomy 4:11), and the "heart of Jerusalem" (Isaiah 40:2).

The heart can reflect the emotions
of anguish (Jeremiah 23:9), wisdom
(Exodus 31:6), evil (Genesis 8:21) and
good (Ezekiel 13:22) inclinations, delight (1 Kings 8:66), pleasure (Psalms
16:9), praise (Psalms 9:2), warmth
(Psalms 39:4), shame (Psalms 69:21),
singing (Psalms 84:3), and charity
(Exodus 35:22).

Statements are made regarding
the heart of a villain (1 Samuel 25:
36), the heart of a king (Proverbs
25:3), the heart of a prince (Jeremiah
4:9), the heart of a fool (Proverbs
12:23), the heart of a widow (Job
29:13), the heart of a man (Proverbs
19:21), and the heart of an understanding person (Proverbs 14:33).

Various adjectives are used to describe the heart, including haughty
(Ezekiel 31:10), frightened (Deuteronomy 28:67), pure (Psalms 24:4),
happy (Proverbs 15:13), fleshy (Ezekiel
11:19), melting (Nahum 2:11), perfect (1 Chronicles 28:9), intelligent
(Proverbs 11:29), broken (Psalms 51:
19), upright (Psalms 97:11), stout
(Psalms 76:6), trembling (Deuteronomy 28:65), listening (1 Kings 3:9),
fat (Isaiah 6:10), oppressed (Isaiah
57:15), pained (Isaiah 65:14), and
uncircumcised (Jeremiah 9:25).

The heart is described as the deci-
sion-making organ (*Leviticus Rabbah*
4:4). A detailed exposition of the
heart's functions and activities is found
in the homiletical commentary on the
phrase "I spoke with my own heart"
(*Ecclesiastes Rabbah* 1:16).

In the Talmud, the Hebrew word
lev (or its Aramaic equivalent *libba*) has
meanings other than heart. *Lev* is used
to denote the stomach (*Gittin* 70a;
Chullin 59a). The word *lev* also refers to the chest or breast (*Moed
Katan* 22b; *Semachot* 9:5; *Sanhedrin*
68a; *Sotah* 1:5). The placing of phylacteries (*tefillin*) "on your hearts"
(Deuteronomy 6:8 and 11:18) is interpreted in the Talmud to mean the left
biceps, in opposition to the left chest
or breast (*Menachot* 37a). Finally, the
Hebrew word *lev* connotes the mind
(*Baba Batra* 12b), in that before a person eats and drinks he has two hearts
(i.e., he cannot make up his mind).

The anatomy of the heart is discussed in the Talmud where large and
small cavities (i.e., chambers) are de-

scribed (*Chullin* 45b). No mention of heart valves is found in the Talmud. It was recognized that the piercing of an animal's heart renders it nonviable. The aorta or "artery of the heart" is also mentioned (ibid.). Diseases of the heart are described in the Talmud under several categories including *ke'ev lev* or "pain of the heart" (*Berachot* 40a and 55a), *chulsha de libba* or "weakness of the heart" (*Shabbat* 10a; *Taanit* 7a; *Berachot* 40a; *Eruvin* 24b), *yukra de libba* or "heaviness of the heart" (*Shabbat* 140a; *Gittin* 69b), *pircha de libba* or "palpitations of the heart" (*Gittin* 69b), and *kircha de libba* or "pressure of the heart" (*Gittin* 69b). Another condition called *goneiach milibbo*, or "groaning from heart pain," is also discussed (*Temurah* 15b). It cannot be determined with certainty whether any of these "heart" ailments in fact refer to organic heart disease in the modern sense. Hence, it is impossible to state whether any of the proposed remedies has scientific validity or justification.[1]

---

1. F. Rosner, "The Heart," in *Medicine in the Bible and the Talmud*, 2nd ed. (Hoboken, NJ: Ktav and Yeshiva University Press, 1995), pp. 93–101.

HEMOPHILIA—The sex-linked transmission of hemophilia was recognized by the talmudic Sages (*Yebamot* 64b). Females carry the defective gene but are clinically healthy and affected males

suffer from this bleeding disorder. The key passage in the Talmud states:

For it was taught: "If she circumcised her first child and he died [as a result of bleeding from the operation], and a second one also died [similarly], she must not circumcise her third child." These are the words of Rebbe [Rabbi Judah the Prince, redactor of the Mishnah, the second-century compilation of Jewish law]. Rabban Simeon ben Gamliel, however, said: "She may circumcise the third child but must not circumcise the fourth child." (*Yebamot* 64b)

Rabbi Judah and Rabbi Simeon do not differ on the question of the maternal transmission of the disease but on the number of repetitive events required to establish a pattern and to remove a subsequent similar event from the category of chance. This is a technical point of talmudic law. Although, in general, three repetitive events are necessary to establish a pattern, in matters of life and death, the view of Rabbi Judah, that two suffice, is upheld. No other form of diagnosis was then available. The codifiers of Jewish law including Alfasi (loc. cit.), Maimonides (*Mishneh Torah, Milah* 1:18), Karo (*Shulchan Aruch, Yoreh Deah* 263:2–3), and others all rule according to the opinion of Rabbi Judah. Some rabbinic authorities thought that males can also transmit this genetic bleeding disorder.[1]

The observations recorded in the Talmud and by the codifiers of Jewish law are incomplete, however. Although families with bleeding disorders were recognized, the question of circumcision of the child whose maternal uncles died of bleeding after circumcision is not considered. A woman whose brothers bled to death after circumcision could well be a carrier. Only the direct maternal transmission of the disease was recognized, whether demonstrated in siblings or maternal cousins.

---

1. F. Rosner, "Hemophilia," in *Medicine in the Bible and the Talmud*, 2nd ed. (Hoboken, NJ: Ktav and Yeshiva University Press, 1995), pp. 43–49.

HEMORRHOIDS—The Lord smites His enemies with hemorrhoids (Psalms 78:66) as He did the Philistines (1 Samuel 5:6–12). Israelites would be similarly stricken if they sin (Deuteronomy 28:27; *Megillah* 25b). The Talmud lists ten things that lead to hemorrhoids: eating the leaves of reeds or of vines; eating unsalted animal palates, fish spines, or insufficiently cooked salted fish; drinking wine lees; or wiping one's anus with lime, clay, or pebbles previously used by others (*Berachot* 55a; *Shabbat* 81a). Fresh grass should not be used to wipe oneself because it may tear hemorrhoids (*Shabbat* 82a). He who sits too long without walking (*Ketubot* 11a) or who

squats to defecate without sitting down may also develop hemorrhoids (*Berachot* 55a; *Shabbat* 81a). Bleeding hemorrhoids may lead to collapse (*Nedarim* 22a). Dates are helpful to treat hemorrhoids (*Ketubot* 10b). [*See also* DEFECATION, FECES, ANUS, and RECTUM]

HEREDITY—The heredity of moral traits is alluded to in the Bible (Exodus 20:5). Epilepsy and leprosy were thought to be inherited disorders and it was recommended that one not marry a woman from a family with epilepsy or leprosy [*see* EPILEPSY]. Before taking a wife, one should examine the traits of her brothers (*Baba Batra* 110a). Hereditary succession is described in detail in the Talmud (ibid., 108a). The righteous and wicked each claim the superiority of their respective ancestry (*Sanhedrin* 38a). There are various types of families: A family of Torah scholars produces scholars, a family of scribes produces scribes, and a family of milk men produces milk men (*Ecclesiastes Rabbah* 4:9:1).

The Talmud recognizes that a father or mother does not engender corresponding limbs in the child, for if this were so, a blind man should beget blind children and an amputee should beget children without legs (*Chullin* 69a). A father transmits to his son comeliness, strength, wealth, long life, and generations before him (*Eduyot* 2:9). There are three partners in the creation of a human being: God, the father, and the mother. The father provides the white (sperm) from which are derived the child's bones and sinews, his nails, the marrow in the head (brain), and the white of the eye. The mother provides the red (menstrual blood) from which are derived skin, flesh, blood, hair, and the black of the eye. God gives the spirit and the soul, beauty of features, sight of the eyes, hearing of the ears, speech of the mouth, the ability to move the hands and walk with the feet, understanding, and discernment (*Niddah* 31a).

Hemophilia and its precise genetic transmission is described in the Talmud (*Yebamot* 64b) [*see* HEMOPHILIA]. The laws of Mendelian genetics were applied by Jacob in the biblical narrative (Genesis 30:32ff.) of the speckled and spotted sheep.[1]

_____

1. Y. Flicks, in *Techumin* (Alon Shevut, Israel), vol. 3 (1982), pp. 461–472.

HERMAPHRODITE—A hermaphrodite (*androginos*) is a person of double sex who may be male or female or both (*Tosefta Bikkurim* 2:7). In some legal matters he is like a man, in some he is like a woman (*Bikkurim* 4:1–5), in some he is like both, and in others he is like neither (*Shabbat* 136a). It was thought that a hermaphrodite can both menstruate and ejaculate (*Niddah* 28a), although most see either white sperm or red menstrual

blood (*Tosefta Niddah* 1:3). Adam was created as a hermaphrodite (*Genesis Rabbah* 8:1; *Leviticus Rabbah* 14:1), based on the biblical verse "Male and female He created them" (Genesis 5:2).

A *tumtum* is a person of doubtful or uncertain or indeterminate sex. The word *tumtum* means "sealed" or "covered over," and such a person's true sex can be determined when he is "split" or cut open. Thus, a cryptorchid is a *tumtum* with undescended testicles. After opening the groin or abdomen (laparotomy), the testicles may be found to be rudimentary or degenerated and the *tumtum* is unable to procreate, like a congenital eunuch. The phrase "all thy males" (Exodus 23:17) excludes the *tumtum* and the hermaphrodite (*Chagigah* 4a). Legally, they are generally equal in Jewish law (see *Baba Batra* 126b for an exception).

HOARSENESS—Esau became hoarse from anger when he learned from his father Isaac that Jacob took not only his birthright but his father's blessing (*Genesis Rabbah* 67:4). [*See also* THROAT]

HOMOSEXUALITY—Homosexuality is condemned in Judaism and characterized in the Bible as an abomination (Leviticus 18:22 and 20:13). It is also considered a form of Egyptian and Canaanite fornication practice and hence forbidden (Leviticus 18:3–5). Those who practice homosexuality are executed by stoning (*Sanhedrin* 54a and 55a). In self-defense, a person may kill his attacker to prevent an act of homosexuality. A third person may even kill the attacker, who is classified as a "pursuer" (*rodef*) (*Sanhedrin* 73a). To avoid and prevent homosexual acts, two unmarried men should not sleep under the same blanket (*Kiddushin* 4:14) and unmarried men should not teach young boys (ibid., 4:13). Homosexuality causes the sun to be in eclipse (*Sukkah* 29a).

The people of Sodom practiced homosexuality (Genesis 19:5). Sodom became the prototype of all depravities (Ezekiel 16:50). "Sodomy" and "Sodomite grapes" (Deuteronomy 32:32) are expressions for immoral, debased behavior. The townspeople of Gibeah also practiced homosexuality (Judges 19:22). A detailed comparison of the immoral practices in Sodom and Gibeah is given by Preuss.[1] Potiphar wanted to commit a homosexual act with the handsome Joseph (Genesis 39:6) but was divinely prevented from doing so (*Genesis Rabbah* 86:3; *Sotah* 13a). "Kings lying in glory in their own houses" (Isaiah 14:18) refers to homosexuality (*Shabbat* 149b). The righteous king Asa banished homosexuals (1 Kings 15:12), as did his son Jehoshofat (ibid., 22:47). [*See also* LESBIANISM, BESTIALITY, and RAPE]

1. F. Rosner (trans.), *Julius Preuss' Biblical and Talmudic Medicine* (Northvale, NJ: Jason Aronson, 1993), pp. 234–235.

HONEY—Honey was used in antiquity as a substitute for sugar and is an essential element for life (*Sirach* 39:26). Only a sated soul tramples on a honeycomb (Psalms 25:7). One should eat honey only to satiation (Psalms 25:16). Eating too much honey is not good (Psalms 25:27). He who consumes a lot of honey at one time on an empty stomach in the summertime snaps his heart (or stomach) strings (*Chullin* 59a). Faint people are refreshed by honey (1 Samuel 14:27). If one is afflicted with a ravenous hunger on Yom Kippur one is given honey and other sweet things to restore one's strength (*Yoma* 83b). Honey is especially good for children (Isaiah 7:15). Honey stimulates the appetite and satisfies (*Yoma* 83b).

Israel is said to be the land of milk and honey (Exodus 3:8, 3:17, 13:5, and 33:3; Leviticus 20:24; Numbers 13:27 and 14:8; Deuteronomy 6:3, 11:9, 26:9, and 27:3; Joshua 5:6; Jeremiah 32:22). One rabbi saw a trail of milk and honey sixteen miles long and sixteen miles wide (*Megillah* 60a). Other rabbis also saw flowing honey in abundance (*Ketubot* 111b). The words of Torah are compared to honey in that they are sweet (Psalms 19:11) like honey (*Song of Songs Rabbah* 1:2:3;

Deuteronomy Rabbah 1:6). Honey was applied on sores or scabs for healing purposes (*Shabbat* 77b; *Baba Metzia* 38b) in addition to being eaten as a food (*Shabbat* 78a). One rabbi had an ass laden with honey, which he used to apply to camel's sores caused by the chafing of the saddle (*Shabbat* 154b). The animal is also given putrefied honey to eat (*Shabbat* 154a). Barley flour in honey was consumed for stomach pains (*Yoma* 83b) and for weakness or faintness (*Gittin* 69b). White honey was part of a recipe against *barsam* (*Chullin* 105b). Rue in honey was used to treat a berry like excrescence (*Abodah Zarah* 28a). A honey-containing potion was also recommended for the illness called *unklai* (ibid., 29a). Honey was thought to be helpful to the eyes if consumed after meals (*Yoma* 83b). Orally consumed honey may be harmful to wounds (*Baba Kamma* 85a). *Anomalin* is a mixture of wine, honey, and pepper used as a cooling drink in the bathhouse (ibid., 30a). Some honey drinks can be intoxicating (*Nazir* 4a).

Honey is divinely permitted for human consumption even though it is derived from an "unclean" animal (*Bechorot* 7b). Honey combs exude honey or the honey can be removed from them manually (*Shabbat* 19b and 143b; *Betzah* 36a; *Uktzin* 3:11). Loaves of honey may not be removed from the beehive on the Sabbath (*Shabbat* 95a). Beehives are full of honey in the summer but not in the winter (*Shabbat* 43b; *Betzah* 36a). A beehive is regarded as landed property, that is attached to the ground, for legal purposes (*Baba Batra* 80b). If one buys the annual issue of a beehive, he takes the first three swarms. The seller may then emasculate the remaining bees using mustard, to enable them to devote themselves entirely to producing honey (ibid., 80a).

The honey from Ziphim (see Joshua 15:55 and Psalms 54:2) was special (*Sotah* 58b; *Machshirin* 5:9). Honey is one of the seven liquids that render produce susceptible to ritual uncleanness (*Machshirin* 6:4). Honey on the body constitutes an interposition regarding ritual immersion (*Menachot* 21a). A woman in the city of Sodom was once daubed with honey and bees came and consumed her (*Sanhedrin* 109b). Herod preserved the body of a young maiden in honey (*Baba Batra* 3b). "Rich" unleavened bread kneaded with honey may not be suitable for the Passover seder (*Pesachim* 35a), although wheat cakes streaked with honey serve as a remedy for heart palpitations (*Gittin* 69b).

HORSES—A horse puts its weight on its forefeet (*Shabbat* 93b) and rests on its hind legs (*Zavim* 4:7). A horse dozes by taking sixty respirations while standing (*Sukkah* 26b). Six things were said of a horse: It loves promiscuity and battle, has a proud spirit, despises sleep, eats much, and excretes little

(*Pesachim* 113b). Although a horse responds to its master in battle (*Sanhedrin* 63b), it stands still when it urinates and can thereby endanger its rider during a battle (*Jerushalmi Pesachim* 4:31). The urine of horses is thin (dilute) and not like milk (*Bechorot* 7b). Scabs or sore spots on horses caused by chafing of the saddle were treated with honey (*Shabbat* 77a).

Horses are employed for work (*Shabbat* 94a; *Abodah Zarah* 16a) such as pulling chariots (*Sanhedrin* 21b) and for riding (*Chagigah* 15a; *Sanhedrin* 46a). Horses are housed in stalls in horse stables (*Sanhedrin* 21b) and their hoofs are trimmed (*Moed Katan* 10a). Some horses had a fox's tail suspended between their eyes (*Shabbat* 53a) or bells attached to their bodies (*Pesachim* 50a) to ward off the evil eye. No one may ride on the king's horse (*Sanhedrin* 22a and 95a). In the past a deceased king's horse had its sinews severed (Joshua 11:6) so that it could not be ridden by anyone else (*Abodah Zarah* 11a). This act is prohibited in Judaism as cruelty to animals.[1]

Jewish writings speak of white, black, and red horses (*Song of Songs Rabbah* 1:9:4), Persian horses (*Lamentations Rabbah* 1:13:41; *Song of Songs Rabbah* 8:9:3), horsemen (*Sanhedrin* 21b and 42b; *Megillah* 27a), horse guards (*Baba Batra* 8a), horse whips (Proverbs 26:3), horse surgeons (*Numbers Rabbah* 9:5), and even wooden musical toy horses (*Kelim* 16:7). A white horse is a favorable omen in a dream (*Sanhedrin* 93a). One should not live in a town without horses (*Pesachim* 113a). A mule may not be mated with a horse (*Chullin* 79a) because of the prohibition against mixing different species.

1. F. Rosner, *Modern Medicine and Jewish Ethics*, 2nd ed. (Hoboken, NJ: Ktav, 1991), pp. 353–373.

HOSPITALS—Jews have always had brotherhoods or societies that concerned themselves with charitable deeds, mainly the burial of the dead and the visitation of the sick. Such a *chavruta* is explicitly mentioned in the Talmud (*Moed Katan* 27b). No formal hospitals were established until the Middle Ages, but King Uzziah, in biblical times, had a home for lepers (2 Kings 15:5; 2 Chronicles 26:21). King Azariah also established leprosariums when he was stricken with leprosy (2 Kings 15:5). Hospitality houses were also known since the time of Abraham the Patriarch, who built one for strangers (*Genesis Rabbah* 54:6). Early Jewish hospitals beginning in the thirteenth century are described elsewhere.[1]

1. H. Jungmann and F. Rosner, "Hospitals," *Encyclopedia Judaica*, vol. 8 (Jerusalem: Keter, 1972), pp. 1033–1039.

HUNCHBACK—A man once bragged he could straighten the hump of a hunchback. The latter retorted: If you could do that, you would be called a great physician and command large fees (*Sanhedrin* 91a). A hunchback priest (Leviticus 21:20) is unfit to serve in the Temple because of his unsightly appearance (*Bechorot* 43b). A child with a crooked spinal column (*Niddah* 24a) probably refers either to meningomyelocele or scoliosis. [*See also* SPINAL COLUMN]

HUNGER—A person's eyes become sunken from hunger (Midrash Psalms 73:7). Hunger may cause one's skin to turn greenish (*Ruth Rabbah* 3:6) and one's sperm to decrease (*Gittin* 70a). Poor people are always hungry and do not know it because they become accustomed thereto (*Megillah* 7b). One is obligated to feed them (Isaiah 58:7). Weakness of the heart may occur in hungry people (*Shabbat* 10a; *Taanit* 7a), for which a folk remedy with wine and meat is recommended (*Eruvin* 29b). Extreme hunger may be associated with hunger pangs and finally delirium and death (*Sanhedrin* 63b). King David's hungry entourage was fed all types of foods (2 Samuel 18:28–29). Dropsy caused by hunger is called "swollen" (*Shabbat* 33a).

If a person is seized by a ravenous hunger (bulimia) on Yom Kippur, a fast day, one may feed him honey and all kinds of sweet things to restore his endangered health. If necessary, one may even feed him from prohibited foods (*Yoma* 83a–b). Honey seems to be a good antidote for bulimia (1 Samuel 14:29). A man who ate fig cakes and raisins (1 Samuel 30:12) was extremely hungry and may have suffered from bulimia (*Tosefta Shabbat* 8:30). When Rabbi Yochanan suffered from bulimia, he sat under a fig tree (i.e., ate figs) and became healthy (*Ecclesiastes Rabbah* 7:11). [*See also* FASTING and FAMINE]

HYSSOP—Hyssop is a small, bushy, aromatic plant. Whole twigs were used in rites of purification of people ritually impure because of contact with a corpse (Numbers 19:18). The sprinkling of the waters of lustration was performed with hyssop (ibid., 19:6). So too the purification of lepers (Leviticus 14:4; Psalms 51:9). The paschal lamb offering was preceded by the application on the lintels and doorposts of hyssop dipped in blood (Exodus 12:22).

Different types of hyssop exist, including ordinary hyssop, wild hyssop, stibium hyssop, Roman hyssop, and Greek hyssop (*Sukkah* 13a; *Chullin* 62b; *Negaim* 8:6). Hyssop can be grown in a courtyard (*Niddah* 51a). It is sold in bundles (Leviticus 14:4; *Niddah* 26a). Hyssop buds do not absorb water (*Niddah* 13b).

Medically, Greek hyssop is a medicine and not a food (*Shabbat* 109b). For curing a stomach (or heart) ailment called *unklai*, the patient should eat several herbs including hyssop (*Abodah Zarah* 29a). Hyssop is also used for fuel (*Sheviit* 8:1). The cedar is the tallest tree and the hyssop the most lowly, yet both are equal in the eyes of God (*Exodus Rabbah* 17:2; *Numbers Rabbah* 19:3). Therefore, the Jews humbled themselves like the hyssop when they repented for the sin of the Golden Calf (*Exodus Rabbah* 1:36).

HYSTERIA—Hysterical muteness is well known in ancient Jewish writings (*Song of Songs Rabbah* 2:41; *Chagigah*

3a). Hysterical paralysis is also described from ancient times.[1] *Hystero* means "uterus" and, therefore, love-sick people were said to be afflicted with hysteria (2 Samuel 13:1ff.; *Sanhedrin* 75a). The Palestinian Talmud calls this illness *racham*, meaning "love," which is related to the word *rechem*, meaning "uterus," and corresponds to hysteria in the ancient sense of the word.

---

1. F. Rosner (trans.), *Julius Preuss' Biblical and Talmudic Medicine* (Northvale, NJ: Jason Aronson, 1993), p. 307.

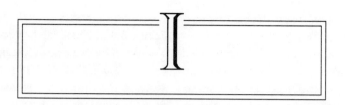

ILLNESS—Abraham introduced the world to old age, Isaac to suffering, and Jacob to illness (*Genesis Rabbah* 65:9 and 97:1). Until Jacob there was no illness (Genesis 48:1; *Baba Metzia* 87a; *Sanhedrin* 107b). Until Elisha, no sick person ever recovered (*Baba Metzia* 87a). Elisha died of his third sickness (2 Kings 13:14; *Sanhedrin* 107b). Six things help the sick to recover from illness: cabbage, beets, dry *sisin* herbs, tripe, womb, and liver. Some also say small fish (*Abodah Zarah* 29a). Six things are a good prognostic sign for a sick person: sneezing, perspiration, open bowels, seminal emission, sleep, and a dream (*Berachot* 57b). Ten things cause exacerbation of illness: eating beef, fat roast meat, poultry, roast egg, pepperwort, cress, milk, or cheese; shaving; and bathing (ibid.). Some add nuts and large cucumbers (*Abodah Zarah* 29a).

Eighty-three sicknesses depend on the gall and all can be rendered ineffectual by eating one's morning bread with salt and drinking a jugful of water (*Baba Metzia* 107b). Morning bread is an antidote against heat and cold, winds, and demons and the evil eye.[1] The most common cause of illness and death is a cold, which may result from one's own negligence (ibid.). Some sages say that most people have themselves to blame for their illness and death (*Leviticus Rabbah* 16:8; *Jerushalmi Shabbat* 14:14). A change in one's diet or lifestyle is the beginning of sickness (*Baba Batra* 146a). One may become ill from eating onions (*Eruvin* 29b). Garlands or plants cure illness (*Shabbat* 66b). Hot blankets are used to relieve chills and cold compresses to relieve fever (*Niddah* 36b).

A sick person requires guarding (*Berachot* 54b). Visiting the sick is a meritorious act and a religious obligation.[2] For a dangerously ill patient, the Sabbath may be desecrated (*Betzah* 22a). If one is deathly ill, one recites the *viduy*, or confession prayer (*Shabbat* 32a). A sick person recovers from illness when his sins are forgiven (*Nedarim* 41a). If a person falls ill, he should not tell anyone the first day so that he does not have bad luck (*Berachot* 55b). One should not inform a sick person of the death of a close relative (*Moed Katan* 26b).

A diagnostic test using a hard-boiled egg is described (*Nedarim* 50b) and was used by the physician Mar Samuel on himself (*Yebamot* 116b). Divine healing of illness (Psalms 103:3) is desirable, but many illnesses have a fatal outcome. A person who recovers from illness recites a special blessing of thanksgiving (*Berachot* 54b). [*See also* DEATH, FEVER, VISITING THE SICK, DEMONS, EVIL EYE, ASTROLOGY, and specific illnesses and diseases].

1. F. Rosner (trans.), *Julius Preuss' Biblical and Talmudic Medicine* (Northvale, NJ: Jason Aronson, 1993), pp. 139–141.
2. F. Rosner, *Medicine in the Bible and the Talmud*, 2nd ed. (Hoboken, NJ: Ktav and Yeshiva University Press, 1995), pp. 176–181.

INCANTATIONS—The medical effectiveness of incantations was never in doubt in classic Jewish sources.[1] Incantations to heal a scorpion's bite are permitted even on the Sabbath, as are snake or scorpion charming to prevent injury or harm by them (*Shulchan Aruch, Yoreh Deah* 179:6–7). Maimonides points out that such incantations are absolutely useless but are permitted because of the patient's dangerous condition, so that he not become distraught (*Mishneh Torah, Akum* 11:11). One whispered a spell to heal eye illnesses (*Tosefta Shabbat* 7:23). Rabbi Chaninah healed Rabbi Yochanan by uttering an incantation (*Song of Songs Rabbah* 2:16). A bone stuck in the throat can be dislodged by an incantation (*Shabbat* 67a). When Elisha ben Abuya entered a synagogue and saw children making progress in the Torah, he uttered incantations over them (*Song of Songs Rabbah* 1:4:1). An incantation against the demon of blindness is described in the Talmud (*Pesachim* 112a; *Abodah Zarah* 12b) as is an incantation to heal someone bitten by a mad dog (*Yoma* 84a). Incantations are recited over oil contained in a vessel (*Sanhedrin* 101a).

The main question concerning the permissibility of incantations in Judaism is whether or not they represent a form of forbidden heathen practice, in that Jews are commanded not to go in the ways of Amorites (Leviticus 18:3). Some talmudic sages declare that if one whispers a spell over a bodily illness, one is deprived of everlasting bliss, i.e., the world to come. These sages further prohibit a person from calling another to recite a biblical verse to calm a frightened child (*Jerushalmi Shabbat* 6:8b).

On the other hand, the Talmud clearly states that whatever is used for healing purposes is not forbidden on account of the ways of the Amorites (*Shabbat* 67a). This rule is codified by Asher Ben Yechiel, known as Rosh. Rashba states that the prohibition on account of the ways of the Amorites is limited to those practices specifically enumerated in the Talmud (*Tosefta Shabbat*, chs. 7 and 8).

Zimmels lists a variety of diseases cured by charms as found in the Responsa literature, including certain eye diseases, headache, infertility, and epilepsy.[2] He also describes the custom of transference, whereby an illness can be transferred to an animal or a plant by a certain procedure, with or without the recitation of an incantation. For example, patients with jaundice were told to put live fish under their soles to transfer the jaundice to the fish. In more recent times, pigeons are placed on the abdomen of jaundiced patients to transfer the illness to the pigeons.[3] [*See also* ASTROLOGY, DEMONS, EVIL EYE, EXORCISM, MAGIC, SORCERY, and AMULETS]

---

1. F. Rosner (trans.), *Julius Preuss' Biblical and Talmudic Medicine* (Northvale, NJ: Jason Aronson, 1993), pp. 144–146.
2. H.J. Zimmels, *Magicians, Theologians, and Doctors* (London: Goldston & Son, 1952), pp. 140–142.
3. F. Rosner, "Pigeons As a Remedy (*Segulah*) for Jaundice," *New York State Journal of Medicine* (1992), pp. 189–192.

INCENSE—The burning of incense in a pan is part of a variety of Temple services (*Pesachim* 59a; *Yoma* 14b, 25a, and 34a). The procedure is described in detail (*Yoma* 47a and 53a; *Tamid* 6:3). The priestly family of Abtinas was in charge of its preparation (*Ketubot* 106a). To stop an outbreak of plague, Aaron the High Priest offered incense (Numbers 17:12). The odor of incense is more powerful and fragrant than women's perfume (*Yoma* 39b). For this reason, incense is put under corpses to neutralize the odor (*Moed Katan* 27b; *Tosefta Niddah* 9:16).

A person being led out to execution is given frankincense in wine to benumb his senses (*Sanhedrin* 43a). The holy frankincense used in the Temple may not be prepared for secular use (Exodus 30:34–38).

INCEST—Incest is biblically prohibited (Leviticus 20:17). The abominations described in the Bible (ibid., 18:27) refer to incest (*Yebamot* 21a). One must rather be killed than commit incest (*Pesachim* 25b; *Yoma* 82a; *Ketubot* 19a; *Sanhedrin* 74a). Incest is one of the sins for which leprosy is inflicted as punishment (*Arachin* 16a). Another punishment is exile (*Shabbat* 33a; *Avot* 5:9). The most famous biblical case of incest is Lot with his daughters (Genesis 19:32ff.). An incestuous relationship with one's father or mother is a capital crime (*Sanhedrin* 50b and 53a). The punishment of execution by stoning or burning depends on which relative one commits incest with. There are first- and second-degree types of incest (*Yebamot* 20a and 21a). Because of the stringent legal requirements for imposing a sentence of capital punishment, it was extremely rare for a death penalty to be carried out, even once in seventy years (*Makkot* 7a).

Cohabitation with a hermaphrodite relative is not punished as incest (*Tosefta Bikkurim* 2:5), but the law against homosexuality is applied (*Tosefta Yebamot* 10:2). Pregnancy resulting from artificial insemination of sperm from a married man or a forbidden relative is not considered adultery or incest, respectively.[1] [*See also* ADULTERY, HOMOSEXUALITY, and MARRIAGE, FORBIDDEN]

---

1. F. Rosner, *Modern Medicine and Jewish Ethics*, 2nd ed. (Hoboken, NJ, and New York: Ktav and Yeshiva University Press, 1991), pp. 85–121.

INFLAMMATION—Metal instruments that cut the skin, especially iron instruments (*Chullin* 77a), may cause inflammation (infection) (*Shabbat* 134a). Wounds touched by hands become inflamed (*Abodah Zarah* 28b). Eye inflammations may be treated even on the Sabbath (ibid., *Betzah* 22a). Green leaves are applied to inflamed eyes (*Shabbat* 108b). [*See also* WOUNDS]

INJURIES—A bruise or injury from which blood exudes but is not expelled (ecchymosis) is called a *chabura*

(wound or injury) (*Shabbat* 107b). To stop a bleeding wound or injury, one applies cress with vinegar (*Abodah Zarah* 28a). Cain inflicted many wounds on his brother Abel before he killed him (*Sanhedrin* 37b). Wounds on the back of the hand or foot are considered dangerous (*Abodah Zarah* 28a). David injured Goliath with his slingshot (1 Samuel 17:49). A fall from a roof can cause multiple injuries (*Exodus Rabbah* 28:9). A red-hot portable stove once fell on a woman's leg and she died from the injury (*Chagigah* 4b). Other fatal injuries are also discussed (*Baba Batra* 175b). A fall from a coach (nowadays a bus or car) can fracture limbs and cause other injuries including blindness (*Leviticus Rabbah* 31:4). Dislocations or sprains occurred to Job (Job 31:21–22). Jaw dislocation disqualifies an animal from being offered in the Temple (*Bechorot* 6:10). Broken bones are discussed in the section FRACTURES.

Penetrating abdominal injuries occur with attempted disembowelment (2 Maccabees 14:39–46). Ehud thrust his sword into Eglon's abdomen (Judges 3:21–22). If someone is stabbed with a sword or lancet, he should drink strong wine and fat meat roasted on coals (*Gittin* 70a). If one is struck by an arrow or a spear, one should apply the herbal remedy *samtar* (*Yebamot* 114b). If one injures one's fellow man, one must pay financial remuneration (Exodus 21:19). If a man accidentally strikes a pregnant woman, she may miscarry (Exodus 21:22). [*See also* WOUNDS, BLEMISHES, DEFECTS, and specific body organs]

INSOMNIA—Insomnia occurs in the unsatisfiable (*Sirach* 34:20) and in the very wealthy (Ecclesiastes 5:11). The wicked are punished with insomnia (Deuteronomy 28:67). King Ahasuerus could not sleep (Esther 6:1). Nor could King Darius after he threw Daniel into the lion's den (Daniel 6:19). King David complained of insomnia (Psalms 77:5). Aggrieved people such as Job have nightmares and cannot sleep (Job 7:4), perhaps due to severe bone pain (Job 30:17). Jacob did not sleep at night (Genesis 31:40). Sleep does not exist for God (*Sotah* 18a) as stated in the Bible (Psalms 121:4), although, anthropomorphically, God is said to sleep (Psalms 44:24). [*See also* SLEEP]

INTESTINES—The biblical term *mai'ayim* for intestines (2 Samuel 20:10) also refers to the abdomen (Genesis 15:4) and the womb (Genesis 25:23). The small and large intestines are two of the ten organs of digestion (*Ecclesiastes Rabbah* 7:3). If one drinks abundantly with meals, one is protected from intestinal illnesses (*Berachot* 40a). The latter should not be neglected (*Sotah* 4b). A change in diet is the beginning of bowel troubles (*Ketubot* 110b). Perforation of the

intestines (*Moed Katan* 22a; *Chullin* 48b) is not necessarily fatal since they can be sealed with mesenteric fat (*Chullin* 49b) or with mucus (*Chullin* 50a). Barley bread shrinks the intestines and causes blockage (*Sanhedrin* 81b), whereas cucumbers make the intestines expand (*Abodah Zarah* 11a). Aged wine is food for the intestines; fresh wine is harmful (Psalms 104:15; Proverbs 31:4–7). Spleen or leeks is good for the bowels (*Berachot* 44b).

Intestinal illnesses described in the Bible and Talmud are mostly diarrhea or worms. The causes and treatments of diarrhea are discussed in the section DIARRHEA. Treatment for intestinal worms include garlic (*Baba Kamma* 82a), hedge mustard (*Gittin* 69b), and pennyroyal (*Shabbat* 10b). Bowel complaints are painful and difficult to tolerate (*Shabbat* 11a). Such patients are often righteous (*Shabbat* 118b) and are forgiven for their sins and do not go to Gehenna (*Eruvin* 41b). People with bowel diseases may die suddenly (*Eruvin* 41b). An expert physician treated the Temple priests who suffered from intestinal ailments (*Shekalim* 5:1–2; *Jerushalmi Shekalim* 5:48). Dates are good for intestinal illnesses (*Ketubot* 10b). One can also massage the abdomen with wine and oil, even on the Sabbath (*Shabbat* 134a and 147b; *Sanhedrin* 101a).

Scurvy starts in the mouth and extends to the intestines (*Abodah Zarah* 28a). Diphtheria or croup (*askara*) is a punishment for slander and begins in the bowels and ends in the throat (*Shabbat* 33b). An illness of the large bowel called *kolos* (colitis?) is dangerous and should be treated by drinking pulverized cress in aged wine (*Jerushalmi Shabbat* 14:14; *Jerushalmi Abodah Zarah* 2:40). King Jehoram's illness was an intestinal ailment (2 Chronicles 21:14–18), either dysentery or cancer of the rectum.[1] Antiochus was stricken with pain in his bowels (2 Maccabees 9:5ff.), which Preuss suggests was an abscess from bowel perforation. The Israelites who complained about the manna (Numbers 11:5) were punished with some type of intestinal ailment (*Leviticus Rabbah* 18:4; *Numbers Rabbah* 7:4).

Animals with duplication of the intestines are described (*Chullin* 58b). Animal intestines were used to make harp strings (*Abodah Zarah* 47a). The intestines of a ritually slaughtered animal may be consumed (*Chullin* 33a). [*See also* ABDOMEN, STOMACH, DIARRHEA, and WORMS]

---

1. F. Rosner (trans.), *Julius Preuss' Biblical and Talmudic Medicine* (Northvale, NJ: Jason Aronson, 1993), pp. 183–184.

INTOXICANTS—Dates were thought to intoxicate. Therefore, he who eats dates should not teach (*Ketubot* 10b). If a priest eats figs from Keilah or drinks honey with milk, he may become intoxicated thereby (*Nazir* 4a). If he then enters the Temple, he violates the prohibition against strong drink (Leviticus 10:9). Maimonides also considers milk to be an intoxicant (*Mishneh Torah, Biyat Mikdash* 1:3). Beer made from asparagus or cabbage sprouts imbibed on an empty stomach can also intoxicate (*Berachot* 51a). [*See also* BEER, DRUNKENNESS, and WINE]

ISOLATION—In biblical times, patients with flux (gonorrhea), both male and female, and those defiled by the dead were isolated or quarantined outside the camp (Numbers 5:3). In talmudic times, they were allowed only in the outermost of the three concentric camps (*Taanit* 21b; *Kelim* 1:8). Patients with *tzaraat* (leprosy) were also isolated (Leviticus 13:4). Patients with *raatan* were shunned and lived in isolation (*Ketubot* 77b). A healed leper remained isolated for seven days before rejoining the community after an elaborate purification process (Leviticus 14:8). [*See also* PLAGUE]

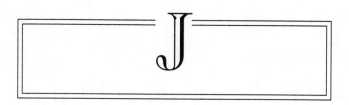

JAW—The Hebrew word *lechi* refers both to jaw and to cheek. Samson slew a thousand Philistines with the jawbone (*lechi*) of an ass (Judges 15:15). Human facial features include a fully developed chin or jawbone (*Niddah* 23b). The five corners of the beard are two at each jaw (angle and point) and one at the chin (*Sifra*, Leviticus 19:27). He who smites an Israelite on the jaw is as though he has assaulted the Divine Presence (*Sanhedrin* 58b). If the upper or lower jaw of a priest protrudes, he is unfit to serve in the Temple (*Bechorot* 40a). If the lower jawbone of an animal is gone, one can keep it alive by putting food directly into the gullet (*Chullin* 55b). An animal's jaw is also called the bone of the mouth (*Bechorot* 40b). Jaw bars were made for injured animals (*Shabbat* 54b). The jaws of slaughtered animals were given to the priests as gifts (*Yebamot* 99b). Dislocation of the jaw renders an animal unfit to be offered in the Temple (*Bechorot* 6:10).

He who walks with his chin or jaw turned sideways is considered to be haughty (*Derech Eretz Rabbah* 11:15). Putting one's hand on the chin hides the fact that one is yawning (*Berachot* 24b).

The treatment for a dislocated jaw in humans is permissible even on the Sabbath because of possible danger to life (*Abodah Zarah* 28b). [*See also* FACE and NECK]

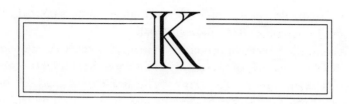

KIDNEYS—The kidneys (*kelayot*) have an indentation or hilum (*charitz*) and the "white below the loins" (calyces and pelvis) that connects to the inner parenchyma of the kidneys (*Chullin* 55a). The kidneys are covered by a double membrane (fat and fibrous). The perinephric fat (Leviticus 3:4) is outside both membranes. Animals have a lot of perinephric fat (Isaiah 34:6). The veins of the kidneys are prohibited as fat (*Chullin* 93a). The kidneys and perinephric fat of certain sacrifices in the Temple were burned on the altar (Leviticus 3:16; *Pesachim* 64b).

Absence of a kidney or an extra kidney was recognized in talmudic times (*Bechorot* 39a). An animal with both kidneys removed is said to be viable (*Chullin* 3:2). Small shrunken kidneys render an animal *terefah* (nonviable) (*Chullin* 55a–b). So, too, if a kidney is putrefied from pus or infection up to the calyces and pelvis (ibid.). A diseased kidney does not regenerate (*Chullin* 128b). A perforation or clear water (cysts?) in the kidney is not a life-threatening defect (*Chullin* 55b). Kidney stones in animals are first re-corded in the posttalmudic Codes of Jewish law (*Yoreh Deah* 44:4). Kidney juice is efficacious in healing ear disorders (*Abodah Zarah* 28b).

The Bible attributes pleasure and sensation to the kidneys (Proverbs 23: 16). Metaphorically, Job's kidneys withered within him (Job 19:27). The kidneys are the source of wisdom (Job 38:36). They are tested by God (Jeremiah 11:20), who stays far from the kidneys of the wicked (ibid., 12:2). The kidneys advise and counsel (Psalms 16:7; *Genesis Rabbah* 61:1; *Ecclesiastes Rabbah* 7:19; *Berachot* 61b). [*See also* URINE, URINATION, and BLADDER]

KING HEZEKIAH'S BOOK OF REMEDIES—King Hezekiah of Judah, descendant of King David of Israel, reigned for twenty-nine years in Jerusalem (2 Kings 189:2ff.). He was considered to have been completely righteous to the point that God wished to appoint him as the Messiah (*Sanhedrin* 94a). To Hezekiah and his school is attributed the writing of the books of Isaiah, Proverbs, Song of Songs, and Ecclesiastes (*Baba Batra* 15a). God afforded personal protection to Hezekiah because of his righteousness (*Genesis Rabbah* 87:4). Six virtues are recorded of Hezekiah: He is called wonderful, counselor, prince, mighty, everlasting father, and prince of peace (Isaiah 9:5; *Ruth Rabbah* 7:2). Through prayer, Hezekiah turned Sennacherib's sweeping victory into complete defeat (2 Kings 18:9–13 and 19:14ff.). Hezekiah and his companions recited *Hallel* (Praise to God) when Sennacherib attacked them, and the Holy Spirit responded (*Pesachim* 117a).

One of the most famous talmudic passages concerning King Hezekiah describes six acts that he performed without the prior consent of the sages, three of which they approved and three of which they disapproved (*Pesachim* 56a; *Berachot* 10b). One of the acts that met with the sages' approval was his concealment of "The Book of Remedies." What was "The Book of Remedies" and why did Hezekiah conceal it? Many famous rabbis ascribe the authorship of "The Book of Remedies" to King Solomon. Among them are Rashi (1 Kings 5:13), Nachmanides (introduction to the book of Genesis), Radak (2 Kings 20:4), Rashba (Responsa 1:413), and Yaakov Emden (*Iggeret Bikkoret* p. 26a). Some believe an anonymous writer composed "The Book of Remedies" and others

attribute its authorship to the Sons of Noah.[1]

In his commentary on *Pesachim* 56a, Rashi states that Hezekiah concealed "The Book of Remedies" because people "were not humbled by their illnesses but were healed immediately." In *Berachot* 10b, Rashi states "so that people plead for mercy [from God] to be healed." In other words, Hezekiah hid "The Book of Remedies" because people were cured so quickly and effortlessly that illness failed to promote a feeling of contrition and humility and a recognition that God is the true Healer of the sick. Others, such as Rashba, support Rashi's view.

Maimonides, on the other hand, gives two reasons why Hezekiah concealed "The Book of Remedies" and refutes the reason given by Rashi. Maimonides states that the book contained remedies based on astrological phenomena and magical incantations that might lead people to use them for idolatrous purposes (*Guide for the Perplexed* 3:37); hence, Hezekiah concealed it. Secondly, Maimonides states that the book contained prescriptions for the preparation of poisons and their antidotes. When corrupt people used this information to kill their enemies by poisoning, Hezekiah concealed the book. Then Maimonides cites but strongly refutes the interpretation of Rashi by asserting that just as a person thanks God for the bread

He gives to cure his hunger, so too he thanks God for the remedies He gives to cure his illness.

Tosafot Yom Tov, in his Mishnaic commentary, states that since "The Book of Remedies" was apparently widely accepted among the Jews until Hezekiah concealed it, it seems logical to assume that it was probably written by sages of Israel. Why therefore, asks Tosafot Yom Tov, does Maimonides assume that it was written by astrologers? Furthermore, if it was an astrological work, Hezekiah should have burned it. The latter question is answered by Tiferet Yisrael, who explains that Hezekiah did not burn it so that it could still be used in a situation of grave danger. Rashba (Responsa 1:413) states that the fact that the book was only concealed and not burned shows us clearly that its contents were not contrary to religion. Tiferet Yisrael also gives his interpretation for the concealment of "The Book of Remedies," viz., in it were written amulets with astrological figures and planets. In order to prevent these from being used for idolatry, Hezekiah hid the book.

Zimmels concludes that there are five interpretations concerning the contents of "The Book of Remedies":[2] a) various natural remedies (Rashi, Rashba, and others); b) exorcisms and incantations (Josephus, *Antiquities* 8: 25); c) astrological images (Maimonides); d) antidotes for drugs (Mai-

monides); e) various remedies, among them those of occult virtue (Nachmanides and Emden).

Finally, there are three basic reasons offered as to why Hezekiah hid "The Book of Remedies." Rashi states that people lost their faith in God the Healer because they were speedily healed by taking the remedies cited in the book. Rashba, Maharsha (*Berachot* 10b), and others agree with Rashi. Maimonides asserts that Hezekiah hid it either because it was an astrological work whose use bordered on idolatry, or because corrupt people referred to it to concoct poisons to kill their enemies. It is not clear whether Hezekiah concealed the book prior to his own famous illness (vide infra) and, if not, whether he considered using it to cure himself.

---

1. F. Rosner, "The Illness of King Hezekiah and His 'Book of Remedies.'" in *Medicine in the Bible and the Talmud*, 2nd ed. (Hoboken, NJ: Ktav and Yeshiva University Press, 1995), pp. 79–89.
2. H.J. Zimmels, *Magicians, Theologians, and Doctors* (London: Goldston & Son, 1952), pp. 179–180.

KING HEZEKIAH'S ILLNESS—

King Hezekiah's serious illness, his prayer to God, the Divine promise of a prolongation of his life, and Hezekiah's thanksgiving (Isaiah 38:1ff.; 2 Kings 20:1ff.; 2 Chronicles 32:24ff.) are described in detail in the Talmud

(*Berachot* 10a). Hezekiah was afflicted with a deathly illness as punishment for the fact that he remained unmarried. Hezekiah protested when he was punished (*Semachot* 47a). He made excuses for himself by saying that he foresaw that the children that would be his offspring would be wicked. Naturally, this excuse was not considered valid since very person must first fulfill his obligation of procreation and leave the rest in the hands of God. Hezekiah's prayer to God for healing was answered (*Leviticus Rabbah* 10:5).

Another source (*Deuteronomy Rabbah* 1:13) explains why fifteen years were added to Hezekiah's life when he recovered from his illness. The sages of the Talmud (*Yebamot* 50a) are in disagreement as to whether the fifteen years were originally allotted to him at his birth and then curtailed at his illness, or whether the fifteen years were in fact added to his life. Maimonides, in a responsum on longevity, uses the story of Hezekiah's illness, among other things, to prove that the length of one's life is not necessarily predetermined and that one can extend the duration of one's life by prayer and the like.[1]

The nature of Hezekiah's illness is not clear, although most scholars assume that it was leprosy. Other suggestions include an abscess, a throat abscess, pestilence, plague, syphilis, carbuncle, tonsillitis, and influenza.[2] According to the Midrash (*Genesis Rabbah* 65:9 and 97), Hezekiah suffered from more than one illness. Whatever the nature of Hezekiah's illness, he was cured by Divine intervention after he prayed for mercy—and not only was he cured but fifteen years were added to his life.[3]

---

1. F. Rosner, "Moses Maimonides' Responsum on Longevity," *Geriatrics*, 23 (1968):170–178.
2. F. Rosner (trans.), *Julius Preuss' Biblical and Talmudic Medicine* (Northvale, NJ: Jason Aronson, 1993), pp. 341–342.
3. F. Rosner, "The Illness of King Hezekiah and His 'Book of Remedies,'" in *Medicine in the Bible and the Talmud*, 2nd ed. (Hoboken, NJ: Ktav and Yeshiva University Press, 1995), pp. 79–89.

KISSING—In the biblical narrative, Jacob kissed his grandsons (Genesis 48:10). Joseph fell upon his deceased father's body and kissed him (Genesis 50:1), implying that Joseph never kissed his father Jacob during his lifetime (*Kallah Rabbati* 3:19). Laban kissed his nephew Jacob (Genesis 29:13) because he thought that Jacob was carrying precious gems in his mouth (*Genesis Rabbah* 70:13). He also kissed his children (Genesis 13:55). Moses kissed Jethro (Exodus 18:7). The king kissed Absalom (2 Samuel 14:33) and Barzilai (ibid., 19:40). Esau kissed his brother Jacob when they met (Genesis 33:4). Moses and Aaron kissed each other in the wilderness (Exodus

4:27) because they rejoiced at each other's greatness (*Exodus Rabbah* 5:10). Samuel kissed Saul after he anointed him king (1 Samuel 10:1). Orpah kissed her mother-in-law Naomi when she bade her farewell (Ruth 1:14). Jacob kissed Rachel (Genesis 29:11) because she was a blood relative. These kissings are in part explained in the homiletical literature (*Genesis Rabbah* 7:12; *Exodus Rabbah* 5:1; *Ruth Rabbah* 2:21), which asserts that all kissing is indecent except in three cases: the kiss of high office (Saul and Samuel), the kiss of reunion after separation (Aaron and Moses), and the kiss of parting (Ruth and Orpah). Some add: also the kiss of kinship (Jacob and Rachel).

Kissing is usually on the mouth (Genesis 21:40). Samuel kissed Chanan bar Abba on his mouth (*Jerushalmi Berachot* 1:3). Ulla used to kiss his sisters on the hand (*Abodah Zarah* 17a). The Medes kiss only on the hand and not on the mouth (*Genesis Rabbah* 74:2; *Berachot* 8b). A man kissed Rabbi Yochanan's foot out of respect (*Ketubot* 49b). Rabbi Akiba's wife kissed his feet when he returned after twenty-four years of Torah study (*Ketubot* 63a). Rabbi Chama kissed Rabbi Papi's feet out of thanks (*Sanhedrin* 27b). Kissing idols is prohibited (*Sanhedrin* 60b). The divine kiss of death is the easiest form of death and is like drawing a hair out of milk (*Berachot* 8a). This is how Moses died (*Baba Batra* 17a).

KNEE—The knees, or *birkayim*, are bent in prayer before the Lord (Isaiah 45:23). Daniel kneeled three times daily in prayer (Daniel 6:11). One also bends the knees to drink water at rivers (Judges 7:6). Knees weaken when one is fearful (Ezekiel 7:17). The knees knock together when the Lord's judgment is near (Nachum 2:11). The Lord, however, firms up feeble knees (Isaiah 35:3). Babes are dandled on their mothers' knees (Isaiah 66:12). Delilah made Samson sleep on her knees (Judges 16:19). Both the human and animal knee is known as *arkuba* (Daniel 5:6; *Yebamot* 12:1). An animal knee has an upper posterior curving part and a lower anterior curving part (*Chullin* 76a). The human knee is like the ankle joint of ruminants but the animal knee joint is located very high up. The human *arkuba* has only bones and sinews but no flesh (*Chullin* 128b). The knee is said to be comprised of five bones (*Oholot* 1:8), two on each side and the knee cap in the middle (*Tosefta Oholot* 1:6). Among the abnormalities that disqualify a priest from serving in the Temple are *kashan* and *kishan*, which are *genu varum* (bowleg) and *genu valgum* (knock-knee). His knees knock together when he walks (*Bechorot* 7:6). Also disqualified is an *iklan*, "whose knees do not touch when the soles of the feet are placed together" (ibid.). Knee bands were worn by certain people (*Shabbat*

63a). [*See also* LEG, ANKLE, THIGH, and TOES]

KORDIAKOS—The Talmud discusses the case of a man suffering from *kordiakos* who asks that a bill of divorce be written for his wife (*Gittin* 7:1). The talmudic sage Samuel interprets *kordiakos* as "being overcome by new wine from the vat" (*Gittin* 67b). Most of the commentaries on the Talmud state that *kordiakos* is an alcohol-induced confusion of the mind. Rashi states that *kordiakos* is the name of the demon that rules in a person who drinks much wine from the vat. Maimonides, himself a physician, says that *kordiakos* is "an illness that occurs as a result of filling of the chambers of the brain, and the mind becomes confused therefrom; it is one of the varieties of falling sickness [i.e., epilepsy]." Bertinoro affirms that the individual afflicted with *kordiakos* is one whose mind is confused because of the demon that reigns in someone who drinks new wine. Tosafot Yom Tov states that the demon is called *kordiakos*. Tiferet Yisrael considers *kordiakos* to be an illness in which the intellect of the person is confused. The same occurs in someone who is "drunk like Lot" (see Genesis 19:31–38). Other commentaries on the aforementioned talmudic passage, including *Tosafot Rid* and *Shiltei Gibborim*, also state that *kor-*

diakos is a bad spirit that prevails over a person who drinks wine from the vat. Such a person is confused, his mind is not clear, and he does not have an intact intellect.

Elsewhere in the Talmud (*Gittin* 70b), Resh Lakish compares a man with *kordiakos* to one who is asleep, whereas Rabbi Yochanan compares him to a madman. Resh Lakish does not put a man with *kordiakos* on the same footing as a madman because for the latter there is no cure, whereas an individual with *kordiakos* can be treated with red flesh broiled on the coals and diluted wine (ibid., 67b). Rabbi Yochanan does not compare him to one who is asleep because a sleeper needs no therapy, whereas a person with *kordiakos* does.

The Jerusalem Talmud also discusses *kordiakos* (*Gittin* 1:1; *Terumot* 1:1) and categorically states that *kordiakos* does not mean folly or idiocy. Both Babylonian and Jerusalem Talmuds describe *kordiakos* as a syndrome characterized by confusion, dizziness, and mental incompetence following imbibition of wine from a new vat of wine. The syndrome is temporary and reversible with specific therapy of red meat and dilute wine.[1]

---

1. F. Rosner, "*Kordiakos*," in *Medicine in the Bible and the Talmud*, 2nd ed. (Hoboken, NJ: Ktav and Yeshiva University Press, 1995), pp. 60–64.

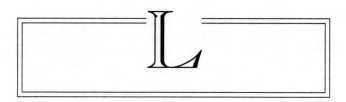

LACTATION—Woman's milk is the main nourishment of infants (*Shabbat* 143b). Cows are sold for the sake of their milk (*Baba Batra* 78b). Cow's milk is used to nourish infants and adults (ibid.). A blind child knows its mother by the smell and the taste of the milk (*Ketubot* 62a). Although a cow desires to suckle more than a calf wishes to suck (*Pesachim* 112a), no dam gives suck to a strange animal unless it has a child of its own (*Bechorot* 24a). Adults also drink human milk (*Keritot* 22a) but this practice is frowned upon. The origin of breast milk in a nursing woman, according to Rabbi Meir, is the decomposition of menstrual blood, which turns into milk (*Bechorot* 6b; *Niddah* 9a); that is why a nursing woman does not menstruate. The same occurs in nursing animals. According to other talmudic sages, the amenorrhea in a nursing woman is due to the pain of parturition and the breast milk is formed directly from blood (*Bechorot* 20b). A woman's milk is formed in globules when it is discharged from the breast and, contrary to spittle, cannot be reabsorbed (*Niddah* 56a). Milk of a clean (i.e., kosher) animal is white and that of an unclean animal is greenish in color (*Abodah Zarah* 35b). The milk of a clean animal, other than the whey, curdles—but the milk of unclean animals does not curdle (ibid.). One may milk an animal for healing purposes (*Machshirin* 6:8).

A nursing woman normally suckles her child for twenty-four months but sometimes for four or five years (*Ketubot* 60a; *Niddah* 9a). A woman is obligated to her husband to suckle her child (*Ketubot* 59b). A nursing mother whose husband died within eighteen or twenty-four months of the birth of their child should not remarry until the completion of the eighteen or twenty-four months (*Ketubot* 60a and 60b). Were she to marry sooner and become pregnant, the child would be prematurely taken from her breast. Nursing mother's milk deteriorates only after three months following conception (ibid.). A mother may bend over on the Sabbath and nurse a child born eight months after conception even if the child is nonviable because of the danger to the child who might otherwise die of starvation before his time and to the mother who may become ill due to accumulation of superfluous milk in her breasts (*Yeba-mot* 80a).

Although the milk of an unclean breast is for adults forbidden in the Pentateuch (*Bechorot* 6b), an Israelite child may be regularly breast-fed by an idolatress or an unclean breast. He may be suckled even on the Sabbath (*Yebamot* 114a) because his life would otherwise be endangered.

If a woman is given a child to suckle, she should not suckle together with it either her own child or the child of any friend of hers. While in charge of the child she must not eat things injurious for her milk (*Ketubot* 60b). The Talmud then describes what foods are injurious to a nursing woman. On the other hand, wine is said to be beneficial for lactation (*Ketubot* 65b).

For a more detailed presentation of lactation and suckling, wet nurses, infant nursing from an animal or bottle, and related topics and for precise bibliographic citations, the interested reader is referred to Preuss' book. [*See also* MILK]

1. F. Rosner (trans.), *Julius Preuss' Biblical and Talmudic Medicine* (Northvale, NJ: Jason Aronson, 1993); pp. 404–410.

LACTATION IN MALES—Lactation in males (galactorrhea) is de-scribed in the Talmud, which discusses "the milk of a male" (*Chullin* 113b) and asserts that such milk is ritually clean (*Machshirin* 6:7). A case is described in which it once happened that a man's wife died and left a child to be suckled and he could not afford to pay a wet nurse, whereupon a miracle was performed for him and his teats opened like the two teats of a woman and he suckled his son (*Shabbat* 53b). This man certainly had galactorrhea, albeit by Divine intervention.

The Midrash states (*Esther Rabbah* 6:5) that Mordechai raised his niece Esther because when her mother was pregnant her father died and soon after her birth her mother also died (*Megillah* 13a). Elsewhere, the Midrash asks:

> Did Mordechai actually feed and sustain Esther? Said Rabbi Judan: On one occasion he went round to all the wet nurses but could not find one for Esther, whereupon he himself suckled her. Rabbi Berachiah and Rabbi Abbahu in Rabbi Eleazar's name said: Milk came to him and he suckled her [always, and he never sought a wet nurse]. When Rabbi Abbahu taught this publicly, the congregation laughed. Said he to them: Yet is it not a Mishnah? [*Machshirin* 6:7, "The milk of a male is clean."] (*Genesis Rabbah* 30:8)

Another Midrash is of the opinion that the wife of Mordechai suckled Esther and that he himself was only the male nurse (Midrash Psalms 22:23).

LAMBS—A lamb with a hole in its windpipe can be cured by the insertion of a reed tube to close the hole (*Chullin* 57b). This seems to be the earliest description of a tracheotomy in Semitic sources.[1] A lamb with a double ear is considered to be blemished and may not be offered in the Temple (*Bechorot* 6:9). After childbirth, a woman brought a lamb and a pigeon as offerings in the Temple (Leviticus 12:1–8). When a lamb is born, its lips appear first in the vulva (*Bechorot* 35a). Sperm-producing "threads" are visible in the testicles of lambs prior to the thirtieth day of life (*Chullin* 93b). The marrow of a lamb's thighbone is considered to be a delicacy (*Tosefta Pesachim* 4:10).

Unprotected lambs are devoured by wolves (*Exodus Rabbah* 5:21). Lambs in the meadows outside town are not brought home every evening into town (*Pesachim* 47b). The Talmud describes young lambs (*Sanhedrin* 11a), stuffed lambs (*Pesachim* 74b), and cells in which lambs were kept (*Yoma* 15b; *Arachin* 13a). The sages argue whether or not lambs are better than goats (*Pesachim* 57a–b). Both are suitable for the paschal offering (*Pesachim* 69b) and are roasted for that purpose (*Horayot* 10b). Lambs can be carried on one's shoulders (*Pesachim* 69b).

LAMENESS—Legend relates that when Noah emerged from the Ark, a lion pushed him so that he limped (*Leviticus Rabbah* 20:1). The same happened to a Pharaoh when he sat on Solomon's throne (*Ecclesiastes Rabbah* 9:2). When Jacob wrestled with the angel (Genesis 32:32), he became lame or "bent on one side" like Levi bar Sisi (*Taanit* 25a). Jonathan's son Mephiboshet fell and became lame (2 Samuel 4:4) in both feet (ibid., 9:13). Because of his lameness, he could not saddle his ass (ibid., 19:27). Balaam was lame in one foot and Samson in both feet (*Sotah* 10a). Stuttering and stammering are considered "lameness of the tongue" (Micah 4:6; Zephaniah 3:19). When the Jews stood at Mount Sinai, there were no lame among them (*Song of Songs Rabbah* 4:7:1). When the Messiah comes, even the lame will be cured (Isaiah 33:23). In the future world, God will heal the lame (*Genesis Rabbah* 95:1; Isaiah 35:6).

A lame priest cannot serve in the Temple (Leviticus 21:18). A lame animal may not be offered as a sacrifice (Malachi 1:8). A lame shepherd cannot run after his goats (*Shabbat* 32a). A lame person usually becomes a watchman (*Tosefta Baba Kamma* 9:2). A person lame in one leg is exempt from making the required pilgrimages to Jerusalem on the three festivals (*Chagigah* 3a). The ceremony of the suspected adulteress is not carried out if she or her husband is lame (*Numbers Rabbah* 9:4:2).

---

1. F. Rosner (trans.), *Julius Preuss' Biblical and Talmudic Medicine* (Northvale, NJ: Jason Aronson, 1993), p. 211.

Lameness is caused by unnatural cohabitation (*Nedarim* 20a). One should accept lameness as a divine decree (*Berachot* 58b). He who feigns lameness will eventually become lame (*Peah* 8:9). A lame child may or may not eventually be able to walk (*Chagigah* 6a). A great tall and lame man lectured in Nehardea (*Shabbat* 59b). A lame man once participated in a Roman festival (*Abodah Zara* 11b). [*See also* PARALYSIS]

LEECHES—It is forbidden to drink water from rivers or pools directly with one's mouth for fear of swallowing a leech (*Abodah Zarah* 12b), which may then cause swelling of the abdomen (*Bechorot* 44b). If a person swallows a leech, he should drink vinegar (*Abodah Zarah* 12b) or use the *pishpash* bug, which is a remedy against leeches (*Jerushalmi Berachot* 9:13). [*See also* BLOODLETTING and CUPPING]

LEEKS—Garden grown leeks and field (i.e., wild) leeks (*Kilayim* 1:2; *Uktzin* 3:2) serve as food for humans and animals (*Sheviit* 7:1) and are stored in warehouses (*Abodah Zarah* 40b). Leeks are tied in bundles both for private use and for sale in the market (*Sheviit* 8:3). Leeks are classified as a vegetable related to garlic and onions (*Nedarim* 58b), with which they can be pickled (*Terumot* 10:10). Shredded leek placed inside a fish is a tasty dish (*Betzah* 17b). Syrian leek (*Chullin* 97b), added to fish (*Jerushalmi Betzah* 2:61), can be served with poppy and plums (*Jerushalmi Berachot* 6:10). Leeks from Geba in Samaria are also mentioned in the Talmud (*Kelim* 17:5). The sharpness of radishes is neutralized by leeks (*Pesachim* 116a). Onions and leeks impart their strong flavor in a vegetable stew (*Chullin* 97b). Leek roots and top parts are described (*Uktzin* 1:2). One should begin to eat leeks from their leaves and not the top side (*Betzah* 25b). Leeks should be eaten on Rosh Hashanah as a symbol of prosperity and fertility (*Horayot* 12a; *Keritot* 6a). The Jews in the desert missed the leeks they ate in Egypt (Numbers 11:5).

Therapeutically, leek consumption is recommended for patients with chronic fever (*Gittin* 67b) and jaundice (*Shabbat* 109b–110a). Mashed leeks are part of a remedy for lung bleeding (*Gittin* 69). Cut leek and chicken meat serves as an antidote for snake bites (*Tosefta Shabbat* 15:14). Leek juice is part of a remedy for *tzemirta* (bladder stones?) (*Gittin* 69b). Leek is also said to be good for the intestines but bad for the teeth (*Berachot* 44b). Therefore, it should be swallowed without chewing. Spittle formed by chewing leek is like molten lead (*Taanit* 27b), meaning that it produces heartburn if swallowed.

LEG—The word *regel* refers both to the foot and the leg (*Yebamot* 103a). Foot-driven machines were used to water the land (Deuteronomy 11:10). Feet lead a person to places that he chooses (*Sukkah* 53a). A person is master over his mouth, his hands, and his feet (*Genesis Rabbah* 67:3). Hillel was once asked to teach a man the entire Torah while standing on one foot (*Shabbat* 31a). God protects man from dashing his foot against a stone (Psalms 91:12). The Israelites find no resting place for the soles of their feet among the nations (Deuteronomy 28:65). Delicate women do not walk on their feet but are carried (ibid., 28:56). To stamp with one's feet or to walk on one's toes is a sign of haughtiness (*Derech Eretz Rabbah* 2:8). The heel is called *ekev* (Genesis 26:26). The lower legs below the knee are called *keraayim* (Leviticus 11:21) and the shinbone is called the *lechta* of the lower leg (*Yebamot* 103a). Legs are also known as *shokayim* and allegorically called "pillars of marble" (Song of Songs 5:15). Prostitutes uncover their legs (Isaiah 47:2; *Berachot* 24a). God does not take pleasure in the legs of people but rather in them that fear Him (Psalms 147:10–11).

The foot has thirty bones, the lower leg has two, and the upper leg has one (*Oholot* 1:8). Nahum's legs were mutilated (*Taanit* 21a). King Asa suffered from gout in his feet (1 Kings 15:23). Surgical treatment of foot wounds is described (*Abodah Zarah* 10b) as are amputations of the toes (Judges 1:6–7) and feet (2 Samuel 4:12). A variety of foot and leg abnormalities disqualify a priest from serving in the Temple (*Bechorot* 159). Flat-footed people live in watery marshes (*Shabbat* 31a). Broken legs are placed in plaster (*Exodus Rabbah* 27:9) or set by manipulation (*Shabbat* 22:6). A diseased leg afflicted with leprosy may become gangrenous (*Kiddushin* 30b; *Keritot* 3:8). A leg deformity may make a man walk on the upper side of his foot (*Yebamot* 103a). A bunion on the sole of the foot is called *tzinit* and is treated by the application of a hard, rough coin (*Shabbat* 65a). The soles of the feet are hard and therefore not considered as skin (*Negaim* 6:8).

If one intentionally breaks a person's leg, even at his request, one must pay restitution (*Baba Kamma* 8:7). So, too, one is liable for damage caused by one's foot or one's ox's foot (*Baba Kamma* 3a). Amputees wore wooden legs (*Chagigah* 4a) or artificial shoes or feet (*Shabbat* 65b; *Yoma* 78b; *Yebamot* 103a) with inner padding or a stool to help in locomotion (ibib.). Such prostheses were made by hollowing out logs of wood (*Shabbat* 11b). Leg guards made of leather were also used (*Kelim* 26:3). [*See* AMPUTEE and PROSTHESES]

Foot washing is described in the Bible in relation to Abraham (Genesis 18:4), Lot (ibid., 19:2), the Egyptians (ibid., 24:32), and the Gibeonites (Judges 19:21). One also washes the feet upon returning from a journey (2 Samuel 11:8) and every evening before retiring (Song of Songs 5:3).

Domestic footstools (*Kelim* 16:1) with three or four legs (ibid., 22:3) are used as a footrest (*Chagigah* 14a; *Sanhedrin* 38b). Footstools for a throne are built either before (*Chagigah* 12a) or after the throne (Leviticus Rabbah 36:1). [*See also* ANKLE, THIGH, KNEE, and TOES]

LENTILS—Jacob gave Esau bread and lentil pottage (Genesis 25:34). Beans and lentils are nutritionally beneficial (2 Samuel 17:29; Ezekiel 4:9). Healthy people eat lentils (*Jerushalmi Baba Kamma* 8:6). Raw and fully cooked lentils are edible; partially cooked ones are not (*Betzah* 26b). Farmers are happy if the lentil crop is successful (*Pesachim* 3b). Lentils represent a cheap food (*Yebamot* 118b; *Ketubot* 67b). Lentils can be made into groats (*Chullin* 6a) or into bread (Ezekiel 4:9; *Eruvin* 81a). Lentil brew is a popular drink (*Abodah Zarah* 38b). Lentils are boiled together with their shells (*Shabbat* 76b). One blows on them to test their quality (*Machshirin* 1:6). Since lentils are plucked, sandy matter or refuse comes with them (*Baba Batra* 94a). Water poured over a bowl of lentils separates the refuse on top from the edible part that remains below (*Betzah* 14b).

Therapeutically, lentils have aphrodisiac properties (*Yoma* 18a). They prevent a person from developing *askara* (diphtheria?), which is a disease that kills by asphyxiation (*Berachot* 40a). Lentil cakes and vinegar is a remedy for the febrile illness *achilu* (*Gittin* 70a). Lentils are part of a compound remedy for mouth abscesses (*Gittin* 69a) and for lung bleeding (ibid.). On the other hand, the daily consumption of lentils can lead to a bad mouth odor (*Berachot* 40a). The therapeutic benefits of lentils are also described by Galen, Dioscorides, Pliny, Aretaus, and Hippocrates.[1]

Eating lentils is a custom of mourning among Jews (*Genesis Rabbah* 63:14; *Baba Batra* 16b). The minimum size of a reptile that ritually defiles is the size of a lentil (*Shabbat* 27a, 28a, 83b, and 93b; *Betzah* 19a; *Chagigah* 11a; *Chullin* 128b; *Meilah* 16b; *Niddah* 43b; *Oholot* 1:7). The Egyptian lentil is intermediate in size (*Kelim* 17:8). In an animal, an ear perforation as large as a lentil is considered a blemish (*Bechorot* 37b). A fetus membrum, when sex becomes distinguishable, is the size of a lentil (*Niddah* 25a).

1. F. Rosner (trans.), *Julius Preuss' Biblical and Talmudic Medicine* (Northvale, NJ: Jason Aronson, 1993, p. 158.

LESBIANISM—Lesbianism as such is not mentioned in the Bible but is considered as an Egyptian practice that should not be followed (Leviticus 18:3). "Women committing immorality with women" (*Niddah* 42b) refers to lesbianism. Queen Vashti refused to come to King Ahasuerus (Esther 1:12) because she had an immoral purpose in mind, perhaps lesbianism (*Megillah* 12b). Rav Huna considers lesbians to be prostitutes and, hence, forbidden to marry priests (*Shabbat* 65a). Other rabbis consider lesbianism only as obscene but without legal consequences (*Yebamot* 76a). Samuel's father forbade his daughters from sleeping together, to prevent lewdness (*Shabbat* 65a–b). [*See also* HOMOSEXUALITY, BESTIALITY, and RAPE]

LETTUCE—Lettuce is sweet except for the stalk, which is bitter (*Genesis Rabbah* 95). Lettuce can serve as the bitter herb at the Passover seder (*Pesachim* 39a), where it is dipped in salt water before being consumed (ibid., 14a). The white leaves of lettuce are not eaten but protect the edible part (*Uktzin* 2:7). Both garden lettuce and wild lettuce (*Kilayim* 1:2) can be pickled (*Lamentations Rabbah* 1:1:14). Lettuce aids in the digestion of food (*Abodah Zarah* 11a). Lettuce was never lacking on the table of Rabbi Judah the Prince (*Berachot* 57b; *Abodah Zarah* 11a). The emperor sent him leeks and he sent lettuce in return (*Abodah Zarah* 10b).

LICE—One of the biblical plagues was lice (Exodus 8:12). The affliction on the crown of the head described by the prophet (Isaiah 3:17) is said to refer to swarms of lice (*Lamentations Rabbah* 4:15:18). For bladder calculi, lice were placed into the urethral opening (*Gittin* 69b). The use of lice to treat urinary retention in the nineteenth century is described by Preuss.[1] [*See also* WORMS]

---

1. F. Rosner (trans.), *Julius Preuss' Biblical and Talmudic* Medicine (Northvale, NJ: Jason Aronson, 1993), p. 229.

LIFE—Life is sacred and of infinite value. He who saves a life is as if he saves a whole world (*Sanhedrin* 37a). To save a life, all biblical and rabbinic laws are waived (*Yebamot* 114a; *Yoma* 83a; *Eruvin* 44b; *Ketubot* 5a and 15b) except for the cardinal three: idolatry, murder, and forbidden sexual relationships such as incest and adultery (*Ketubot* 19a; *Abodah Zarah* 27b). There are precedences in the saving of lives when all cannot be saved (*Horayot* 13a; *Numbers Rabbah* 6:1). "The treasures of life" (*Chagigah* 12b) refers to the fountain of life (Psalms 36:10). The necessities for life include wines, oils, and various kinds of flour (*Baba Batra* 91a). The seat of life is the nose (i.e., respiration) (*Ecclesiastes Rabbah* 12:2) as stated in the Bible (Genesis 7:22). The seat of intrauterine life is the navel, from which the embryo develops (*Sotah* 45b). The stages of life are depicted (*Ecclesiastes Rabbah* 1:2:1).

The transitory nature of life is described as follows: Life is like a bird that flies past and its shadow passes with it. Life is like a shadow cast by a wall or a date palm (*Genesis Rabbah* 96:2; *Ecclesiastes Rabbah* 1:2:1 and 6: 12:1). The phrase "a time to be born and a time to die" (Ecclesiastes 3:2) has many interpretations (*Ecclesiastes Rabbah* 3:1:1ff.). Life is compared to a store where credit can be obtained but dues must be paid to collectors (*Avot* 3:16). One forfeits one's life as expiation for futile thought (*Avot* 3:4), for breaking off one's Torah study (ibid., 3:7), or for forgetting it (ibid., 3:8). The futility of life (*Eruvin* 13b) and temporal and eternal life (*Shabbat* 33b) are discussed. The life of the over-compassionate, the hot tempered, and the too fastidious is miserable (*Pesachim* 113b). So, too, hut dwellers and desert travelers lead a miserable life (*Eruvin* 55b). Life can be extended by good behavior [*see* LONGEVITY and OLD AGE]. It can also be shortened by bad behavior (*Avot* 2:11 and 3:10; *Berachot* 55a).

LIONS—The lion is the king of the wild animals (*Chagigah* 13b; *Song of Songs Rabbah* 3:10:4). Some kings are likened to lions (*Sanhedrin* 94b). King Darius threw Daniel into a den of lions (Daniel 6:19) and he survived.

Ordinarily, a man who falls into a den of lions and is not seen again is presumed to be dead (*Berachot* 33a; *Yebamot* 121a). The lion has six names (*Sanhedrin* 95a): *ari* (Genesis 49:9), *kefir* (Judges 14:5), *lavi* (Genesis 49:9), *laish* (Isaiah 30:6), *schachal* (Psalms 91:13), and *schachaz* (Job 28:8). The roar of pain of a fiery lion's whelp when it lost a hair was heard for miles (*Sanhedrin* 64a). A lion's roar can make a person's teeth fall out from fright (*Chullin* 59b). Woe is to a person who throws his garment between a lion and a lioness when they are copulating (*Sanhedrin* 106a).

A lion tears its prey and devours it (*Pesachim* 49b; *Taanit* 8a; *Sanhedrin* 90b). This includes asses that were fed to the lions (*Menachot* 103b). Most lions attack with their claws (*Chullin* 53a). Lions injure the public (*Abodah Zarah* 16a) in that they may devour people (ibid., 26a). A lion usually does not attack two people together (*Shabbat* 15b). A man was once miraculously saved from a lion (*Berachot* 54a). A curse is to say to someone: "May a lion devour you" (*Eruvin* 53b) or your grandfather (*Ketubot* 72b).

Milk of a lioness can cure patients with consumption (tuberculosis?) (*Baba Kamma* 80a; Midrash Psalms 39:2). A lion's pregnancy is said to last three years (*Bechorot* 8a; *Genesis Rabbah* 20:4). In Noah's Ark, lions were nourished by fever (*Sanhedrin* 108b). When Noah left the Ark, a lion pushed him and maimed him (*Genesis Rabbah*

30:6 and 36:4; *Leviticus Rabbah* 20:1). One may see a lion in one's dreams (*Berachot* 56b). A famous proverb says that it is better to be a tail unto lions than a head unto foxes (*Avot* 4:15; *Sanhedrin* 37a). Another proverb says: Be strong as a lion to do the Lord's will (*Avot* 5:20).

LIPS—The lips are known as *sefatayim*. The upper border is called the red of the lip (*Tosefta Negaim* 2:13). Lovers say to each other "Thy lips are like a thread of scarlet" (Song of Songs 4:3) and "Your lips are like lilies" (ibid., 5:13; Job 27:4). Job vows that his lips will not speak evil (Job 27:4). A "man of lips" (Job 11:2) is one who boasts and "words of the lips" (2 Kings 18:20) refers to gossip. To have "uncircumcised lips" (Exodus 6:12) implies poor speech. The prophet's lips quivered (Habakkuk 3:16). The lips of a deceased scholar move gently in the grave if a teaching of his is discussed or reported in his name (*Yebamot* 97a), as is required in Jewish law (*Megillah* 15a). The lips of two famous talmudic sages trembled as one admired the extensive Torah knowledge of his colleague and the latter admired the other's keen intellect (*Eruvin* 67a).

A split lip (harelip) is cause for ridicule (*Baba Kamma* 117a). To "shoot out the lip" (Psalms 22:8) and to "split the lip" (*Derech Eretz* 2:1) means to scorn or ridicule someone. To "pucker the lips" (Proverbs 10:10) is to gesticulate with spite. "The lips of the aged are loose" (*Shabbat* 152a) means that the lower lip hangs loosely down. The meaning of the word *nib* (of the lips) (Isaiah 57:19) is uncertain. Spinning flax causes the lips to fissure (*Ketubot* 61b).

A priest whose upper lip protrudes over the lower lip is unfit to serve in the Temple (*Bechorot* 7:5). An animal whose lips are pierced, split, or otherwise injured is unfit to be offered in the Temple (*Bechorot* 6:4) because only blemish-free animals may be offered (Leviticus 22:20).

LIVER—The liver lies below the diaphragm (*Chullin* 46a) and is adjacent to the fifth rib (*Sanhedrin* 49a). Asahel and Abner's livers were pierced with spears (2 Samuel 2:23 and 3:27) through the fifth rib (*Sanhedrin* 49a). The left lobe of the liver is the caudate or "extra" lobe (Leviticus 3:4 and 3:15). One of the three major blood vessels (inferior vena cava?) connects the heart to the liver (*Chullin* 45b). If a needle enters the liver via the large vessel an animal can survive, but if it pierces the intestine the animal is not fit for human consumption (*Chullin* 48b).

The liver is the source of blood (*Bechorot* 55a). The liver exudes blood but does not absorb it (*Chullin* 110b). If it is dipped in vinegar or in boiling water, it no longer exudes blood (ibid., 11a). The seat of anger is in the liver

(*Exodus Rabbah* 9:8; *Leviticus Rabbah* 4:4; *Berachot* 61b). If a drop of gall falls into the liver, the anger is assuaged (*Berachot* 61b). The liver may also be the seat of love (Proverbs 7:23).

Liver flukes or worms may occur if one eats raw or fat meat or beef or certain cabbage seeds on an empty stomach and then drinks water. Various remedies are described (*Shabbat* 109b). A wormy liver is not necessarily dangerous (*Tosefta Chullin* 3:10). The normally red liver of an animal may be green (jaundice?) (*Chullin* 56b). An animal whose liver is gone can survive with only a small liver remnant (ibid., 46a). Hemoptysis from the lung can be cured but hematemesis due to liver disease cannot be cured (*Gittin* 69a). Eating liver can either help a patient overcome illness (*Berachot* 57b) or make it more severe (*Abodah Zarah* 29a).

If a man vows not to eat meat, he is forbidden to eat liver (*Nedarim* 54b). Homiletically, God made Pharaoh's heart hard like liver (*Exodus Rabbah* 13:3). The phrase "He looks at the liver" (Ezekiel 21:26) means to inspect the liver as a form of divination (*Lamentations Rabbah Proem*). [*See also* BILE, *YERAKON*, and GALL-BLADDER]

LOINS—The loins represent that part of the trunk where one wears a belt. To "gird one's loins" (2 Kings 4:29) means "to put on one's belt," often in preparation for a journey. It also means "to prepare for battle" (Job 38:3). Because of fright, the joints of the loins of a famous king loosened (Daniel 5:6). A scribe carries an ink horn on his belt or loins (Ezekiel 9:2). A mourner puts sackcloth on his loins (Genesis 37:34). Breeches extend from the loins to the thighs (Exodus 28:42). Pain in the loins makes one feel as if caught in a net (Psalms 66:11). Labor pains in parturient women include pain in the loins (Isaiah 21:3; Nahum 2:11). Pain in the loins was treated by rubbing oneself with wine and vinegar or with oil, especially rose oil (*Shabbat* 14:4). "To come forth from the loins" means "to sire children" (Genesis 35:11). Animals' strength resides in the loins (Job 40:16). The fat in the loins of animals is prohibited for human consumption (*Chullin* 45a and 93a).

LONGEVITY—Normal lifespan is seventy years—eighty if one is strong (Psalms 10:10). Before the deluge, people lived for hundreds of years (Genesis 5:1ff.). Men who lived very long indeed include Adam, Mesuthaleh, Shem, Jacob, Amram, Achiya the Shilonite, and Elijah (*Baba Batra* 121b). Abraham lived 175 years (Genesis 25:7) and Moses 120 years (Deuteronomy 34:7). One's lifespan is determined at birth. If one is worthy, one is allowed to complete the full period, or years may even be added to one's lifespan (*Yebamot* 50a; *Ecclesi-*

astes Rabbah 3:2:3). To engage in righteousness such as charity allows one to attain old age (*Genesis Rabbah* 59:1ff.). Life can be prolonged by Torah study (*Avot* 2:7 and 6:7; Proverbs 3:1–2 and 9:11), by cleaving to God and His commands (Deuteronomy 30:20), and by honoring one's parents (Exodus 20:12; Deuteronomy 5:16). One prolongs one's life by drawing out one's prayers, one's meals, and one's easing in a privy (*Berachot* 54b–55a). Longevity is achieved by not being impatient, by respect for scholars, by proper Torah study, by not rejoicing at one's friends' disgrace, by not calling one's neighbor by his nickname (*Taanit* 20b), by praying in a proper environment, by sanctifying the Sabbath (*Megillah* 27b), and by not using the synagogue for a shortcut (*Numbers Rabbah* 11:4).

Members of one family in Jerusalem died at eighteen years of age. Following advice from their rabbi, they studied Torah and lived much longer (*Rosh Hashanah* 18a). Although many sources say that longevity depends on merit (*Numbers Rabbah* 19:32; *Ecclesiastes Rabbah* 7:7:2), other sources say it depends not on merit but on destiny (*Shabbat* 156a; *Moed Katan* 28a). [*See also* LIFE and OLD AGE]

LUNGS—The lungs of an animal are called the wings (*Leviticus Rabbah* 18:1). Each wing or lung is divided into lobes. The right lung has three lobes and the left has two. Lobes are separated by indentations. The right lung of ruminants has a "rose lobe" or middle lobe (*Chullin* 46a and ff.). The lung has two membranes, the visceral and parietal pleura (ibid.). The lung absorbs liquids (*Berachot* 61b; *Leviticus Rabbah* 4:4). The voice emanates from the lungs (*Leviticus Rabbah* 18:1) but the larynx brings it out (*Berachot* 61a). Blood from the lungs (hemoptysis) is curable (*Gittin* 69a). Therapy for lung bleeding is a broth made of mangold, leeks, jujube berries, lentils, and cumin together with strong beer (ibid.).

A variety of diseases and defects of the lungs include perforation of both lung membranes (pneumothorax) (*Chullin* 46a), blisters (cysts) on the lungs (ibid., 46b), a hole in the lung (ibid., 48b), a fistulous communication between two adjacent bronchi (ibid.), a fibrous membrane on the lungs (ibid., 47b), obstruction or non-expansion of the lungs, pus in the lungs, lungs that look like liver or a block of wood (pneumonia) (ibid.), a needle in the lung, dried up or atrophic lung (ibid., 55b), a lung that is so dry that it crumbles (caseation) (ibid., 46b), and lobes that adhere to each other. The main vessel leading to the lung is either the trachea or the pulmonary artery (*Chullin* 45b). [*See also* WINDPIPE]

LUST—The serpent in the Garden of Eden infused Eve with lust (*Yebamot*

103b). Coveting a neighbor's wife is biblically forbidden (Exodus 20:14). Even a lustful or covetous look at a woman is reprehensible (*Berachot* 24a). One is forbidden to gaze lustfully even at a woman's small finger (*Shabbat* 64b). Jealousy, lust, and the desire for honor put a man out of the world (*Avot* 4:21). When one finds lust, an epidemic strikes and slays both good and bad people (*Genesis Rabbah* 36:5). Unmarried men of twenty years or older spend their life in lustful thoughts (*Yoma* 29a). Amnon, a son of King David, was lovesick for his stepsister and eventually raped her (2 Samuel 13:1ff.).

The kidneys are said to be the seat of sensation and lust (Proverbs 23:16). Because of yearning, Job's kidneys withered in him (Job 19:27). The lovesick shepherdess is depicted in the Bible (Song of Songs 2:5). Lust for cohabitation is called *chimud* (*Niddah* 20b). Jezebel painted pictures of harlots on her frigid husband's chariot to sexually arouse him (*Sanhedrin* 39b). Viewing animals copulate may excite sexual passions (*Yebamot* 76a). A man with a strong lust for a woman was not allowed by the sages to illicitly fulfill his desire, although physicians recommended this "sex therapy" to cure him

of his lovesickness (*Sanhedrin* 75a). A person who cannot control his sexual desire should go to a place where he is not known and dress in dark clothes, but not sin (*Moed Katan* 17a). One must struggle against carnal lusts and temptation as did Joseph when Potiphar's wife tried to seduce him (Genesis 39:12).

LUZ BONE—At the bottom of the spine is a bone resembling an almond (Ecclesiastes 12:5) called *luz* (coccyx). This bone is indestructible (ibid., *Leviticus Rabbah* 18:1). Only during the Flood when God intended to annihilate mankind (Genesis 6:7) did He destroy the *luz* bone (*Genesis Rabbah* 28:3). The Talmud also speaks about the small bone at the end of the spine (*Berachot* 28b). An in-depth analysis of the *luz* bone and the legends surrounding it is available.[1] The *luz* bone should not be confused with the city or district called Luz (Genesis 28:19; Judges 1:23; *Sukkah* 53a; *Sotah* 46b; *Sanhedrin* 12a).

1. E. Reichman and F. Rosner, "The Bone Called *Luz*," *Journal of the History of Medicine and Allied Sciences,* vol. 51 (1996), 52–65.

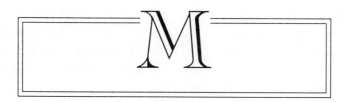

MAGIC—Magical incantations were recited to ward off the evil eye (*Berachot* 55b). Magical practices and necromancy are biblically prohibited (Deuteronomy 8:10–11) and are discussed in the Talmud (*Sanhedrin* 65b). Bewitched oil used for magical purposes is also described (*Sanhedrin* 101a). Women sometimes practiced magic with their hair (*Jerushalmi Sanhedrin* 7:26). A woman once used magic and witchcraft in order not to bear children. The Talmud identifies her as Yochani, daughter of Ratibi (*Sotah* 22a). A magical incantation against the demon of the lavatory is also mentioned (*Shabbat* 67a). Dropsy can be caused by magic (ibid., 33a).

Healing by magic supplements the literature on incantations and amulets as remedies. The efficacy of three knots to arrest an illness, five to heal it, and seven to help even against magic is described in the Talmud (*Shabbat* 66b). The nail from the gallows of an executed person is efficacious against the illness called *ababitha* (*Jerushalmi Shabbat* 6:8). In Jewish law, judges need to acquire a knowledge of magic in order to properly adjudicate a criminal case involving magic (*Sanhedrin* 17a). One who performs magic is liable to death (*Sanhedrin* 67a). Eliezer caused cucumbers to grow by magic (ibid., 68a). Demons, exorcism, and spells are also discussed in the Talmud (*Chullin* 105b; *Abodah Zarah* 38b). [*See also* ASTROLOGY, DEMONS, EXORCISM, EVIL EYE, INCANTATIONS, SORCERY]

MANDRAKES—One of the earliest references to the conception-promoting properties of mandrakes *(duda' im)* is the biblical narrative of Reuben and his mother Leah (Genesis 30:14) who did not give them to her sister Rachel when she asked for them, on the condition that Jacob cohabit with her, Leah, during that night. Jacob agreed and Leah bore Jacob a fifth son (Genesis 30:17) and later a sixth. According to Preuss,[1] the *duda' im* perhaps brought the favor of her husband back to Leah, for the one night that Rachel conceded to her must have been followed by many more, as the subsequent births demonstrate. The mandrakes, however, did not provide her with fertility, for she had never lost her ability to conceive. The correction of the infertility of Rachel as a result of the use of the *duda' im* is similarly difficult to accept. The fact that the pregnancies of both women resulted from the hearkening by God to their prayers cannot be used as evidence for or against the efficacy of the mandrakes, because according to religious interpretation, no medication is effective without God giving His blessing thereto—and, on the other hand, even God employs natural means to effect healing.

As a result, Preuss does not accept the exegetics of the hypothesis that *duda' im* represents a remedy against infertility. He is also not disconcerted by the biblical phrase "The mandrakes emit an aroma" (Song of Songs 7:14), for it is a long way from the efficacy of an aroma as a sexual excitant, an action that is undisputed since time immemorial, to the presupposed influence on the sterility of a woman.

Very difficult to understand is the botanical identification of *duda' im*. It is usually accepted that it is a plant that grows or blossoms or ripens "in the days of the wheat harvest." Most biblical commentators translate *duda' im* as "mandrakes." Rashi states that *duda' im* are a type of plant that in Arabic is called "Jasmin." Ibn Ezra asserts that *duda' im* have a good aroma, as it is written *"duda' im* give forth

fragrance" (Song of Songs 7:14). They resemble the human form for they have the likeness of a head and hands. Ibn Ezra concludes by saying that he does not know why they promote conception.

Hertz quotes the 1611 King James authorized version of the Bible where the word *duda' im* is translated "love apples." The fruit, continues Hertz, is of the size of a large plum, quite round, yellow, and full of soft pulp. The fruit is still considered in the East to be a love charm. This explains Rachel's anxiety to obtain it.

Nachmanides disputes Rashi's interpretation and states that Reuben only wanted his mother to benefit from the good aroma because she became pregnant with the help of God, not through medical means. Reuben brought his mother the leaves (i.e., the fruit) of the mandrake, which look like apples and are aromatic. He did not, however, bring the root, which has the likeness of a head and hands and which is said to promote conception. (If the latter is true, concludes Nachmanides, it happens as an unusual and unnatural occurrence that he, Nachmanides, a prominent physician, did not find mentioned in any medical text.)

Ba' al Haturim points out that the Hebrew word *duda' im* has the same numerical value as the Hebrew word *ke'adam*, "like man," i.e., it has human likeness. *Malbim* states that *duda' im* promote conception and that Reuben's intent was for his mother to have more sons since he did not wish to be an only son. Hirsch considers *duda' im* to be wild flowers. *Seforno* interprets *duda' im* to be aromatic plants that prepare the womb for the fetus. *Duda' im* or more potent aphrodisiacs were eaten, especially on Fridays, to increase the love between two young lovers.

In explaining the above biblical passage concerning mandrakes, the Talmud (*Sanhedrin* 99b) asks: What are *duda' im*? Rab said *yabruchi* (mandrakes); Levi said *sigli* (cypress); Rabbi Yonathan said *sabiski* (mandrake flowers). Rashi, in the Talmud, asserts that it is not clear what *yabruchi* is. *Sigli* and *sabiski* are other types of *yabruchi*. *Sigli* is a root of certain plants and it is a type of aromatic herb. The ancestry of these plants is called *sigli*. *Sabiski* is also a type of aromatic herb. *Torah Temimah* states that *yabruchi, sigli,* and *sabiski* are all types of flowers that emit good odors, as found elsewhere in the Talmud (*Berachot* 43b): "For *sigli* one recites the blessing: Who hast created aromatic plants." In the Midrash, there are two additional interpretations of *duda' im:* barley and fruits of *mayishim,* which are hackberries or myrtle berries (*Genesis Rabbah* 72:2).

In summary, the biblical term *duda' im* (Genesis 30:14) is interpreted by most classical commentaries to refer to an aromatic plant, probably the mandrake, whose root resembles human form with head, hands, and feet. It has the unusual property of promoting conception and its leaves

(i.e., fruits) resemble apples. [*See also* APHRODISIACS]

1. F. Rosner (trans.), *Julius Preuss' Biblical and Talmudic Medicine* (Northvale, NJ: Jason Aronson, 1993), p. 462.

MANGOLD—Mangold heals sick patients (*Berachot* 57b). Mangold is good for internal inflammation (*Gittin* 69b). Mangold juice heals a sore throat (*Berachot* 36a). Mangold broth is good for the stomach (or heart), for the eyes, and for the intestines (*Berachot* 39a). Eating mangold protected the Babylonians from developing *raatan* (leprosy?) (*Ketubot* 77b). A folk remedy is "radish against fever and mangold against cold" (*Abodah Zarah* 28b).

MANNA—Manna is the dew of heaven (Genesis 27:28; Exodus 16:13; *Genesis Rabbah* 66:3). It was given by God to the Israelites for forty years in the desert on the merit of Moses (*Megillah* 13a; *Taanit* 9a; *Leviticus Rabbah* 27:6; *Numbers Rabbah* 1:2) and ceased upon his death (*Genesis Rabbah* 62:4). God blessed the Sabbath (Genesis 2:3) with manna and hallowed it through manna (*Genesis Rabbah* 11:2). The Israelites found in the manna the taste of every kind of food (*Yoma* 75a). To young men it tasted like bread, to old men like honey wafers, to babies like mothers' milk, and to the sick like fine flour

mingled with honey (*Exodus Rabbah*
5:9; *Yoma* 75b; *Numbers Rabbah* 19:
22). The manna was ground for the
righteous (*Chagigah* 12b). It was like
coriander seed and the color of bdel-
lium (Numbers 11:20; *Yoma* 75a). A
double portion was given on Fridays
(Exodus 16:22; *Berachot* 39b). Manna
is one of the ten things created on the
eve of the first Sabbath at twilight
(*Pesachim* 54a; *Avot* 5:6). The manna
had many other attributes as well (*Exodus Rabbah* 25:2–10; *Yoma* 75a). It
was sixty cubits high (*Yoma* 76a). Cosmetics for women and pudding ingredients came down with the manna
(*Yoma* 75a) as did precious stones and
pearls, which the women stored away
(*Exodus Rabbah* 33:8).

Yet in spite of everything, the Israelites complained about the monoto-
nous diet of manna (Numbers 11:1ff.)
and were threatened by Moses with
punishment (Numbers 11:20). Moses
instituted the first blessing of the Grace
after meals at the time when manna
descended for the Jews (*Berachot* 48b).
For forty years when the Jews ate
manna, none of them had to defecate
because it was transformed for them
into flesh (*Numbers Rabbah* 1:24).
One bottle of manna was concealed
(Exodus 16:33) at the time the Holy
Ark was hidden (*Horayot* 12a; *Yoma*
52b).

MAR SAMUEL—Mar Samuel, perhaps the most renowned physician in

the Talmud, was probably as great a
physician as he was a rabbinic scholar.
His knowledge of medicine spans many
specialties, including ophthalmology,
gynecology, pediatrics, anatomy, toxi-
cology, urology, gastroenterology,
bloodletting, therapeutics, and more.
His eye salve was in great demand
because of its efficacy. As with other
physicians of antiquity, Samuel considered bloodletting to be a universal
panacea, prescribing it even as a prophylactic measure. His recommendations in hygiene and general therapeutics were legion. He was physician to
Rabbi Judah the Prince, and probably
also to King Shapur I. His familiarity
with astronomy was no less profound
than his knowledge of medicine and
his expertise in talmudic law.

Born in Nehardea in Babylon, Mar
Samuel is described as "short and big-
stomached" (*Nedarim* 50b). He was
called *Yarchinah* (*Baba Metzia* 85b),
meaning "astronomer" and was nick-
named *Arioch* (*Kiddushin* 39a; *Menachot* 38b; *Shabbat* 53a; *Chullin* 76b),
meaning "king" or "judge" or "powerful." He was also called *Shakud*,
meaning "industrious scholar" (*Ketubot* 43b). He never ceased studying
(ibid., 77a). His expertise as astronomer, talmudist, and physician is detailed elsewhere.[1] His knowledge of
medicine seems to have been all-
encompassing. His famous eye salve
that cured Rabbi Judah the Prince
(*Baba Metzia* 85a) and his prophylactic regimen to prevent eye infections

(*Shabbat* 108b) are well known. Mar Samuel discusses the stages of childhood leading to puberty (*Niddah* 65a) and details the secondary sex characteristics (*Niddah* 47a). He describes tachycardia (*Nedarim* 45b), esophageal injuries (*Gittin* 70b), nasal polyps (ibid.), and various intestinal diseases (*Nedarim* 37b; *Berachot* 44b and 62b).

His toxicological knowledge is reflected by his recognition of poisonous snakes (*Abodah Zarah* 31b) and the fatal outcome of most poisonings (*Gittin* 70a). He made numerous statements concerning obstetrics, gynecology, and fetal development (*Niddah* 25a, 26b, 64b, and 66a; *Chagigah* 14b; *Shabbat* 128b and 129a). He describes eczema of the face (*Shabbat* 133b) and scabs on the body (*Nedarim* 81a).

Mar Samuel discusses bloodletting at great length. He correctly points out that excessive phlebotomy is harmful and can endanger a person's life. He advises a person to eat a little prior to and after bloodletting, to rest for a while after venesection, and to decrease the frequency as one becomes older (*Shabbat* 129b). He also had extensive knowledge of anatomy (*Bechorot* 45a; *Chullin* 43b, 44a, 45b, and 76a), therapeutics (*Shabbat* 109a and 147b; *Baba Metzia* 113b), urology (*Yebamot* 75b; *Shabbat* 137b), neurology (*Chullin* 45a), and general medicine (*Gittin* 67b; *Nedarim* 41a). Mar Samuel, rabbi, physician, astronomer, and one of the most important Babylonian talmudists, was an intellectual giant.

1. F. Rosner, "Mar Samuel the Physician," in *Medicine in the Bible and the Talmud*, 2nd ed. (Hoboken, NJ: Ktav and Yeshiva University Press, 1995), pp. 216–229.

MARRIAGE—Early marriage is a deterrent to illicit sex. One should marry between ages eighteen and twenty-four, although some rabbis married much earlier (*Kiddushin* 30a). Men sometimes married off their sons at twelve years of age (*Lamentations Rabbah* 1:1:2). A man is obligated to marry off his sons and daughters (ibid., 30b). He who marries off his children shortly after their puberty, before they fall prey to sin (*Derech Eretz Rabbah* 2:56), has a house of peace (Job 5:24). If one has a wife, one can study Torah with purity of thoughts (*Yoma* 72b). If one is still unmarried at twenty years of age, one lives a life of sin (*Yoma* 29a). A man who has no wife lives without joy, blessing, goodness, or peace (*Yebamot* 62b; *Genesis Rabbah* 17:2; *Ecclesiastes Rabbah* 9:9:1). The biblical prophets were all married (1 Samuel 8:2; Isaiah 8:18; Ezekiel 24:18; Hosea 1:2) as were the talmudic rabbis. One exception was Ben Azzai, who was in love with the Torah (*Yebamot* 63b). A High Priest had to be married in order to serve in the Temple (*Yoma* 2a).

He who has no wife is as if heaven excommunicated him (*Pesachim* 113b) and he does not wish to be called "human" (*Yebamot* 63a) since God created Adam and Eve and called them "human" (Genesis 5:1). One of the reasons why the sons of Aaron died prematurely (Numbers 3:4) was their celibacy (*Leviticus Rabbah* 20:9). One's marriage partner is from the Lord (Proverbs 19: 14). The Lord serves as matchmaker since the time of creation (*Genesis Rabbah* 68:3–4; *Leviticus Rabbah* 8:1). He couples every individual with a kindred soul (*Numbers Rabbah* 3:6). Forty days before an embryo is formed, a heavenly voice proclaims that so-and-so will marry so-and-so (*Moed Katan* 18b; *Sanhedrin* 22a).

It is in the nature of man to go in search of a woman and not the reverse (*Kiddushin* 2b). More than a man's desire to marry is the woman's desire to be married (*Yebamot* 113a; *Ketubot* 6a; *Gittin* 50a). A woman prefers married life with a bad husband rather than widowhood (*Ketubot* 75a; *Kiddushin* 7a). A man engaged to be married should do so quickly to avoid temptation and heartache (Proverbs 13:12). For a virgin, the usual period of engagement is twelve months, for a widow four weeks (*Ketubot* 5:2). The Talmud mentions the marriage canopy (*Shabbat* 137b), the bridal or marriage chamber (*Ketubot* 48b; *Pesachim* 101a), and marriage outfits (*Ketubot* 50b and 68a).

Certain blemishes found after the marriage can invalidate it (*Kiddushin* 50a; *Ketubot* 75a). A marriage contracted while the man is drunk is legally invalid (*Even Haezer* 44:3) since

he is classified as temporarily mentally ill (*Choshen Mishpat* 235:22). If a man falsely tells his wife that he is a perfume maker and he turns out to be a tanner, the marriage can be invalidated (*Tosefta Kiddushin* 2:4).

Men with hypospadias *(petzua daka)* who are incapable of procreation may not marry Jewish women (Deuteronomy 23:2). Marriage of men to men is prohibited (*Tosefta Yebamot* 2:5; *Tosefta Bikkurim* 2:4). Therefore, a hermaphrodite cannot marry a man but his marriage to a woman is legally binding. A deaf-mute can marry a woman through affirmative gestures since he cannot recite the proper marriage formula (*Yebamot* 14:1).

MARRIAGE, CONJUGAL RIGHTS— A woman is entitled to sexual gratification as part of the husband's obligations to his wife (Exodus 21:10) to maintain marital harmony and domestic peace. These conjugal rights of the wife are known as *onah*. A man cannot vow to deny his wife her conjugal rights (*Ketubot* 5:6). It is improper for a man to cohabit with his wife while fully clothed *(Ketubot* 48a). No cohabitation should occur without the wife's consent (*Eruvin* 100b). If a man loses his ability to perform his conjugal duties, he should dissolve his marriage unless his wife is content even without cohabitation (*Yebamot* 64a). A scholar should not remain away from his wife to study Torah more than thirty days (*Ketubot* 5:6; *Genesis Rabbah* 76:7) unless she consents to a longer period (*Ketubot* 62b).

MARRIAGE, FORBIDDEN—Cohabitation with or marriage to close relatives such as a mother, sister, sister-in-law, daughter, daughter in-law, or aunt and their like, is biblically forbidden (Leviticus 18:8–16). These are abominable Egyptian practices (Leviticus 18:3). Many more second degree relatives are rabbinically forbidden. Excluded from the prohibition are marriages of first cousins, uncle and niece, and stepsister with stepbrothers. Under specific circumstances, a man is allowed/obligated to marry his sister-in-law; this is called levirate marriage (Deuteronomy 25: 5–10). A priest may not marry a divorced or profaned woman (Leviticus 21:7). A high priest is also forbidden to marry a widow (ibid., 21:14) and may only marry a virgin (ibid., 21:13). A man may not remarry his divorced wife if she married another man in the interim (Deuteronomy 24:1–4). Other forbidden matings are discussed in their respective sections: see ADULTERY, INCEST, HOMOSEXUALITY, and LESBIANISM.

MARRIAGE, GENEALOGY—One should try to marry the daughter of a scholar and marry one's daughter to a scholar (*Pesachim* 49b). If not, let him marry the daughter of a great man of the generation or the head of the synagogue, charity treasurer, or teacher (ibid.). If a scholar marries into a priestly family, he brings honor upon it (ibid., 49a). Priests can marry Israelites (*Sanhedrin* 32a). Babylonian Jews married Palestinian Jews (*Ketubot* 111a). He who wishes to take a wife should inquire about the character of her brothers (*Baba Batra* 110a). One should not marry into a family of epileptics or lepers because these illnesses were thought to be hereditary (*Yebamot* 64b).

MARRIAGE, LEVIRATE—Jewish law requires a man to marry his childless deceased brother's widow and to name the firstborn son after the deceased brother. This process is called *yibbum* (Deuteronomy 25:5–10). Thus, the brother's house is built up (*Chagigah* 5a) and the ancestral property remains in the family (Numbers 36:7). If the man refuses to fulfill his levirate marriage obligation, his sister-in-law takes off his shoe and spits before him as part of the *chalitzah* ceremony (Deuteronomy 25:9). The purpose of levirate marriage is thus to prevent the dispersal of land ownership and its transfer to another family or tribe. Even in talmudic times, levirate marriage was not universally practiced (*Yebamot* 39b; *Bechorot* 1:7) and today *chalitzah* is the preferred option.

MASTURBATION—The prohibition against adultery (Exodus 20:13) also implies a prohibition against masturbation with hand or foot (*Niddah* 13b). "Your hands are full of blood" (Isaiah 1:15) refers to those who masturbate with their hands (*Niddah* 13b). They are compared to blood shedders or murderers (*Niddah* 13ba). Men who masturbate should figuratively have their hands cut off (*Niddah* 13a). The deluge came upon the world because people expended their sperm on the ground (Genesis 6:12–13). Onanism (Genesis 28:9) refers to coitus interruptus (*Yebamot* 341). Since Onan's expulsion of semen for naught was displeasurable in the eyes of the Lord (Genesis 28:10), the Talmud concludes that both coitus interruptus and masturbation are forbidden (*Niddah* 13a).

Masturbation can occur in stages (*Sanhedrin* 55a). Young people who sit alone may come to sin by masturbating (*Berachot* 63b). Camel riders who ride with saddles are exposed to "warming their flesh" (*Niddah* 14a). A popular saying states: He masturbates with a pumpkin, his wife with a cucumber (*Megillah* 12a). King Asa's mother practiced idolatry (1 Kings 15:13; 2 Chronicles 15:16), which is interpreted to mean that she masturbated with her idol (*Abodah Zarah* 44a). The Bible cites another example of masturbation as part of the heathen cult (Ezekiel 16:17). [*See also* CHASTITY, VIRGINITY, INCEST, ADULTERY, and MARRIAGE]

MEAT—Originally, meat consumption to satisfy one's appetite was prohibited. Permission was granted by God to Noah (Genesis 9:3) and to the Israelites (Deuteronomy 12:15) as a general dispensation to slaughter and eat animals (*Deuteronomy Rabbah* 4:9). Meat consumption in moderation is advised (Proverbs 27:27) but not in excess (ibid., 23:20–21). A rebellious son becomes liable when he eats a gluttonous amount of meat (*Sanhedrin* 70a). The Jews in the desert who demanded meat died as a result of their gluttonous overeating of quail meat (Numbers 11:33). Priests in the Temple suffered from diarrhea because they ate meat from the offerings constantly and walked barefoot on the marble floors (*Shekalim* 5:1–2; *Avot de Rabbi Nathan* 35:5). Thus, a person should only eat meat when he has a special desire for it (*Chullin* 84b), although rich people may consume meat daily (*Yebamot* 63a). Meat should be consumed on joyous occasions (*Pesachim* 109a) and on the Sabbath and Festivals. Meat for the Sabbath meals must be cooked or roasted before the Sabbath (*Shabbat* 19b). Meat may be specially designated for Passover consumption (*Pesachim* 53a).

Meat is salted or grilled to allow the blood to flow out (*Chullin* 111b; *Pesachim* 74b). Meat was sometimes washed in vinegar to contract the blood vessels and bind the blood (*Pesachim* 74b). Raw meat was sometimes eaten (*Pesachim* 41a) but was generally considered loathsome and repulsive (*Sanhedrin* 39a). Meat was sometimes pickled (*Sanhedrin* 70a), occasionally boiled, but mostly roasted (*Pesachim* 41a). Most people eat meat with bread but Persians eat chunks of roasted meat without bread (*Eruvin* 29b). Meat is cut on tables (*Berachot* 8b) and sold in meat shops (*Ketubot* 15a). One can cut one's hand while carving meat (*Jerushalmi Niddah* 9:41)

A mourner may partake of meat and wine (*Taanit* 13a) but Jews do not eat meat on the day before the Ninth of Av fast that commemorates the destruction of the Temple (ibid., 30a). A woman can vow not to eat meat (*Ketubot* 72b). Consecrated meat that is unclean may not be eaten (*Yebamot* 82a) based on Leviticus 7:19–20. The prohibitions of meat and milk (Exodus 23:19 and 34:26; Deuteronomy 14:21) mean that meat and milk may not be served or consumed together (*Shabbat* 13a), nor may meat and milk be seethed together (*Pesachim* 44b; *Nazir* 37a; *Sanhedrin* 4b; *Kiddushin* 57b; *Temurah* 33b).

Meat is much more nourishing than vegetables or grains (*Nedarim* 49b). Fat meat is said to be beneficial for the whole body (*Pesachim* 42b). A pregnant woman who eats meat and drinks wine has robust children (*Ketubot* 60b). It is considered very generous to provide meat for poor people (*Ketubot* 67b) and for guests (Genesis 18:7; *Berachot* 58a). The High Priest is not fed a variety of foods, including meat,

just prior to Yom Kippur for fear that he may fall asleep (*Yoma* 18a–b). For fever, a person should eat very red meat; for a chill, very fat meat (*Gittin* 67b). For weakness of the heart, Abaye recommended roast meat (*Eruvin* 29b). If one eats raw or fat meat on an empty stomach and then drinks water, one suffers from *arketha* (*Shabbat* 109b). After bloodletting, one should eat meat (*Shabbat* 129a). Eating fat meat gives strength to the body and light to the eyes (*Pesachim* 42a). Fat meat consumption may lead to nocturnal pollution (*Tosefta Zavim* 2:5). Sickness may return if a patient eats beef, fat meat, roasted meat, poultry, etc. (*Berachot* 57b).

MEDICAL INSTRUMENTS—Preuss[1] calls attention to the *makdeach*, or small drill of physicians (trephine) for opening the skull, which is called a "medical instrument" in the Talmud (*Oholot* 2:3). A drill for teeth is also mentioned (*Kiddushin* 24b). A large knife or *sakkin* was used for circumcision and for postmortem cesarean sections (*Arachin* 7a). Zipporah used a flint or stone to circumcise Moses' sons (Exodus 4:24) and Joshua used stone knives for this purpose (*Genesis Rabbah* 31:8). By law, any sharpedged object is suitable for circumcision (*Chullin* 16b) except for a sharp reed, which is dangerous. Shards, sharp stones, and sharp reeds were used to cut the umbilical cord (*Chullin* 1:2).

Mothers used sharp stones to cut their own babies' navels (*Leviticus Rabbah* 5:1; Midrash Psalms 8:5).

Instruments for bloodletting include the *kusilta* or lancet (*Abodah Zarah* 27a; *Kelim* 12:4), the *masmar* or nail (i.e., pointed instrument) (*Kelim* 12:4), the *keren* or cupping horn (*Shabbat* 154b), and cupping glasses (ibid.). One should not use cupping glasses for drinking (*Makkot* 16b). A splinter or thorn was removed with a sewing needle (*Shabbat* 17:1) using warm water (*Abodah Zarah* 28b). Since the removal of a splinter produces a small wound, a son should not remove a splinter from his father if another person is available to do so (*Sanhedrin* 84b) because the infliction of a wound on one's parent is biblically prohibited and considered a capital crime (Exodus 21:15). A newborn infant with an imperforate anus is rubbed with oil and the anal skin cut crosswise with a barley grain but not with a metal instrument that may cause inflammation (*Shabbat* 134a), especially an iron implement (*Chullin* 77a). A barley grain is also used to cut the edges of a penile fistula to help it heal (*Yebamot* 76a).

Surgeons wore leather aprons (*Kelim* 26:5) and used operating tables (*Tosefta Shekalim* 1:6). They also had instrument and bandage boxes containing scissors, razors, and knives (*Kelim* 16:8). Also described are scalpels, planes, drills (*Kelim* 13:4), forceps (*Kelim* 13:8), medicine boxes (*Jerushalmi Berachot* 5:9), instrument boxes (*Kelim* 12:3 and 15:1), and a large ladle of physicians (*Kelim* 17:12). A *kisem*, or toothpick, was used to clean one's teeth (*Betzah* 4:6; *Tosefta Betzah* 3:18). Reeds were used for the same purpose and for circumcision (*Chullin* 16b; *Jerushalmi Shabbat* 8:11) but were considered dangerous because of bleeding. Also mentioned is a chamber pot for excrements (*Kelim* 17:2) and a wooden spice box (*Kelim* 2:7).

Barber's clippers and scissors, swords, knives, sickles (*Kelim* 13:1), notch-free slaughtering knives (*Chullin* 17b), and many other instruments and utensils are mentioned in the Talmud, but it is not clear whether these were used for surgical or other medical purposes.

---

1. F. Rosner (trans.), *Julius Preuss' Biblical and Talmudic Medicine* (Northvale, NJ: Jason Aronson, 1993), pp. 191–192

MELANCHOLY—According to Josephus (*Antiquities*, vol. 10, ch. 2:1), King Hezekiah was afflicted with a deep depression when he became ill because he was childless. The Talmud states that he voluntarily refrained from procreating because he foresaw that his children would be wicked (*Berachot* 10a) [*see* KING HEZEKIAH'S ILLNESS]. Preuss suggests that both Nebuchadnezzer (Daniel

4:29–34) and Saul (1 Samuel 16:14) may have suffered from melancholy but considers that unlikely.[1]

Dates are helpful for melancholy or bad thoughts (*Ketubot* 10b). "Heaviness of the heart" *(yukra de libba)* for which remedies are prescribed (*Shabbat* 140a; *Gittin* 69b) may refer to depression or melancholy. [*See also* MENTAL ILLNESS]

---

1. F. Rosner (trans.), *Julius Preuss' Biblical and Talmudic Medicine* (Northvale, NJ: Jason Aronson, 1993), pp. 311–312.

MELONS—The Jews in the desert yearned for the melons they ate in Egypt (Numbers 11:5). Ashes from roasted, dried, pulverized melon leaves, sprinkled on an anal sore, help heal it (*Abodah Zarah* 28b). Cut melons left uncovered overnight should not be consumed lest a poisonous animal ate from them (*Abodah Zarah* 30b). The same is true of watermelons, or sweet melons that have been bitten (*Terumot* 8:6). Eating melons may aggravate an illness (*Abodah Zarah* 29a). The Talmud describes sweet melons (*Terumot* 2:6), cucumber melons (*Kilayin* 1:2), rotten melons (*Terumot* 3:1; *Uktzin* 2:3), and melons with offensive smells (*Yebamot* 89a). [*See also* POMEGRANATES]

MENSTRUATION—Menstruation is called "the manner of women" (Genesis 31:35) and the climacteric is its cessation (Genesis 18:11). A menstruant woman is called *dava*, meaning "unwell" (Leviticus 20:18); *zava*, meaning "a woman with issue" (Leviticus 15:19); or *niddah*, meaning "menstruant" (Ezekiel 18:6). An entire tractate of Talmud (*Niddah*) is devoted to this subject. A menstruant woman is biblically unclean for seven days (Leviticus 15:19) and imparts ritual uncleanness (ibid., 15:20) even if she bleeds for less than seven days. A man who cohabits with a menstruant woman is liable to a heavenly death penalty (ibid., 20:18) and is flogged by rabbinic decree (*Makkot* 3:1). Such cohabitation is an immoral heathen practice (Leviticus 18:3) and may result in the birth of leprous or otherwise abnormal infants (*Leviticus Rabbah* 15:5).

Menstruating women have to be "separated" from their husbands (Leviticus 15:25) and the Talmud cites a "house of unclean women" (*Niddah* 7:4). Married women wore different clothes during their menses (*Ketubot* 65b) and some put on no makeup (*Shabbat* 64b). Most women have regular menses (*Niddah* 64a), usually every thirty days (ibid., 15a). The shortest interval between menses is eleven days (ibid., 72b). Menses is usually heralded by signs and symptoms such as yawning, sneezing, trembling, coughing, or abdominal pain (ibid., 63b). Menses may be brought on by jumping, carrying a heavy load, illness (*Tosefta Niddah* 9:1), sudden fright (*Niddah* 71a; *Megillah* 15a), sexual excitement or lust (*Niddah* 20b), or the anticipation of coitus (ibid., 66a).

Since the fourth century, Jewish women consider any intermenstrual bleeding as "blood from the fountain" that ritually defiles and requires seven clean (i.e., bloodless) days before the woman immerses in a ritual bath for purification (*Niddah* 67b). The Egyptians were smitten with the plague of blood (Exodus 7:19ff.) because they refused to allow Jewish women to ritually immerse after their menstruation (*Exodus Rabbah* 9:10; *Numbers Rabbah* 10:2; *Esther Rabbah* 5:1). Blood from the bladder or a vaginal wound does not defile since it is not of uterine origin (*Niddah* 59b). Certain sages became specialists in identifying the source of blood from its aroma and color (ibid., 20b). Uterine blood can be red, black, saffron-colored, or like earthy water (ibid., 19a). There may be geographical differences in blood color (ibid., 20a). An elaborate procedure was used to determine whether a red stain on a woman's clothing or bed sheets is blood or a colored dye [*see* FORENSIC MEDICINE].

When a woman cohabits with her husband after the ritual bath, she is most fertile (*Niddah* 31b; *Leviticus Rabbah* 14:5) and is again beloved by her husband as when they were first married (*Niddah* 31b). Menses cease

with the beginning of pregnancy since the blood is converted to milk (*Niddah* 9a). Pregnancy can occur even before the onset of menses (ibid., 45a; *Sanhedrin* 69b). One should not marry an adult woman who has never menstruated since she is considered infertile (*Niddah* 12b).

Physicians are called to diagnose and treat vaginal bleeding (*Niddah* 22b). A speculum can be used to examine for blood and to determine its source (ibid., 66a). A variety of folk remedies for vaginal bleeding are described in the Talmud (*Shabbat* 110a–b). Vaginal bleeding from a miscarriage or following childbirth is discussed elsewhere [*see* ABORTION and CHILDBIRTH]. [*See also* DEFLORATION and RITUAL BATH]

MENTAL DEFICIENCY—Although deaf people may have normal intelligence, deaf-mutes are usually mentally deficient (*Chagigah* 2b). They have weak understanding (*Yebamot* 113a) and cannot reflect well (*Machshirim* 6:1). The term *shoteh* for fool or imbecile means "to roam about," i.e., "absent-minded." Imbeciles are considered mentally deficient but not insane. They do not have full adult intellect and are legally equated with minors and deaf-mutes.[1] Intermittent loss of intellect can occur in an intoxicated person suffering from *kordiakos* (*Gittin* 7:1) who is temporarily confused. One's intellect weakens with advancing age (2 Samuel 19:36; *Shabbat* 152b). One cannot cite proof from the action of imbeciles (*Niddah* 30b) as was once attempted in a case where a child was found dead and the mother was suspected (*Ketubot* 60b). A person can be sane at times and mad at other times (*Rosh Hashanah* 28a). [*See also* MENTAL ILLNESS]

1. F. Rosner (trans.), *Julius Preuss' Biblical and Talmudic Medicine* (Northvale, NJ: Jason Aronson, 1993), pp. 315–317.

MENTAL ILLNESS—Mental illness or insanity *(shiga'on)* is Divine punishment for wrongdoing (Deuteronomy 28:28 and 28:34; Zechariah 12:4). A madman who claims he is a prophet is a false prophet (Jeremiah 29:26). Babylonian King Nebuchadnezzer was mad in that he ate grass like oxen and his nails grew long like bird's claws (Daniel 4:30). King Saul was terrified (1 Samuel 16:16), raved in his house (1 Samuel 18:10), stripped off his clothes, and lay naked (ibid., 19:23–24). King David feigned madness (ibid., 21:14). These are detailed elsewhere.[1]

The mentally ill go out at night alone, spend the night in the cemetery, and tear their garments and other things (*Chagigah* 3b; *Sanhedrin* 65b; *Niddah* 17a). A fool repeats his folly like a dog who returns to its vomit (Proverbs 26:11; *Leviticus Rabbah*

16:9). A person does not transgress unless a spirit of folly enters him (*Sotah* 3a). This includes immoral sexual behavior by wife or husband (*Bechorot* 5b). A lunatic may have periods of clear or sound state of mind (*Yebamot* 31a). An intoxicated person behaves like a madman (*Megillah* 12b) because when wine enters the body, understanding leaves (*Numbers Rabbah* 10:8). The Aramean army suffered from auditory hallucinations (2 Kings 7:6).

Mad people were put in prison (Jeremiah 29:26). The Talmud says that there are no medications for madmen (*Gittin* 70b). A woman who killed a baby in order to remarry was said to be mad (*Ketubot* 60a–b). [*See also* MENTAL DEFICIENCY]

1. F. Rosner (trans.), *Julius Preuss' Biblical and Talmudic Medicine* (Northvale, NJ: Jason Aronson, 1993), p. 311–313.

MICE—Mice are ritually unclean animals (Leviticus 11:29). They are considered pests (1 Samuel 6:5) and may be the source of plagues.[1] Mice gnaw at fruit and are, therefore, repulsive (*Sukkah* 36b). A group of mice once united and killed a cat (*Baba Metzia* 97a). Mice even eat sacred books (*Shabbat* 14a). Mice eat leavened bread (*Pesachim* 10a and 13a). If one eats from that which a mouse has eaten, one forgets one's studies (*Horayot* 13b). Corpses are guarded from mice before burial (*Berachot* 18a; *Shabbat* 151b, *Genesis Rabbah* 34:12) A mouse was once found in a spice box (*Betzah* 36b; *Shabbat* 121b). If a mouse falls into a keg of beer, one should not drink from it (*Abodah Zarah* 68b). If a mouse nibbles on a melon, one should not eat from it (*Chullin* 9a). Sea mice and land mice exist (*Chullin* 126b; *Niddah* 43b). A hybrid mouse of part flesh and part earth was believed to exist (*Chullin* 126b; *Sanhedrin* 91a). Mice are caught in mousetraps (*Kelim* 15:6).

---

1. F. Rosner (trans.), *Julius Preuss' Biblical and Talmudic Medicine* (Northvale, NJ: Jason Aronson, 1993), p. 156.

MIDWIFE—The biblical term for midwife is *meyaledet* (Genesis 35:17 and 38:28; Exodus 1:19). Pharaoh instructed the two midwives Shifra and Puah to drown all newborn male Hebrew infants (Exodus 1:15). They refused (ibid., 1:17). Tradition states that these two midwives were Yocheved, mother of Moses, and Miriam her daughter or Elisheva her daughter-in-law (*Exodus Rabbah* 1:13). Shifra was so named because she cleaned (*shafar*) the babies (*Sotah* 11b) and Puah was so named because she had only to call (*poah*) the woman in labor and the child came forth (*Ecclesiastes Rabbah* 7:1). These midwives feared God (Exodus 1:17) and went to the rich to collect water and food for the poor (*Exodus Rabbah* 1:15). A mid-

wife was present at the confinement of Rachel, who died during childbirth (Genesis 35:17). During the twin birth of Tamar, the midwife tied a red thread to the hand of the child that put its hand out first (Genesis 38:28). The word of a midwife about which of two twins is born first is accepted without question (*Genesis Rabbah* 85:13; *Kiddushin* 73b). Women stood around the high priest Eli's daughter-in-law during childbirth. It is not clear if they were midwives (1 Samuel 4:20).

The talmudic term for midwife is *chachama* (wise woman) or *chaya* (*Chullin* 4:3). One may summon a midwife to deliver a baby on the Sabbath (*Shabbat* 128b), even from a distant location beyond the Sabbath limit (*Eruvin* 45a; *Rosh Hashanah* 23b). For her own confinement, a midwife needs another midwife (*Exodus Rabbah* 1:16; *Sotah* 11a). In the absence of a midwife, a maidservant can deliver a baby (*Jerushalmi Ketubot* 5:30). A proverb says that while the midwife and the woman in labor are arguing, the child is lost (*Genesis Rabbah* 60:3). A midwife requires guarding against evil spirits (*Berachot* 54b) The heads of Babylonians are said to be round because they lack skillful midwives (*Shabbat* 31a). A midwife who touches a dead fetus in a woman is ritually unclean for seven days (*Numbers Rabbah* 19:1; *Chullin* 71a; *Niddah* 42b), but only by rabbinic decree (Chullin 72a).

An Israelite should not act as a midwife to a heathen woman because she would be delivering a child to idolatry (*Abodah Zarah* 26a). Extreme caution should be observed in the use of heathen midwives for Jewish women (*Tosefta Abodah Zarah* 3:4; *Abodah Zarah* 26a). Fees for midwives are mentioned in the Talmud (*Abodah Zarah* 26a). [*See also* PREGNANCY and CHILDBIRTH]

MILK—The Bible repeatedly asserts that Israel is a land flowing with milk and honey. This Divine blessing is graphically depicted in the Talmud (*Ketubot* 111b). Resh Lakish saw the flow of milk and honey at Sepphoris extend over an area of sixteen square miles (ibid., *Megillah* 6a). It is a blessing or sign of prosperity if there is an "abundance of milk" (Isaiah 7:22), if one's "pails are full of milk" (Job 21:24), if there is "enough goats' milk" (Proverbs 28:27), if the "hills flow with milk" (Joel 4:18), or if "honey and milk are under your tongue" (Song of Songs 4:11). Not only are suckling animals (1 Samuel 7:9) and human infants (Isaiah 28:9) nourished with milk but adults too drink milk (Ezekiel 25:4; Judges 4:19 and 5:25), sometimes mixed with wine (Song of Songs 5:1), and sometimes free of charge (Isaiah 55:1). The word milk is also used in allegorical or figurative ways (Song of Songs 5:12; Lamentations 4:7; Isaiah 60:16). For example, the phrase "His teeth are white from milk" (Genesis 49:12) is said to refer

to a man's honesty (*Kallah Rabbati* 53b). The words of the Torah are compared to milk (*Song of Songs Rabbah* 1:2:3; *Taanit* 7a).

The consumption of meat and milk together is prohibited, based on the thrice-repeated biblical admonition not to seethe a kid in its mother's milk (Exodus 23:19 and 34:26; Deuteronomy 14:21). One talmudic sage allows the consumption of fowl flesh with milk (*Yebamot* 14a), exempting fowl meat from the general prohibition (*Shabbat* 130a; *Chullin* 116a; *Bechorot* 10a; *Pesachim* 24b and 44b). The flesh of fish and locusts is not included in the prohibition of meat and milk (*Chullin* 103a). The rules and regulations relating to this prohibition are exhaustively discussed elsewhere.[1]

Milk is useful medicinally. It is used in eye salves (*Shabbat* 77b). Goats' milk is curative for patients with "chest attacks" (*Ketubot* 60a). Milk combined with certain foods such as preserved figs and honey may have intoxicating properties (*Yoma* 76a; *Nazir* 4a). Milk increases semen production (*Yoma* 18a). Woman's milk is the main nourishment of infants (*Shabbat* 143b), although cows' milk is also used for infants (*Baba Batra* 78b) and even for adults (*Keritot* 22a). Milk can also be harmful. One who underwent bloodletting should abstain from milk (*Nedarim* 54b; *Abodah Zarah* 29a). Milk can aggravate an illness (*Berachot* 57b; *Avodah Zarah* 29a). After consuming fish, cress, and milk, one should not lie down to sleep (*Moed Katan* 11a).

Many laws pertaining to milk are found in classic Jewish sources. Thus, human milk is ritually clean (*Ketubot* 60a) but can contract uncleanness as a liquid and convey uncleanness to other liquids and foods (*Keritot* 13b), whether or not its flow is desired (*Machshirin* 6:8). Dried milk on the skin constitutes an interposition and must be removed before a ritual bath can be valid (*Shabbat* 120b; *Pesachim* 65b; *Zevachim* 35a; *Menachot* 21a). A calf born after the mother gave milk exempts from the law of the firstling (*Bechorot* 16a and 20b). Additional rules and laws pertaining to milk are detailed elsewhere.[2] [*See also* LACTATION]

---

1. S. Y. Zevin (ed.), *Encyclopedia Talmudit*, vol. 4 (Jerusalem, 1956), s. v. *basar bechalav*, pp. 690–727.

2. S. Y. Zevin (ed.), *Encyclopedia Talmudit*, vol. 15 (Jerusalem, 1976), s. v. *chalav*, pp. 154–192.

MOLE—A mole can be used to identify a corpse, although moles may undergo postmortem change (*Yebamot* 120a). A hairy mole on the face of a woman may disfigure her (*Ketubot* 75a). A mole on the genitalia of a child or minor can be mistaken for pubic hair (*Niddah* 46a). A man once recognized his sister by the mole on her shoulder (*Lamentations Rabbah* 1:46). A white mole may be an early stage of leprosy (Leviticus 13:3). [*See also* SKIN]

MOURNING—A mourner rends his garments as a sign of mourning (*Moed Katan* 26b) and places sackcloth on his loins (Genesis 37:37). A mourner is forbidden to wear shoes (*Pesachim* 4a), to bathe (*Berachot* 16b), to cut his nails (*Moed Katan* 18a), to cut his hair (ibid., 14b), and to use cosmetics (ibid., 20b; *Ketubot* 4b). Oil embrocations are also omitted during mourning (Daniel 10:3). Striking one's thigh is a sign of mourning (Ezekiel 21:17). Tamar put ashes on her hair as a sign of mourning (2 Samuel 13:19). A High Priest does not wear torn garments nor let his hair grow when he is in mourning (Leviticus 10:6 and 21:10).

Pagan custom was to cut oneself (Jeremiah 16:6), especially on the hands (Jeremiah 48:37), and to shave off one's beard (Isaiah 15:2) as a sign of mourning. Such cutting is prohibited in Judaism (Leviticus 19:28). It is a custom of mourning among Jews to eat lentils (*Genesis Rabbah* 63:14). The mourner's meal is not served on ornamental trays but in plain baskets (*Moed Katan* 27a). Mourners wore black garments (*Baba Metzia* 59b). Tears of mourning are worst if one mourns for the loss of a grown-up child (*Shabbat* 151b; *Lamentations Rabbah* 2:15). For a close relative, the initial deep mourning period is seven days (*Nazir* 15b; Genesis 50:10; *Deuteronomy Rabbah* 9:1). Public mourning is described (*Moed Katan* 24b and 28b). Recent mourning differs from ancient mourning and public mourning differs from private mourning (*Yebamot* 43b). [*See also* BURIAL, COFFIN, CORPSE, DEATH, and GRAVE]

MOUTH—The Hebrew world *peh* for mouth also refers to the lips and the oral cavity. Man is master over his mouth, hand, and foot (*Genesis Rabbah* 67:3)—except for Balaam, in whose mouth God put words (Numbers 22:35). One eats with the mouth (Ezekiel 4:14), breathes with the mouth (Job 15:3a), yawns with the mouth (*Tosefot, Niddah* 63a), and speaks with the mouth (Psalms 19:15). The mouth articulates words (*Berachot* 61a). The mouth of the Lord also speaks (Isaiah 1:20), but only with Moses did he speak "mouth to mouth" (Numbers 12:8). One also kisses with the mouth [*see* KISSING]. To "split open the mouth" (Lamentations 2:16 and 3:46) means to deride or scoff at someone. To "enlarge one's mouth" (Ovadiah 1:12) means to speak proudly or arrogantly.

Bad mouth odors, as emitted by the giant Goliath (*Song of Songs Rabbah* 4:24) and an adulteress (*Numbers Rabbah* 9:21), are offensive. A woman who suffers from a bad mouth odor can have her marriage annulled by her husband (*Ketubot* 75a). Lengthy fasting can produce offensive mouth odors (*Genesis Rabbah* 42:1; *Avot de Rabbi Nathan* 6:3), as can the daily consumption of lentils (*Berachot* 40a). The same occurs in people who eat raw vegetables in the morning (*Berachot* 44b) or who fail to walk after eating and lie down to sleep before the food is digested (*Shabbat* 41a). Even Mar Samuel had no remedy for this situation (*Baba Metzia* 113b). Spinning Roman flax also causes the mouth to emit a foul odor (*Ketubot* 61b). Fish and meat salted together produce a foul aroma in the mouth (*Pesachim* 112a). The saliva in the mouth is sweet to help neutralize food (*Numbers Rabbah* 18:22). To counteract a bad mouth odor one should eat peppers (*Shabbat* 90a), chew on mastic (*Tosefta Shabbat* 12:8), rub the teeth with a dry powder (ibid.), or consume ginger and cinnamon (*Shabbat* 65a).

Several remedies are recommended for an abscess in the mouth (*Gittin* 69a). Several prominent talmudic sages suffered from stomatitis (*tzafdina*) (*Abodah Zarah* 28a; *Yoma* 84a; *Baba Metzia* 85a), which caused gum bleeding (*Yoma* 84a). Its causes and remedies are also described (ibid.). The same illness is described in the Midrash as an affliction of the teeth and gums (*Genesis Rabbah* 33:2 and 96:2; *Ecclesiastes Rabbah* on 11:2). One of the signs of the *raatan* illness (leprosy?) is salivation from the mouth

(*Ketubot* 77b), perhaps from lesions within the mouth. The illness *askara* (diphtheria?) affects primarily children (*Taanit* 27b) but also adults (*Sotah* 35a). Death occurs by asphyxiation (*Leviticus Rabbah* 18:4) and is very painful (*Berachot* 8a and 40a). An epidemic killed thousands (*Yebamot* 62b). Preventive measures are suggested (*Bechorot* 40a). One treatment for this illness is bloodletting (*Yoma* 84a).

Malformations of the mouth include harelip, for which a person may be ridiculed or laughed at (*Baba Kamma* 117a). A constricted or contracted mouth (*balum*) is considered a blemish that renders an animal unfit to be offered in the temple (*Bechorot* 40b).

The homiletical literature states that among the things created by God at sunset on Friday night (*Avot* 5:6) are the mouth of the earth (Numbers 16:30), the mouth of the well (Numbers 20:7–11), and the mouth of Balaam's ass (Numbers 22:28). Further, in the hereafter the mouth and the stomach will contend with each other *(Genesis Rabbah* 100:7). [*See also* FACE, LIPS, and FOREHEAD]

MULES—A mule is a hybrid of a horse and a donkey. Adam is said to have crossed two different animals from which came forth the mule (*Pesachim* 54a). One rabbinic opinion is that the mule was created on Sabbath eve at twilight and is not the result of cross-breeding (*Pesachim* 54a). A mule may only be mated with another mule and not with a horse or ass (*Chullin* 79a). A mule is not fruitful and does not procreate (*Genesis Rabbah* 38:6; *Shabbat* 67a; *Baba Batra* 91a). A mule can inflict serious injury on another animal (*Chullin* 7b) or on people (*Yoma* 49a). The Talmud speaks of red mules and white mules (ibid.) and mule drivers' markets (*Chagigah* 9b). Mules pull wagons (*Baba Batra* 77b; *Chullin* 79a). They kneel to urinate (*Eruvin* 100b; *Bechorot* 22a). The dung of a white mule is one of many folk remedies for vaginal bleeding (*Shabbat* 110a–b). [*See also* ASSES, HORSES, and GOATS]

MUSIC THERAPY—The history of Jewish music from biblical to modern times and the significant restriction of musical expression since the destruction of the Temple are described in detail elsewhere.[1,2] Two major talmudic sources are the basis for the prohibition against secular music nowadays (*Sotah* 48a; *Gittin* 7a). Jewish law prohibits listening to vocal and instrumental music both as a sign of mourning following the destruction of the Temple and because secular music leads to inappropriate gaiety, frivolity, and debauchery. Exceptions to this ban on music include festive occasions of a religious nature such as weddings or the celebration of the Festival of Tabernacles. Another exception is the singing of praises and hymns to God, since the goal of such singing is to approach the Creator and to strive for moral perfection to know God.

On the other hand, Maimonides prescribes music therapy for the preservation of body health and for the cure of psychiatric illness such as melancholy. He recognizes the relationship of the soma to the psyche and asserts that mental and physical health are dependent upon each other. Both are necessary to obtain wisdom and to strive for the acquisition of the knowledge of God. If music therapy is needed to achieve that goal, Maimonides permits it.[3] He thus foresaw the modern medical demonstration that music therapy is useful for the treatment, rehabilitation, education, or training of people suffering from physical, mental, or emotional disorders.

1. C. Roth (ed.), *Encyclopedia Judaica*, vol. 12 (Jerusalem: Keter, 1971), pp. 554–678.

2. A. Khan, "Music in Halakhic Perspective," *Journal of Jewish Music and Liturgy*, vol. 9 (1986–87), pp. 55–72.

3. F. Rosner, "Moses Maimonides on Music Therapy and His Responsum on Music," *Journal of Jewish Music and Liturgy*, vol. 16 (1993–94), pp. 1–16.

MUSTARD—Mustard needs sweetening before it is ready for consumption (*Genesis Rabbah* 11:6; *Leviticus Rabbah* 11:7; *Ecclesiastes Rabbah* 1: 12:1; *Song of Songs Rabbah* 1:1:7). Regular monthly consumption of mustard keeps sickness away but eating it every day may weaken the heart (or stomach) (*Berachot* 40a). Tongues with mustard are considered a delicacy (*Baba Metzia* 86b). Mustard is food for doves (*Shabbat* 128a) and was carried in baskets (ibid., 91b). Mustard consumption may produce tears (*Lamentations Rabbah* 2:15). Hedge mustard may induce semen flow (*Yoma* 18a). Hedge mustard was also used as a substitute for pepper (*Eruvin* 28b).

Mustard strainers are described in the Talmud (*Kelim* 14:8 and 25:3). One may not strain mustard grain through its own strainer on Festivals nor sweeten it with a glowing coal (*Shabbat* 134a). Flour may not be put in mustard on Passover lest the flour become leaven (*Pesachim* 40b). Mustard must be kept away from beehives since they injure each other and the bees may be rendered sterile (*Baba Batra* 18a, 19a, 25a, and 80a). Mustard seed plants are subject to the law of the corner (*Niddah* 51a). Mustard and Egyptian mustard are not considered diverse species (*Kilayim* 1:2; *Pesachim* 39a). Mustard is grown in small fields (*Kilayim* 1:9). It may not be sown near a cornfield since it harms the corn, but may be sown close to a vegetable field (*Kilayim* 1:8). Mustard seeds stored in an earthenware vessel are ritually unclean (*Chullin* 25a). Priestly dues may be eaten only roasted and with mustard (*Chullin* 132b).

MUTILATION—The mutilation of a human corpse is prohibited as a desecration of the body created in the image of God.[1] A mutilated or decomposed corpse can be identified by the nose and the cheeks (*Jerushalmi Yebamot* 16:15) Mutilating leprosy resulted in limb amputations (*Keritot* 3:8). Legend relates that Nahum was born blind, with mutilated hands and legs and boils all over his body (*Taanit* 21a). In biblical times, Israel's enemies cut off the noses and ears of the Jews (Ezekiel 23:25). [*See also* AUTOPSY, AMPUTEE, CASTRATION, TORTURE, and ANIMALS, CRUELTY TO]

---

1. F. Rosner, *Modern Medicine and Jewish Ethics* 2nd ed. (Hoboken, NJ, and New York: Ktav and Yeshiva University Press, 1991), pp. 313–333.

MYRRH—Pure myrrh is one of the choicest spices (Exodus 25). Myrrh gives off its perfume when near a fire and makes the hands smart (*Song of Songs Rabbah* 1:13:1 and 3:6:2). Flowing myrrh is the foremost or chief of the spices (*Numbers Rabbah* 14:12; *Esther Rabbah* 6:3) and, therefore, people sing about it (*Genesis Rabbah* 91:11). The shepherdess carries a bundle of myrrh between her breasts and proudly shows it to her friend (Song of Songs 1:13). Myrrh is one of the eleven ingredients in the incense prepared by the house of Abtinas (*Song of Songs Rabbah* 3:6:4). Maidens at the court of King Ahasuerus beauti-

fied themselves with oil of myrrh for six months (Esther 2:12; *Megillah* 13a). Some sages interpret this oil to be *stata* (oil of myrrh), whereas others say it refers to oil from one-third-ripe olives (*Moed Katan* 9b; *Megillah* 13a; *Menachot* 86a). Rich girls used oil of myrrh as a depilatory because it not only removes hair but makes the flesh soft (*Shabbat* 80b; *Pesachim* 43a). Licentious girls placed myrrh and balsam in vials in their shoes. When handsome young men passed, the girls splashed them with the fragrant spices to arouse their passions (*Yoma* 9b; *Shabbat* 62b). Myrrh gum is thick and adheres to glass vessels (*Shabbat* 15b; *Mikvaot* 9:5).

MYRTLE—The myrtle tree and its branches have a pleasant aroma but a bitter taste (*Esther Rabbah* 6:5). Myrtle is a fragrant wood (*Berachot* 43a–b) and the branches are cut for their aroma (*Eruvin* 40a). Shops were decorated with roses and myrtle for their fragrant aroma (*Abodah Zarah* 12b), and bridal canopies or overhead awnings of myrtle were erected for wedding ceremonies (*Ketubot* 17b; *Shabbat* 150b). People danced with myrtle twigs before a bride (*Ketubot* 17a). A man once betrothed a woman with a myrtle branch (*Kiddushin* 12b). Another man did the same with a mat of myrtle twigs (ibid.).

Myrtle is one of ten kinds of cedar trees (*Rosh Hashanah* 23a; *Baba Batra* 80b). The myrtle tree is crowded with leaves and is therefore called a thick tree (*Exodus Rabbah* 2:5; *Leviticus Rabbah* 30:8). It has thick boughs (Leviticus 23:40), meaning its branches completely cover its trunk (*Sukkah* 32b). The Egyptian myrtle has seven leaves in each nest (*Sukkah* 33a). Three myrtle branches are used as one of the four species utilized on the holiday of the Tabernacles (*Leviticus* 23:40; *Sukkah* 34a). Stolen or withered myrtles are not valid for this purpose (*Sukkah* 32b).

Therapeutically, fresh myrtle is part of a remedy for plethora (*Gittin* 68b). Myrtle leaves were used to remove large insects or worms from the brain of sufferers from *raatan* (*Ketubot* 77b). Myrtle is an ingredient in the preparation of perfumed soap (*Shabbat* 50a). Myrtle branches are put on coffins to honor the dead (*Betzah* 6a; *Niddah* 37a). "God stood among the myrtle trees" (Zechariah 1:8) refers to the righteous, such as Esther (*Megillah* 13a).

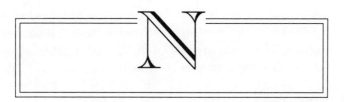

NAILS—Every finger has a nail; every limb or organ with a nail also has a bone (*Niddah* 6:2). A fully developed fetus has hair and nails (*Yebamot* 80b). One old talmudic sage had lustrous and rosy nails like those of a child (*Jerushalmi Rosh Hashanah* 2:58). Every part of a corpse imparts ritual defilement except the teeth, hair, and nails (*Oholot* 3:3). A person in mourning does not cut the fingernails (*Moed Katan* 18a). A woman captured in war either lets her nails grow (Deuteronomy 21:12) or pares them (*Yebamot* 48a). The emotionally disturbed Nebuchadnezzar let his nails grow long and curved like birds' claws (Daniel 4:30). If one pares one's nails without washing the hands, one may suffer fear at a later time (*Pesachim* 112a). A knife was used to cut fingernails (*Tosefta Kelim* 3:12). It is wrong to discard one's fingernails lest a barefoot person walk on them and become hurt or a pregnant woman suffer by treading on them. Righteous people burn or bury them (*Niddah* 17a; *Moed Katan* 18a).

When Potiphar's wife tried to seduce Joseph (Genesis 39:12), he resisted by pressing his fingernails into his hands as he saw his father's image before him (*Genesis Rabbah* 87:6–7). The Talmud also says that to avoid immoral acts, one should bore one's nails into the ground (*Shevuot* 18a). Jews who were persecuted by Hadrian had needles stuck under their nails (*Song of Songs Rabbah* 2:7). To test whether or not a slaughtering knife is notch free, it is examined with one's fingernail (*Chullin* 17b). One may not slaughter an animal with one's fingernail if it is attached to the person's finger (ibid., 15b). The nipping of birds for certain sacrifices, however, was performed with the fingernail (*Chullin* 20a). [*See also* FINGERS and TOES]

NAKEDNESS—Ham saw his father Noah's nakedness when the latter was drunk (Genesis 9:22). Priests wore linen trousers to cover their nakedness (Exodus 28:42). They also walked up a ramp rather than climb steps to the altar so that their nakedness would not be visible (Exodus 20:23). Vashti refused to appear naked before her husband Ahasuerus and the entire royal court (*Esther Rabbah* 3:13). Rabbi Simeon ben Yochai and his son lived hidden from the Romans for thirteen years. To preserve their clothes and not offend God by their nakedness, they buried themselves in sand all day so that their skin became raw and cracked (*Genesis Rabbah* 79:6). When tears fell on their skin, they cried out in pain (*Shabbat* 33b).

Nakedness is considered a grievous evil (*Ecclesiastes Rabbah* 5:12:1). Walking naked on the street is objectionable and abominable (*Yebamot* 63b). One may not stand nude in the presence of the Divine Name (*Shabbat* 120b). He who stands naked before a lamp may develop epilepsy (*Pesachim* 112b). One may not look at a king when he is naked or bathing (*Sanhedrin* 2:5) because it may harm the public awe of the king.

NAVEL—The world *tabbur* for navel refers to the middle point, as in the middle of the earth (Ezekiel 38:12). A deep lying navel is compared to a pit (*Avot de Rabbi Nathan* 31:3). An embryo in its mother's womb develops from its navel (*Sotah* 45b) since the navel is the central point of intrauterine life (*Song of Songs Rabbah* 7:3). The Sanhedrin is compared to the navel because its place was in the center of the Temple like the navel is the center of the abdomen (*Numbers Rabbah* 1:4). When a baby is born, its mouth

opens and the navel closes (*Yebamot* 71b). The umbilical cord or "navel string" is tied and/or cut even on the Sabbath (*Shabbat* 129b), based on biblical verses (Ezekiel 16:4). Either the midwife (*Exodus Rabbah* 23:8) or the mother herself (*Leviticus Rabbah* 5:1) cuts the cord.

Legend relates that the tongues of the scouts who spoke evilly about the land of Israel (Numbers 14:37) extended to their navels as Divine retribution (*Sotah* 35a). For abdominal pain, heat is applied to the navel (*Shabbat* 66b). During menstruation, a woman may feel pain around her navel. If a person is buried under a pile of rubble on the Sabbath, one clears the debris up to the navel to determine whether the person is dead or alive (*Yoma* 85a; *Jerushalmi Yoma* 8:45). After death, metallic vessels were placed on the navel to prevent the body from swelling (*Semachot* 1:2). A mourner rends his garments down to the navel (*Moed Katan* 26b). [See also ABDOMEN, INTESTINES, STOMACH, etc.]

NAZARITE—A Nazarite is a person who vows for a specific period (usually thirty days) to abstain from partaking of grapes or any of its products, from cutting his hair, and from touching a corpse (Numbers 6:3–9). At the end of his Nazariteship, he brings an offering and cuts his hair (*Nedarim* 1:1; *Taanit* 11a; Numbers 6:18). An entire tractate of Talmud (*Nazir*) is devoted to this subject, including the assumption of Nazarite vows, the different types of Naziriteship, the observance and breach of the obligations to abstain from wine, shaving the hair, contact with the dead, and the order of purification on the completion of the Nazarite's term.

A Nazarite for life (*Nazir* 4b) is exemplified by Samson (Judges 13:5) and Samuel (1 Samuel 1:21). Samson's strength was dependent on his Naziriteship (*Numbers Rabbah* 14:9). Absalom was also a lifelong Nazarite (*Nazir* 4b). He polled his hair (2 Samuel 14:26) and was hanged by his hair (2 Samuel 18:9). A lifelong Nazarite may lighten his hair with a razor if it becomes too heavy (*Numbers Rabbah* 10:17).

Joseph is said to have been a Nazarite (*Genesis Rabbah* 98:20). A Nazarite may cleanse his hair and part it but may not comb it because his hair may thereby be pulled out (*Shabbat* 50b and 81b). He may not shampoo his head with clay for the same reason (*Betzah* 35b). A Nazarite is considered a sinner because he denies himself that which the Torah permits (*Taanit* 11a; *Nazir* 19a and 22a; *Sotah* 15a) and asceticism is not a Judaic practice or concept (*Nazir* 4b). A Nazarite is also called holy (Numbers 6:5; *Taanit* 11a). The Torah section dealing with a Nazarite is directly contiguous to the section dealing with a suspected adulteress to teach that priests, kings, and princes, as well as ordinary citizens, should avoid excessive wine imbibition, which may lead to lewdness, so as not to disgrace themselves (*Numbers Rabbah* 10:1–4). [*See also* ASCETICISM]

NECK—A beautiful neck (*tzavar*) is like the Tower of David (Song of Songs 4:4) or like a tower of ivory (ibid., 7:5). The skin of the neck is usually smooth. Rebecca placed a kid's skin on the "smooth of the neck" of Jacob so that his father could not distinguish him from his hairy brother Esau (Genesis 27:16). Moses was accused by his critics of having an obese neck (*Genesis Rabbah* 51:6). Victorious generals placed their feet on the necks of the captured enemy as a sign of victory (Joshua 10:24). A yoke was placed on the neck of the conquered (Jeremiah 28:10). Neck irons (Kelim 12:1), neck chains, or ropes were used to confine prisoners (*Abodah Zarah* 15b). In Roman times, pieces of gold were hung around the neck (ibid., 11b). In the Bible, the Egyptian Pharaoh hung a gold chain around the neck of his newly appointed viceroy Joseph (Genesis 41:42). Cain killed his brother Abel when he struck him in the neck, perhaps severing his carotid arteries (*Sanhedrin* 37b).

Having one's hand on the neck of one's son means that one has control over him (*Kiddushin* 30a). The Jews are called stiff-necked or obstinate by their leader Moses (Exodus 32:9, 34:9, etc). Someone who is burdened by anxiety and worries is said to have a millstone around his neck (*Kiddushin* 29b). Turning one's back on one's enemy means to show the nape of the neck (Joshua 7:8). The nape of the neck was revealed when a famous rabbi's head covering blew off (*Jerushalmi Betzah* 5:63).

The Talmud says that there are eight bones or vertebrae in the neck (*Oholot* 1:8). Severance of the cervical vertebra is lethal in both man (1 Samuel 4:18) and animal (*Chullin* 113a). A heifer's neck was broken to atone for a murder when the murderer is unknown (Deuteronomy 21:4). Ritual slaughtering is accomplished by severing the carotid arteries, trachea, and esophagus in the neck (*Chullin* 18b). Maimonides' commentary on the Talmud (*Chullin* 2:1) speaks of the pulsating vessels in the neck (i.e., carotids) adjacent to the windpipe.

NEWBORN—When a baby is born, the navel is tied and cut (*Tosefta Shabbat* 15:3). If the child does not cry or breathe, the placenta is rubbed over it and the baby will breathe and cry (*Shabbat* 134a). The prophet Ezekiel describes the handling of a newborn in biblical times, which includes cutting the navel, washing in water, salting, and swaddling (Ezekiel 16:4–5). All these functions may be carried out even on the Sabbath (*Shabbat* 129b).

Salting for cleansing and astringency was an indispensable part of the treatment of the newborn in antiquity.[1] In talmudic times, newborns were bathed in wine (*Tosefta Shabbat* 12:13). Swaddling or wrapping the newborn is known as *lafaf* (*Shabbat* 147b). The straightening of the baby's limbs by manipulation was also performed (*Shabbat* 22:6 and 147b). To rid the newborn of mucus in the mouth, the baby was induced to vomit (*Shabbat* 123a).

In ancient Egypt, the Israelite women went out to the fields to deliver their babies under apple trees. Angels from heaven came and cleansed and manipulated the newborn in the manner of the midwife (*Sotah* 11b), and bathed and anointed the baby (*Exodus Rabbah* 23:8). Either the angel or the mother cut the navel with a sharp stone (*Leviticus Rabbah* 5:1). In one town it was customary to smear the head of newborns with crushed spices so that insects not bite them (*Genesis Rabbah* 34:15). On the other hand, a rooster was once killed because it picked at the pulsating anterior fontanelle of a newborn, which is soft (*Menachot* 37a), thinking it was an insect (*Jerushalmi Eruvin* 10:26). Newborns were kept in small beds or cribs that could be rocked (*Genesis Rabbah* 53:10). Newborns were suckled at their mother's breast [*see* LACTATION].

A newborn with an imperforate anus should be rubbed with oil and the skin cut crosswise with a barley grain to make an orifice (*Shabbat* 134a). A newborn with esophageal atresia (literally: obstructed foodpipe) cannot survive; a baby with a perforated esophagus, however, can survive (*Niddah* 23b). All male infants are to be circumcised on the eighth day of life as a sign of the covenant between God and Abraham (Genesis 17:10–15) [*see* CIRCUMCISION]. Occasionally, newborns had their eyes painted with eye shadow and amulets hung around their necks by their mothers (*Kiddushin* 73b). An infant learns to speak after it eats wheat bread (*Sanhedrin* 70b). Infants develop "milk teeth" (*Kiddushin* 24b). During the time of the Temple, some priests fasted every Wednesday so that *askara* (diphtheria?) should not afflict young children (*Taanit* 27b).

---

1. F. Rosner (trans.), *Julius Preuss' Biblical and Talmudic Medicine* (Northvale, NJ: Jason Aronson, 1993) p. 402.

NOSE—The biblical term for nose is *af* (Psalms 115:6), plural *apayim* meaning "nostrils." The talmudic word for nose is *chotem*. The term *tarfa denechira*, or "membrane of the nose," is also used to denote nostrils (*Berachot* 55b). The nose determines the facial expression; hence a corpse can be identified if the nose is still intact on the face (*Yebamot* 16:3). The nostrils of an embryo are compared to two drippings of a fly close to each other (*Niddah* 25a). Poetically, the nose is compared to the tower of Lebanon (Song of Songs 7:5). *Govah af,* literally "nose in the air," refers to haughtiness (Psalms 10:4). Rabbi Gamliel was called "the nose man" (*Taanit* 29a).

The nasal secretion is called "the fluid of the nose" (*Tosefta Shabbat* 8:28), "that which comes out from the nose" (*Machshirin* 6:5), or "excrement of the nose" (*Baba Metzia* 107b). Nasal secretions neutralize a bad aroma (*Numbers Rabbah* 18:22). A small amount of nasal secretion is beneficial; a lot is harmful (*Baba Metzia* 107b). Dripping from the nostrils is a sign of the *raatan* illness (*Ketubot* 77b).

The nose is the organ of respiration. God breathes life into the nostrils (Genesis 2:7) and it remains until the soul departs (Job 27:3). The nose is also the organ of smell (*Berachot* 31b). Idols have noses but cannot smell (Psalms 115:6). A powerful aroma can revive a person who fainted (*Berachot* 43b). A woman feigning loss of smell was found to be a malingerer when a powerful aromatic plant was placed near her (*Baba Batra* 146a). In antiquity the nose was thought to be the organ of anger since an angry person fumes from the nostrils (Job 41:12). A *baal af,* literally "person with a nose," is someone who easily becomes angry (Proverbs 22:24). A hot-tempered person is called *ketzer apayim* (Proverbs 14:17). Bar Kappara dreamt that his nose fell off. The dream was interpreted to mean God removed His anger from him (*Berachot* 56b). The nose also counteracts the sleep-inducing property of the stomach, in that the nose awakens (*Berachot* 61b).

The Talmud portrays a number of defects and disorders of the nose. *Polypus* is said to be either a bad aroma from the mouth (*Tosefta Ketubot* 7:11) or the nose (*Ketubot* 77a), or a large abscess or nasal polyp (*Shabbat* 108b). Unwashed hands touching the nose may produce *polypus* (ibid.) A marriage can be dissolved if either spouse develops a polypus (*Ketubot* 7:10).

Nosebleeds are also described in the Bible and Talmud. Squeezing the nose can induce nose bleeding (Proverbs 30:33). A variety of folk remedies are prescribed "for blood that flows from the nostrils" (*Gittin* 69a). Such blood is ritually clean. The leprosy lesion called *baheret* inside the nose does not impart ritual uncleanness (*Negaim* 6:7). Blemishes of the nose such as *charum* (Leviticus 21:18) or flat-nosedness disqualify priests from Temple service (*Bechorot* 7:3). An animal with a perforated nose cannot be used for an offering in the Temple (*Bechorot* 6:4). Nose rings for humans and animals are also described.[1] [*See also* FACE, LIPS, JAW, and FOREHEAD]

---

1. F. Rosner (trans.), *Julius Preuss' Biblical and Talmudic Medicine* (Northvale, NJ, Jason Aronson, 1993) pp. 295–297.

NUTS—Nuts are harmful to patients convalescing from illness (*Berachot* 57b), especially hazelnuts (*Jerushalmi Gittin* 7:48). Eating nuts may cause recurrence or aggravation of one's illness (*Berachot* 57b; *Abodah Zarah* 29a), although nut rinds are used to treat *raatan* (leprosy?) (*Ketubot* 77b; *Baba Metzia* 83b). It is also unhealthy to eat a lot of nuts on an empty stomach in the summer (*Chullin* 59a).

Nuts and roasted corn were favorite sweets among children (*Song of Songs Rabbah* 1:7). Nuts were cracked open for children (*Ruth Rabbah* 7:11) on the night of Passover to keep them awake (*Pesachim* 109a). A nutcracker (*Yebamot* 81b) or a smith's hammer (*Shabbat* 122b) were used to crack open nuts. Although nutshells are ordinarily refuse (*Shabbat* 89b; *Betzah* 2a), they were used to play games (*Eruvin* 104a), for gambling (*Sanhedrin* 25b), and even for fuel (*Shabbat* 29a). Shopkeepers gave children nuts to encourage their parents to shop there (*Baba Batra* 21b). Shopkeepers' balances were made of nuts (ibid., 89b). Children hollowed out nuts to measure sand or to make scales (*Chullin* 12b; *Kelim* 17:15). Nuts were imported from Perek (*Betzah* 3b; *Abodah Zarah* 74a; *Zevachim* 72b), Alexandria (*Abodah Zarah* 14a), and Greece (*Menachot* 63a).

"I went down to the garden of nuts" (Song of Songs 6:11) is interpreted to mean that the Israelites are compared to a nut tree in many different ways

(*Song of Songs Rabbah* 6:11:1). The nut tree is subject to the laws of *peah* (left over produce for the poor) (*Peah* 1:5). Ten nuts is the minimum for a poor man's tithe (*Eruvin* 29a). Shells and kernels of nuts are also subject to the laws of *Orlah* (*Orlah* 1:8) and the laws of the Sabbatical year (*Sheviit* 7:3). Skins are treated with gallnut to make parchment (*Megillah* 19a; *Gittin* 22a). Gallnut juice can be used as a type of ink (*Shabbat* 104b; *Gittin* 19a). A man once repaid a monetary debt with gallnuts (*Shevuot* 42a).

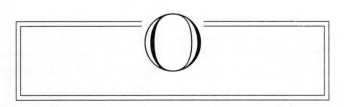

OBESITY—King Eglon was very obese (Judges 3:22). Several talmudic sages had very wide waists (*Baba Metzia* 83b) or were very fat (ibid., 86a). When one sage had his abdomen opened during surgery a basketful of fat was removed from him (ibid., 83a). Legend relates that a theriac to heal snakebites (*Song of Songs Rabbah* 4:5) was made from the excess fat of obese priests (*Baba Metzia* 83b). Obese elderly men gradually lose their axillary hair (*Nazir* 59a).

OIL—The tribe of Asher was blessed with oil (Deuteronomy 33:24), a symbol of lighting up the darkness (*Numbers Rabbah* 2:10). Oil is light unto the world (*Numbers Rabbah* 9:13). Pure olive oil (Exodus 27:20) was used for lighting lamps in the Temple (Numbers 8:2), as commanded by God (*Numbers Rabbah* 15:1–3; *Leviticus Rabbah* 31:1). The Torah is compared to oil: Just as oil gives life and light to the world (i.e., its use for foods and medicines and in industry), so too the words of Torah give life and

light to the world (*Deuteronomy Rabbah* 7:3). Just as oil makes the head and the body feel pleasant, so too the words of the Torah give life and light to the world (*Deuteronomy Rabbah* 7:3). Just as oil makes the head and the body feel pleasant; so too the words of the Torah (*Song of Songs Rabbah* 1:2:3). The ten tribes exported oil to Egypt and brought back foodstuffs (*Lamentations Rabbah* 4:20 and 5:1). Not only was oil used for foods, it was used for greasing utensils (*Demai* 1:3), for softening skin or leather articles such as hides (*Sheviit* 8:9; *Baba Metzia* 38b) or sandals (*Orlah* 2:13), for removing hair (*Megillah* 13a), to pour and rub on the abdomen for abdominal disorders (*Sanhedrin* 101a), for smearing on the place of tree pruning to prevent the sap from running out (*Abodah Zarah* 50b), for anointing bodies after bathing (*Eruvin* 91a), for soaking wicks so that they burn better (*Betzah* 32b), and to rub one's hands after a meal before saying Grace (*Berachot* 42a and 53b).

In the Temple service, oil was poured on the meal offering, mixed with flour (*Sanhedrin* 82), and smeared on wafers (*Zevachim* 91a); and used for the leper's purification (Leviticus 14:12), lamp kindling, and for anointing purposes (Exodus 27:20; *Sheviit* 8:2). Fine oils were donated for Temple service (*Shekalim* 4:3). Ritually unclean oil could not be exported but had to be burnt in the Holy Land (*Sheviit* 6:5). God showed Moses how to make the anointing oil (*Exodus Rabbah* 15:28). Many miracles occurred with anointing oil (*Leviticus Rabbah* 10:8). Moses anointed Aaron between the eyes during each of the seven days of consecration (*Numbers Rabbah* 12:15) by pouring the oil on his head (ibid., 8:9). Aaron carried the anointing oil in a small flask suspended from his girdle (ibid., 4:20). There are two oils of anointment: the oil of priesthood and the oil of kingship (*Song of Songs Rabbah* 1:3:2). Moses rejoiced when he saw the precious oil (Psalms 133:2) run down the beard of Aaron (*Leviticus Rabbah* 3:6; *Song of Songs Rabbah* 1:10:1). David rejoiced when he was anointed (Psalms 16:9) with the anointing oil (*Leviticus Rabbah* 26:9).

Oil is considered a produce (*Eruvin* 27b) and may be superior to wine (*Nazir* 31b). Olive trees were rented for their oil (*Demai* 6:5), olives were crushed to obtain their oil (*Terumot* 1:8), oil was bought and sold commercially (*Baba Batra* 87a), and was usually available from Pentecost onwards (*Gittin* 31b). Oil does not

cause fermentation (*Pesachim* 39b). Roses were preserved in oil (*Sheviit* 7:7). Life's necessities such as wines, oils, and flour should not be hoarded (*Baba Batra* 90b). Oil floats on top of all liquids (*Exodus Rabbah* 36:1; *Numbers Rabbah* 18:16). Oil drips and is not absorbed into the surface of the earth (*Sanhedrin* 104b).

Oil was derived from numerous sources including olives (*Shabbat* 23a, 24b, and 26a; *Horayot* 13a), balsam (*Shabbat* 25b), fish (ibid., 24b and 26a), gourds (ibid.), ricin trees (ibid., 20b and 21a), nuts (ibid., 24b), radishes (ibid.), roses (ibid., 111a), and sesame (ibid., 24b) and poppy seeds (ibid., 23a). To adulterate oil with poppy juice was considered evil (*Ecclesiastes Rabbah* 6:1 and 9:12:1). *Kik* oil is either cottonseed oil or oil from Jonah's *kikayon* tree (Jonah 4:6), probably the ricin tree (*Shabbat* 21a). Also described in the Talmud are oil mills (*Abodah Zarah* 75b), oil presses (*Shabbat* 19a; *Chagigah* 25a; *Abodah Zarah* 75a; *Arachin* 32a; *Niddah* 67a), oil storehouses (*Pesachim* 8a), oil cans (*Taanit* 25a), and oil-measuring cups (*Kelim* 25:3). Although oil is nourishing, it does not delight the soul like wine (Psalms 104:15; *Berachot* 35b). When mixed with mangold juice, oil heals a sore throat (*Berachot* 36a; *Tosefta Berachot* 8:2). Imperforate anus in a newborn is treated by rubbing the area with oil and incising the skin with a barley grain (*Shabbat* 134a). Wounds are treated by oil fomentation (Isaiah

1:6), especially oil of roses (*Shabbat* 14:4). Newborns were anointed with oil (*Kiddushin* 73b). Garlic root ground with oil and salt is good for a toothache (*Gittin* 69a). One rubs the head with oil to treat headache (*Tosefta Shabbat* 12:11). Oil embrocations were used to treat skin diseases (*Jerushalmi Sheviit* 1:38). *Tzafdina* is cured by an oil-containing remedy (*Yoma* 84a). Oil was applied between the eyelids to help close the eyes of a recently deceased person (*Shabbat* 151b).

Homiletically, a good name is better than precious oil (Ecclesiastes 7:1). The name of Bezalel was better than precious oil because the Bible proclaims his fame (*Exodus Rabbah* 48:1). The oil of Hezekiah, which burned in synagogues and Jewish Schools, was responsible for the destruction of the yoke of Sennacherib (*Sanhedrin* 94b). Legally, oil is one of seven liquids that render foodstuffs susceptible to ritual uncleanness (*Machshirim* 6:4). A husband must provide oil and other foods for his wife's sustenance when he is away (*Ketubot* 64b). A poor man applying for help at the threshing floor must be given no less than a quarter *log* of oil (*Peah* 8:5; *Eruvin* 29a). Oil left over in a lamp or dish is forbidden to be used on the Sabbath (*Betzah* 30b). Dough kneaded with wine, oil, or honey may not be suitable for Passover use because it is "rich bread" (*Pesachim* 36a). Wine and oil cannot be tithed for each other (*Bechorot* 54a; *Temurah* 5a). Barrels of oil belong to the finder (*Baba Metzia* 33b) but jars of oil have to be announced (ibid., 25a).

OIL EMBROCATIONS—Oil rubs or embrocations were very popular in the hot climate of the Middle East, particularly following bathing (*Shabbat* 41a). In fact, a bath without an oil rub was considered to be detrimental to one's health (*Shabbat* 40b). The oil was carried to the bathhouse in a flagon (*Jerushalmi Sheviit* 8:38) or in a Galilean pitcher (*Tosefta Kelim* 2:9). Oil was also sold in jugs (*Tosefta Kelim* 10:4). Sometimes, soft olives were sold at the bathhouse entrance (*Tosefta Niddah* 4:8), from which oil was squeezed directly onto the body. Some people poured oil on their heads at home, thus using their hair as an oil receptacle (*Tosefta Shabbat* 16:6). The oil bottle or pitcher was supported on a base (*Jerushalmi Shabbat* 3:6) and warmed on the fireplace (*Jerushalmi Sheviit* 8:38; *Tosefta Shabbat* 3:5). Glass bottles were to be avoided for fear of breakage (*Derech Eretz Rabbah* 10:1). Fragrant oils were used by people who could afford them (*Tosefta Berachot* 6:8; *Tosefta Sheviit* 6:13). An alternate form of oil embrocation was to pour oil on a marble floor and have the person roll on the floor (*Jerushalmi Sheviit* 38; *Tosefta Demai* 1:19; *Tosefta Shabbat* 16:14). Such a method, however, was not considered respectable (*Derech Eretz Rabbah* 10:2).

Oil rubs or embrocations were so widely used that even captives were given clothing, food, and embrocations (2 Chronicles 28:15). Newborn babies were anointed with oil (*Exodus Rabbah* 23:8). One-day-old infants had their small limbs rubbed with oil (*Shabbat* 77b). Even a finger was anointed with oil (*Eduyot* 4:6). Royal children were anointed every day, even on the Sabbath (*Shabbat* 128a). The abdomen was rubbed or massaged with oil to assist in moving one's bowels (*Berachot* 62a). One talmudic sage said that the warm water and oil with which his mother rubbed him during his youth stood him in good stead in his old age (*Chullin* 24b). Hands soiled by food are rubbed clean by oil (*Berachot* 53b). One may anoint a sore even on the Sabbath (*Shabbat* 53b). Rubbing oneself with contaminated oil can produce a rash on the face (*Sanhedrin* 101a). These are all therapeutic applications of oil embrocations. The deceased are anointed with oil and washed in preparation for burial (*Shabbat* 151a; *Yebamot* 74a).

Oil embrocations are also used for pleasure or delight, since oil and perfume gladden the heart (Proverbs 27:9) and the body derives benefit therefrom, whether or not the oil penetrates the body (*Berachot* 57b). At weddings among Babylonian Jews, it was customary to rub oil on the heads of learned men to honor them (*Ketubot* 17b). Although oil is the most commonly used substance, wine and vin-

egar embrocations are also described (*Jerushalmi Maaser Sheni* 2:53). Malodorous perspiration was neutralized with wine vinegar (*Ketubot* 75a). Ordinarily, however, wine and vinegar should not be used for embrocations since they are better used for drinking and cooking (*Sheviit* 8:2). The most commonly used oil for embrocations is olive oil. One can also press olives directly against the body and then rub widely (*Maaserot* 4:1). Precious oils were proudly shown by King Hezekiah to his guests (Isaiah 39:2).

Only during periods of mourning, when all physical comforts are prohibited, are oil embrocations not used (2 Samuel 14:2). Thus, King David (2 Samuel 12:20) and Daniel (Daniel 10:2–3) omitted oil rubs when they were in mourning. Anointing oneself on the Day of Atonement is prohibited (*Shabbat* 86a; *Yoma* 8:1) because one is obligated to afflict oneself on that day by abstaining from food and drink, sex, wearing shoes, and embrocations (Numbers 29:7). So, too, are embrocations prohibited on other fast days such as the Ninth Day of Av (*Tosefta Taanit* 4:1), during the mourning period for a close relative (*Taanit* 13b), as well as in times of great calamity (*Taanit* 1:5).

Holy anointing oil, as used in the Temple, was forbidden to be used for profane purposes (Exodus 30:32) including the anointing of priests or kings. The Tabernacle (Leviticus 8:10) and the Temple vessels were consecrated by anointing oil (*Shevuot* 15a). Anointing with the oil of Heave Offering was also prohibited (*Yebamot* 71a; *Shabbat* 86a; *Niddah* 32a). High priests and kings were anointed with the oil that Moses prepared (Exodus 30:31) in the wilderness (*Horayot* 11b; *Makkot* 11a) at God's behest (*Exodus Rabbah* 15:28). Miracles occurred with this anointing oil that Moses made (*Leviticus Rabbah* 10:8), which was later hidden by Josiah (*Keritot* 5b) and was compared to the dew of Hermon (*Numbers Rabbah* 18:9). [*See also* BATHING]

OLD AGE—At age sixty years one is mature, and at seventy one is hoary; eighty is a sign of added strength and at ninety one is stooped over (*Avot* 5:21). The hoary head is a sign of glory (ibid., 6:8). One must rise for a hoary man (Leviticus 19:32) and respect old men (*Exodus Rabbah* 31:16). Abraham, Joshua, and David were crowned with old age and an abundance of days (*Genesis Rabbah* 69:6). Abraham requested the appearance of old age (*Genesis Rabbah* 65:9) because until Abraham, old and young looked alike (*Baba Metzia* 87a). One's conduct in youth influences how we act in old age (*Genesis Rabbah* 97:1). When a learned man grows old, all flock around him to learn Torah from him (*Deuteronomy Rabbah* 6:3).

In old age, various body organs do not function well (*Leviticus Rabbah* 18:1). Old people may have difficulty in walking (*Chagigah* 2a). In old age, the lips droop, sleep is light and easily disturbed, mental faculties are diminished, one's countenance darkens, strength weakens, the lip bones become more prominent (*Shabbat* 151b–152b), the sense of taste decreases (2 Samuel 19:36), tremors develop (*Chullin* 24b), and axillary hair falls out (*Nazir* 59a). Hearing also decreases in old age (*Shabbat* 152a; *Leviticus Rabbah* 18:1). Barzilai at age eighty could not hear men and women singers (2 Samuel 19:36). Vision is also affected by aging. Excessive crying in the elderly is harmful to vision (*Shabbat* 151a). One talmudic sage had very bushy eyebrows when he became old and they had to be lifted with pincers (*Baba Kamma* 117a). When Isaac was 123 years old (Genesis 27:1), Eli the priest 98 years old (1 Samuel 3:2; 4:15), and Jacob 147 years old (Genesis 48:10), their eyes dimmed and they could not see. Achiya was old when he lost his vision (1 Kings 14:4). Moses is the exception; at age 120 years, his eyes did not dim and his strength did not wane (Deuteronomy 34:7). In towns with hills and valleys, people age prematurely (*Eruvin* 56a). Old age is a particularly dangerous time of life (*Chullin* 21a). The Bible describes old age (Ecclesiastes 11:9 and 12:2) and it is allegorically interpreted (*Ecclesiastes Rabbah* 12:2). When King David became old, he was not warmed even by many layers of clothing (1 Kings 1:1). [*See also* LIFE, LONGEVITY, and HOARY]

OLIVES—Medically, ashes from burned and pulverized stones of unripe olives are applied to scorbutic gums to heal them (*Yoma* 84a). Olive leaves are part of a remedy for plethora (*Gittin* 68b). Frequent consumption of olives makes one forget one's studies, yet the consumption of olive oil has the opposite effect (*Horayot* 13b). Olive oil is used for lighting lamps (*Jerushalmi Berachot* 4:7), as a gargle for pain in the throat (*Berachot* 36a), for embrocations (*Maaserot* 4:1), and for the healing of leprous skin lesions (*Gittin* 86a). Oil of unripe olives rubbed on the skin is soothing (*Sanhedrin* 24a), serves as a depilatory, and smoothes the skin (*Pesachim* 25b and 43a). Olive oil is an essential element for human living (*Sirach* 39:26) and is used in cooking (*Shabbat* 2:2).

Olive trees yield olives for food, olives for drying, and olives for oil that burns brighter than all other oils (*Numbers Rabbah* 8:9). Olives are a relish (*Eruvin* 29a). Olives are picked or plucked (*Baba Batra* 126a; *Yebamot* 116b; *Eduyot* 1:12) during one of the three periods of olive gathering (*Menachot* 86a). Olives are picked in clusters (*Abodah Zarah* 75b) into olive baskets (*Mikvaot* 7:3) from the olive trees (*Peah* 1:7 and 7:1; *Pesachim* 53a; *Baba Batra* 80a). Some olives are pickled

or preserved (*Terumot* 2:6) in jars (*Yebamot* 15b) or barrels (*Baba Metzia* 23b; *Eduyot* 4:6), sometimes with their leaves (*Uktzin* 2:1). Olives are sold (*Demai* 6:6), as is olive wood (*Rosh Hashanah* 22b). Some olives are incorporated into olive cakes (*Abodah Zarah* 39b). Olive presses and olive crushers extract the oil from olives (*Sheviit* 8:6; *Baba Metzia* 117b; *Baba Batra* 28a and 172a; *Chullin* 14b). Olive presses are sold with their accessories (*Baba Batra* 67b). The refuse after the oil has been extracted is discarded (*Baba Batra* 17b). So, too, are olive stones or kernels discarded (*Abodah Zarah* 40b). The Talmud also mentions wild olives (*Baba Metzia* 105a), heaps of olives (*Sanhedrin* 11a), and the olive-boiler's cauldron (*Eduyot* 7:8).

Homiletically, Israel is likened to olives from an olive tree (*Exodus Rabbah* 36:1). The olive tree is said to have brought light to the world in the days of Noah (*Leviticus Rabbah* 31:10). The size of an olive is a legal measure in Judaism for a variety of laws (*Berachot* 39a; *Kelim* 17:8; *Tohorot* 3:4; etc.).

ONANISM—Onan spilled his semen on the ground to avoid impregnating his wife (Genesis 38:9). His act was characterized as "threshing within and winnowing without" (*Yebamot* 34b) and as "ploughing in the garden and pouring out on manure piles" (*Genesis Rabbah* 85:4) in that he practiced coitus interruptus. Onan's brother Er also practiced coitus interruptus and was condemned for it (*Yebamot* 34b). God Himself objects to onanism (Genesis 38:10). Those who practice onanism through external contact (i.e., masturbation) are condemned (*Niddah* 13b). [*See also* MASTURBATION and CONTRACEPTION]

ONIONS—The Jews bemoaned the absence of onions in the desert (Numbers 11:5). Onions are a food staple (*Pesachim* 114a) and are eaten as a vegetable (*Betzah* 25b). He who is easily satisfied is content with an onion (*Pesachim* 114a). One can roast onions (*Shabbat* 19b) and serve them as a relish for bread (*Eruvin* 29a). Medically, onions have aphrodisiac qualities (*Yoma* 18a) and stimulate profuse salivation (*Yebamot* 106a). Onions can cause menstrual bleeding in some women (*Niddah* 63b), although large Persian onions boiled in wine were used to treat abnormal vaginal bleeding (*Shabbat* 110 a–b). Onion peels were applied on wounds (*Tosefta Shabbat* 5:3–4). One is warned against eating peeled onions left unattended overnight (*Niddah* 17a). One should not eat onions after bloodletting (*Abodah Zarah* 29a) because one may faint (*Taanit* 25a). Onions are injurious to the stomach (or heart);

only the wild (Cyprus) onion is healthy for the heart (*Nedarim* 26b and 66a).

Onion seeds (*Terumot* 9:6) are planted in rows (*Kilayim* 3:5–6). Leeks should be grown separately from onions (*Baba Batra* 25a). Small and large onions (*Terumot* 2:5), seedless onions (*Sheviit* 2:9; *Rosh Hashanah* 14a), and summer onions (*Sheviit* 5:4) are harvested and heaped up (*Maaserot* 1:6). They are sold by the bunch (*Peah* 6:10) or by weight (*Arachin* 19a). While the onions grow, their leaves become dark green or blackish (*Sheviit* 6:3; *Nedarim* 58a). Onions have three skins; the innermost one is edible together with the onion (*Chullin* 119b; *Uktzin* 2:4). Onions are subject to the law of corners (*Peah* 6:10; *Niddah* 50a). Onion roots can contract and impart ritual uncleanness (*Uktzin* 1:3). The expression "eat onions (*batzel*) and dwell in the protection (*beztel*) of one's house" (*Pesachim* 114a) means: Do not overspend on food to be able to afford one's house.

OPHTHALMOLOGIST—Tobit traveled to physicians because of corneal erosions but they could not help him (Tobit 2:10). Patients pay their eye doctors even if their eye ailments cannot be healed (*Ketubot* 105a). An ophthalmologist prescribed an eye salve for a woman whose eyelashes fell out as a result of excessive crying (*Lamentations Rabbah* 2:11). The Midrash describes a patient whose eye was removed (*Leviticus Rabbah* 5:6). [*See also* PHYSICIAN and SURGEON]

ORGAN TRANSPLANTS—Organ transplants are sanctioned by most rabbinic decisors because of the overriding consideration of saving the life of the recipient.[1] Biblical, talmudic, and other sources respond to the many Jewish moral and legal questions involved in organ transplantation. In regard to the donor, there are biblical prohibitions against desecrating the dead, deriving benefit from the dead, and delaying the burial of the dead that need to be considered. Furthermore, is consent needed from the deceased or the next of kin? Regarding the recipient, what happens to the old organ if it is removed? Does it require burial or may it be discarded? Who is the "owner" of the transplanted organ, the donor or the recipient? Is the recipient allowed or obligated to risk endangering his life from the surgery to receive an organ transplant? How does one choose the recipient when a scarce organ becomes available? Is it a *mitzvah* or meritorious act to donate one or more organs? Is a live donor allowed or obligated to give up a "spare" organ to save another person's life? These and other questions are answered in lengthy discourses in the Jewish medical ethical literature.[2, 3, 3, 4, 5, 6]

1. F. Rosner, *Modern Medicine and Jewish Ethics,* 2nd ed. (Hoboken, NJ, and New York: Ktav and Yeshiva University Press, 1991), pp. 279–299.
2. N. L. Rabinovitch, "What Is the Halakhah for Organ Transplants?" in *Jewish Bioethics,* F. Rosner and J. D. Bleich, eds. (New York: Hebrew Publishing Co., 1979), pp, 351–357.
3. J. D. Bleich, *Judaism and Healing* (New York: Ktav, 1981), pp. 129–133.
4. Y. Weiner, *Ye Shall Surely Heal* (Jerusalem: Jerusalem Center for Research, 1995), pp. 135–144.
5. I. Jakobovits, *Jewish Medical Ethics* (New York: Bloch, 1975), pp. 285–291.
6. E. N. Dorff, *The Jewish Law Annual,* vol. 12 (Boston: Harwood Academic Publishers, 1997), pp. 65–114.

OVEREATING—People are advised to enjoy meals but to not indulge excessively (*Gittin* 70a). One should eat a third, drink a third, and leave a third empty (ibid.). Overeating or gorging oneself with food may lead to the illness called *achilu* (*Gittin* 70a). Excessive eating and drinking can cause pollution (*Kiddushin* 2b). More people die from overeating than from starvation (*Shabbat* 33a). Eating meat excessively may lead to diarrhea (*Shekalim* 5:1–2). The voracious eating of quail meat by the Jews in the desert resulted in many deaths (Numbers 11:33). Drunkards and gluttons come to poverty (Proverbs 23:21). The rebellious son is usually a glutton and a drunkard (Deuteronomy 21:20). Gluttons used to induce vomiting after a big meal in order to be able to eat more, a practice prohibited by the talmudic sages (*Shabbat* 147b). [*See also* OBESITY]

OXEN—Although the Bible and Talmud are replete with references to oxen, few have medical connotations. An ox with a toothache drank a whole barrel of beer and was relieved of its pain (*Baba Kamma* 35a). An ox with no teeth could not feed itself properly and died (*Baba Metzia* 42b). The fat of an executed ox was used to heal a wound (*Pesachim* 24b). Nebuchadnezzar's madness was manifested by his eating grass like oxen (Daniel 4:29). In the desert after the Exodus from Egypt, the Jews slaughtered oxen as offerings and for food (Leviticus 17: 3–7). The Talmud speaks of a deaf ox, a blind ox, and a small ox (*Baba Kamma* 54b). An ox is said to have a large belly, large hoofs, a large head, and a long tail (*Chullin* 60a).

Female breeding cattle in Alexandria had their wombs removed before being exported to prevent their propagation abroad (*Bechorot* 28a). Although cattle are fit for human consumption (i.e., kosher) because they chew their cud and have cloven hoofs (Deuteronomy 14:6), their internal organs must be examined after ritual slaughtering to be sure they did not suffer from a serious illness or defect (*Chullin* 46a–b) [*see* ANIMALS, DEFECTS and CATTLE].

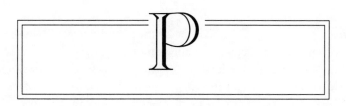

PAIN—The worst type of pain is heart pain, which is characterized as intolerable (*Shabbat* 11a). Bladder stones can produce excruciating pain (*Baba Metzia* 85a). The pain of defloration is vividly described (*Ketubot* 39b). Venesection can also produce pain (*Moed Katan* 28a). Abdominal pain may herald the monthly onset of menses (*Niddah* 9:8). The abdominal pain of gastrointestinal ailments can serve as an atonement for one's sins (*Eruvin* 41b). Job complained of bone pain at night (Job 30:17). Certain depilatory pastes cause pain when they are removed together with the hair (*Moed Katan* 1:7). Bodies are said to experience pain in the grave (*Eruvin* 47b) [*See* GRAVE].

Therapeutically, pain in the ear is treated with kidney juice or other remedies (*Abodah Zarah* 28b). For pain in the chest, sucking goat's milk directly from the udder is permitted even on the Sabbath (*Ketubot* 60a). The antidote for pain in the head, throat, bowels, bones, or throughout the body is Torah study (*Eruvin* 54a). [*See also* HEADACHE].

PALATE—The palate is an organ of speech and taste. Fruit tastes sweet to the palate (Song of Songs 2:3). Job asks, "Does not the palate taste food?" (Job 12:11) The poet says that "My palate speaks the truth" (Proverbs 8:7). In extreme thirst, the tongue may cleave to the palate (Lamentations 4:4). If one remains silent, the tongue may also cleave to the palate (Job 29:10). The Arabs rub the palate of newborns with a chewed date.[1] The Talmud asserts that the consumption of palates of animals leads to hemorrhoids (*Berachot* 55a), especially if the palates are unsalted (*Shabbat* 81a). The pain of defloration was once described "like hard bread on the palate" (*Ketubot* 39b).

---

1. F. Rosner, *Julius Preuss' Biblical and Talmudic Medicine* (Northvale, NJ: Jason Aronson, 1993), p. 88.

PALLOR—Pallor can occur from fear or fright (Jeremiah 30:61), from hunger (*Ruth Rabbah* 3:6), or from sickness as in the case of the suspected adulteress [*see* SOTAH] (*Numbers Rabbah* 9:21). Through fasting, one's blood becomes diminished (*Berachot* 17a). If the fasting is of long duration, the teeth become black and the face pale (*Nazir* 52b). The pallor or livid color of a corpse contrasts with the bright red of a live person (*Ketubot* 103b; *Abodah Zarah* 20b). Pallor in a newborn requires postponement of circumcision. [*See also* YERAKON and CIRCUMCISION]

PARALYSIS—Breaking the neck of an animal causes paralysis (*Chullin* 113a). Alcimus became paralyzed before he died of apoplexy (1 Maccabees 9:55). Philapator was also paralyzed and aphasic as a result of divine punishment (3 Maccabees 2:22). Nabal became drunk at a feast, "became as a stone," and died (1 Samuel 25:38). The phrase "became as a stone" may refer to paralysis or to coma.[1] The Talmud relates that he who feigns an illness such as lameness or paralysis will actually suffer from it (*Peah* 8:9; *Bechorot* 45b).

Several instances of hand "paralysis" or incapacity are discussed by Preuss including the cases of Eleazar (2 Samuel 23:10), Benjaminite soldiers (Judges 20:16), Ehud (Judges 3:15), and Jeroboam (1 Kings 13:4).

---

1. F. Rosner (trans.), *Julius Preuss' Biblical and Talmudic Medicine* (Northvale, NJ: Jason Aronson, 1993), pp. 308–310.

PEAS—Peas are consumed at mealtime as a food staple (*Yoma* 83b). Legumes including peas are served to guests (*Tosefta Peah* 4:8). The poor must be given food for three Sabbath meals including oil, peas, and fish (*Peah* 8:7). Peas alone are inadequate (*Ketubot* 67b). A man who does not live with his wife must provide her with sustenance including peas (or beans) (*Ketubot* 5:8). Fruit was stored in pea stalks (*Eruvin* 87b).

PENIS—The common biblical term for the male genitalia is *ervah*, meaning "shame" or "nakedness" (Leviticus 18:6ff.). Rarely the word *mevush* is used (Deuteronomy 25:11). The Talmud uses the euphemism *panin shel matah*, meaning "lower face" (*Shabbat* 48a). It is forbidden to expose one's genitalia (Genesis 9:22ff.; Exodus 28:42 and 20:23; Ezekiel 22:10; Habakkuk 2:15). The biblical term for penis is *basar*, meaning "flesh" (Genesis 17:13; Ezekiel 16:26). The talmudic terms are *ever*, meaning "organ" (*Baba Metzia* 84a); *etzba*, meaning "finger" (*Pesachim* 112a; *gid*, meaning "tendon" or "nerve"; *amma*, meaning "canal" (*Shabbat* 108b); and *shamash*, meaning "to serve" (*Niddah* 60b). The glans penis is called *rosh hageviya* (*Kiddushin* 25a; *Negaim* 6:7). This term also refers to the penis itself (*Nedarim* 32b). The corona is called *atara*, meaning "crown" (*Shabbat* 137a). In antiquity, the penis was used for purposes of heathen cults (1 Kings 15:13; 2 Chronicles 15:16; Ezekiel 16:17, *Sanhedrin* 65b and 105a; *Abodah Zarah* 44a).

The Bible cites a defect called *kerut shofcha* (Deuteronomy 23:2), which refers either to a man whose penis is "cut into" (hypospadias or epispadias) or "cut off" (*Yebamot* 70a and 76a). Men with the former defect may urinate from the normal urethral opening (if they have one) as well as the abnormal opening on the shaft of the penis (*Yebamot* 76a). Since the sperm of such a man does not "shoot out like an arrow," he may be incapable of procreation (*Tosefta Yebamot* 10:4). One can induce ejaculation to see whether the sperm flows from the normal or abnormal urethral opening (*Yebamot* 76a). A type of plastic surgical repair for such a "hole" in the penis is described (ibid.; *Jerushalmi Yebamot* 8:9). Other defects and various abnormalities of the penis, including duplication of the glans, fissures, perforations, and fistulas (*Yebamot* 75b–76a); a giant penis (*Bechorot* 39b and 44b), and blood from the urethra (*Niddah* 56a) are discussed in the Talmud.

A man whose penis is pierced or cut off may not marry an Israelite woman (Deuteronomy 23:2). His semen flow is sluggish (*Chullin* 48a). The penis can become entangled in the woman's pubic hair during sexual intercourse (*Gittin* 6b; *Sanhedrin* 21a). Holding the penis during urination is condemned (*Niddah* 13a, 16b and 43a). A man once died of a bee sting on the penis (*Moed Katan* 17a). [*See also* TESTICLES, SCROTUM, SPERM, and CIRCUMCISION]

PEPPER—Peppers exist in several varieties including green pepper (*Yoma* 81b), dry pepper (*Shabbat* 50b), long peppers (*Pesachim* 42b; *Megilliah* 7b), and pepper from Nazareth (*Ecclesiastes Rabbah* 2:8:2). Black pepper and white pepper are sweetening condiments (*Shabbat* 90a). Pepper is ground in a pepper mill (*Betzah* 23a; *Eduyot* 3:12), which consists of three separate parts (*Betzah* 23b). The pepper tree's (*Sukkah* 35a) wood and fruit taste alike (*Yoma* 81b). Hedge mustard is used as a substitute for pepper when the latter is not available (*Eruvin* 28b). A merchant once had two hundred camels laden with pepper (*Lamentations Rabbah* 1:1:2).

Medically, chewing pepper improves a bad mouth odor (*Shabbat* 65a and 90a; *Ketubot* 75a) although in some women, this can cause vaginal bleeding (*Niddah* 63b). Long peppers in wine are a remedy for pain in the abdomen (*Leviticus Rabbah* 37:2; *Gittin* 69b) and beneficial for the whole body (*Pesachim* 42b). A mixture of wine, honey, and pepper known as *anomalin* is a cooling drink used in the bathhouse and is also a delicacy served to one's guests (*Abodah Zarah* 30a). Pepper powder was also used as a soap-like material (*Shabbat* 50a).

PERFUME—Perfumes were widely used in antiquity. Miriam, daughter of Nakdimon, spent five hundred gold diners daily on her store of perfumes (*Lamentations Rabbah* 1:16:48). One's beloved carried a bundle of myrrh between her breasts (Song of Songs 1:13). The daughters of Israel used perfume and spices to gladden their husbands all forty years in the wilderness (*Song of Songs Rabbah* 4:14:1). Various types of perfume are described in the Talmud (*Shabbat* 90a). Perfumes were added to flasks of spikenard oil (*Shabbat* 62b). This expensive perfumed spikenard oil (*Tosefta Demai* 1 :26) was not used after the destruction of the Temple, as a sign of national mourning (*Tosefta Sotah* 15:9). The fragrant aroma of the spikenard oil could be appreciated even in garbage dumps (*Sanhedrin* 108a). Spices can be placed on a fire to produce a good smell and for perfuming clothes (*Betzah* 22b).

Perfumed beads were worn as necklaces or suspended from the neck in a small gold or silver container (Maimonides' Commentary on *Sanhedrin* 108a). The spikenard oil was stored in a glass bottle (*Tosefta Shabbat* 8:20) whose neck sometimes broke off (*Kelim* 30:4). When the bottle was opened, the aroma escaped (*Abodah Zarah* 35b). Fragrant oils were also used for embrocations (*Tosefta Sheviit* 6:13), especially after a bath (*Tosefta Berachot* 6:8).

Another fragrant aroma was that of the frankincense of the Temple. It was prohibited for anyone to prepare it for profane purposes (Exodus 30:34–38). The house of Abtinas were experts in its preparation and closely guarded the secret. They forbade their women from using perfumes so as to make people suspect the profane use of incense (*Yoma* 3:11; *Tosefta Yoma* 2:6; *Jerushalmi Yoma* 3:41). The incense to be burned on the Altar was prepared by a *rokeach* or perfume maker (Exodus 30: 35)—usually if not exclusively, a priest (1 Chronicles 9:30: Nehemiah 3:8). Maids may have helped prepare perfume for royalty (I Samuel 8:13).

Women use perfume but men do not because man was created from earth whereas woman was created from Adam's rib (*Genesis Rabbah* 17:8). It is not only inappropriate for a man to use perfume (*Tosefta Berachot* 6:5) but it is offensive for him to do so (*Berachot* 43b). A man is obligated to provide his wife with money for her perfume basket (*Niddah* 66b; *Ketubot* 66b). On the Sabbath, some men used perfumes (*Soferim* 20:1).

Perfume dealers (*Yebamot* 24b; *Kiddushin* 92a) peddled their wares directly in private homes (*Baba Kamma* 82a) or in perfume stores or bazaars (*Tosefta Berachot* 6:8). These spice peddlers also sold fruit (*Masserot* 2:3), although women first asked for perfumes (*Avot de Rabbi Nathan* 18:1). Many husbands were upset with these peddlers because they enticed women to immoral behavior (*Yebamot* 63a). Whole companies of perfume sellers are described (*Baba Metzia* 81a). The Talmud states that the world cannot exist without perfume dealers (*Pesachim* 65a; *Kiddushin* 82b). Anyone who walks into a perfume shop comes out with a pleasant aroma (Proverbs 13:20). Perfume makers use a small mortar with a pestle called *kera* (*Shabbat* 81a) or *regel* (*Jerushalmi Shabbat* 8:11).

Smelling the aroma of a woman's perfume is forbidden (*Shabbat* 62b). The maidens of King Ahasuerus were perfumed for months before being presented to the king (Esther 2:12–13). King Asa's grave was filled with different types of sweet spices (2 Chronicles 16:14), so called because they excite one's passions. Prostitutes placed myrrh and balsam in their shoes, kicking their feet and spraying it on young men passing by who were thereby instilled with passionate desire (*Shabbat* 62b; *Yoma* 9b). Such perfume was also stored in a chicken's stomach (*Lamentations Rabbah* 4:18; *Leviticus Rabbah* 16:11) and went through the young men like the poison of a snake (ibid.). [*See also* COSMETICS and OIL EMBROCATIONS]

PERSPIRATION—Perspiration is a good prognostic sign for sick patients (*Berachot* 57b; *Genesis Rabbah* 20:20). Three types of perspiration are good for the body: the sweat of illness, that of toil, and that of bathing. The sweat of illness heals and nothing compares to the sweat of a bath (*Avot de Rabbi Nathan* 41:4). During baths in the Orient, one drinks water to compensate for perspiration losses (*Shabbat* 40b). He who perspires first leaves the bath first (*Leviticus Rabbah* 14:9). In spite of perspiration in a bath the body does not lose weight (*Genesis Rabbah* 4:4). One sweats a lot in the groin and in the axilla (*Zevachim* 19a). Heavy work to develop a sweat cures the shivers of a chill (*Gittin* 67b). People may become faint during sweating and require time for recuperation (*Shabbat* 9b).

Human perspiration was considered poisonous (*Jerushalmi Terumot* 8:45), except for the sweat from the face. Malodorous perspiration can be neutralized with wine vinegar (*Ketubot* 75a). Hairs may stick together due to perspiration (*Mikvaot* 9:2–3). Profuse sweating may accompany the delirium tremens of alcohol withdrawal [*see* KORDIAKOS]. Absorbent tampons used during cohabitation to prevent conception shrink with perspiration (*Niddah* 3a). Excessive perspiration may disqualify a priest from serving in the Temple (*Ketubot* 75a).

PHYSICIAN—The Hebrew terms for "physician," are *rofe* (plural *rofim*) and *asya*. In the Talmud, these terms do not denote a profession in the modern sense. Rather, *rofe* means "healer," not necessarily a physician. On the other hand, the expression *rofe umman* (*Sanhedrin* 91a; *Tosefta Makkot* 2.5; *Tosefta Baba Kamma* 6:27; and elsewhere) probably refers to either a learned physician or a certified physician.[1]

The term *rofim* is first used in the Bible to denote the Egyptian servants of Joseph who embalmed his father, Jacob (Genesis 50:2). Some of the prophets used the word *rofe* to mean the physician as medical practitioner. Jeremiah thought it unbelievable that no physician lived in Gilead (Jeremiah 8:22). King Asa consulted physicians regarding the disease in his feet, thought to be gout (2 Chronicles 16:12). Job called his friends "physicians of no value," i.e., physicians of vanity (Job 13:4).

The Midrash uses the term in many proverbs: "Physician, physician, heal thine own limp" (*Genesis Rabbah* 23:4); "Honor thy physician before thou hast need to him" (*Exodus Rabbah* 26:7); "Shame on the province whose physician suffers from gout" (*Leviticus Rabbah* 5:6); "A gate that is not opened for good deeds will be opened for the physician," i.e., charity and beneficence keep the doctor away (*Numbers Rabbah* 9:13; *Song of Songs Rabbah* 6:11:1).

Physicians are cited in parables in many places in the Midrash (*Exodus Rabbah* 30:22, 46:4, and 48:5; *Leviti-*

cus Rabbah 13:2; *Numbers Rabbah* 20:14; *Song of Songs Rabbah* 2:3:2; *Lamentations Rabbah* 1:16:51) and Talmud (*Semachot* 14:21). A single example follows as an illustration: If a man had a seizure, came under the care of his physician, and died, he only died because he was in idleness; i.e., work leads to prosperity but idleness leads to death (*Avot de Rabbi Nathan* 11:1).

There are also numerous references to God the Healer throughout the Bible (Psalms 6:3, 41:5, 103:3, and 147:3; Numbers 12:13; Deuteronomy 32:39; Jeremiah 3:22 and 17:14; Isaiah 57:18; etc.). God caused drugs to spring forth from the earth, and with them the physician heals all wounds (*Genesis Rabbah* 10:6). A physician of flesh and blood wounds with a knife and heals with a plaster but the Holy One, blessed be He, heals with the very thing with which He wounds (*Leviticus Rabbah* 18:5, based on Jeremiah 30:17). A physician in Sepphoris possessed the secret of the Ineffable Name (*Ecclesiastes Rabbah* 3:11:3).

A physician applies bandages to the head, hands, and feet of a man who falls from the roof and whose body is bruised (*Exodus Rabbah* 27:9). A qualified physician treats patients with epilepsy (*Leviticus Rabbah* 26:5). If a person was bitten by a snake, one may call for him a physician from a distant place even on the Sabbath, since all Sabbath restrictions are set aside in the case of possible danger to human life (*Yoma* 83b). Physicians compound remedies with which they heal snake bites (*Song of Songs Rabbah* 4:5:1). These statements are self-explanatory.

Other assertions seem to have no scientific validity. A physician can diagnose an intestinal ailment by giving a patient a hard-boiled egg to eat and watching it pass out (*Nedarim* 50a). A physician said that hard pumpkins are injurious to the sick (ibid., 49a). A physician can cure a bodily defect in a betrothed woman (*Ketubot* 74b) or man (ibid., 75a). For pain in the heart, the physicians recommended sucking hot milk from a goat every morning (*Baba Kamma* 80a; *Temurah* 15b). Physicians cured a deathly ill Persian king with the milk of a lioness (Midrash Psalms 39:2).

The Talmud advises: He who has pain should seek a physician (*Baba Kamma* 85a). A physician from afar has a blind eye (or may blind an eye); i.e., he is little concerned about the fate of his patient (ibid.).

A patient pays the physician to cure an ailment without any guarantee that he will be healed (*Ketubot* 105a). A physician can paint the eye of his servant with an ointment and drill his teeth (*Kiddushin* 24b). A woman who wept all night until her eyelashes fell out was told by her physician: Paint your eyes with stibium and you will recover (*Lamentations Rabbah* 2:15). Once again, there seems to be no medical explanation for this epilation secondary to weeping nor for the cure suggested by the Midrash.

Physicians healed Rabbi Tzaddok who was near death from fasting (*Gittin* 56b). Expert physicians attended Rabbi Yochanan and Rabbi Abbahu (*Abodah Zarah* 28a). A doctor who can cure a hunchback (which is impossible) is considered a "great doctor" and can command large fees (*Sanhedrin* 91a). The sages consulted physicians regarding a woman who was aborting objects like red hairs and pieces of red rind (*Niddah* 22b). The physicians explained that she had an internal sore and was shedding the crust or scab. A physician is consulted in cases of claims for restitution for damages for bodily injuries (*Sanhedrin* 78a) and concerning the ability of a convicted criminal to tolerate disciplinary flogging (*Makkot* 3:11). A sick person is fed even on the Day of Atonement at the word of the physicians (*Yoma* 83a). Even if the patient says he does not need food, we listen to the physicians. Conversely, if the physician says the patient does not need it, whereas the patient says he needs it, we hearken to the patient because "the heart knoweth its own bitterness" (Proverbs 14:10). Physicians were consulted in a case where a man had a violent passion for a woman forbidden to him and his heart was consumed by his burning desire, thereby endangering his life (*Sanhedrin* 75a).

The Talmud discusses whether it is preferable for circumcision to be performed by an idolater or a Cuthean in a town where there is no Jewish physician (*Abodah Zarah* 26b–27a, *Menachot* 42a). The Talmud also discusses whether or not one is permitted to follow the advice of a heathen physician (*Abodah Zarah* 27a–28b).

There are specific individuals cited in the Talmud with the title "physician": Minyami, Theodos. Tobiya. Benjamin, Bar Gimte, Rabbi Ammi, and Rabbi Nathan. Minyami the physician said that any kind of fluid is bad for pain in the ear except the juice from kidneys (*Abodah Zarah* 28b). No modern medical concept supports such a statement. Theodos the physician said that no cow or pig leaves Alexandria of Egypt without its uterus being cut out to prevent it from reproducing (*Sanhedrin* 93a; *Bechorot* 28b). The Alexandrians maintained a monopoly on the excellent breed of cows and pigs they had, thus compelling buyers to come to Alexandria. Theodos the physician could also distinguish human from animal skeletons (*Nazir* 52a; *Tosefta Oholot* 4:2). Tobiya the physician is mentioned in the Talmud (*Rosh Hashanah* 1:7) but no medical pronouncement is attributed to him. The same is true of Rabbi Nathan the physician (*Pesachim* 52a).

Abaye described a salve for all pains. The ingredients are not specified. Rabba expounded the recipe in public in Mehoza, whereupon the family (or disciples) of Benjamin the physician tore their garments in despair, fearing their medical practice would diminish (*Shabbat* 133b). Competition among physicians in those days may have been keen. These disciples of Benjamin the physician were thought to be disbelievers in that they said, "Of what use are the rabbis to us?" (*Sanhedrin* 99b). The Jerusalem Talmud cites Bar Gimte the physician (*Betzah* 1:60) and Rabbi Ammi the physician (*Berachot* 2:4).

There are other individuals in the Talmud who certainly had medical expertise although they are not cited as "physicians." The most illustrious of these is Mar Samuel. Others include Rabbi Chiyya, who felt the pulse of his sick colleague (*Berachot* 5b); and Rabbi Ishmael and his disciples, who performed an autopsy on a female corpse. Mar Bar Rav Ashi performed plastic surgery on the penis (*Yebamot* 75b). Rabbi Chaninah was knowledgeable in healing remedies (*Yoma* 49a). Ben Achiya gave remedies to priests with intestinal ailments (*Shekalim* 5:1–2). Rab spent eighteen months with a shepherd to learn eye diseases of animals (*Sanhedrin* 5b). Rabbi Yochanan described a remedy for *tzafdina* that he had learned from a Roman woman (*Abodah Zarah* 28a). Although it is impossible to ascertain with certainty whether the above talmudic sages were physicians, they do demonstrate a considerable knowledge of medicine. [*See also* MAR SAMUEL]

1. F. Rosner (trans.), *Julius Preuss' Biblical and Talmudic Medicine* (Northvale, NJ: Jason Aronson, 1993), pp. 11–33.

PHYSICIANS' FEES—The biblical verse "and heal he shall heal" (Exodus 21:19) is rendered "and he shall pay the doctor's fee" by the Septuagint, the Targum, and the Vulgate.

Healing expenses are one of five items of compensation due by law to an injured party (*Baba Kamma* 8:1). Numerous Jewish sources speak of physicians' fees and compensation. Heirs who are obligated to provide medical care for their chronically ill mother can contract with a physician for an all-inclusive fee (*Ketubot* 52b). Whoever has pain in his eyes should pay the physician money in advance (ibid., 105a). A sectarian once threatened to kick a hunchback and strip him of his hump, to which the hunchback retorted, "If you could do that you would be called a great physician and command large fees" (*Sanhedrin* 91a). A similar statement was made by another hunchback to the same threat (*Genesis Rabbah* 61:7). When Vespasian had physicians feed Rabbi Tzaddok to restore the latter's health, his son said to him, "Father, give the physicians their reward in this world" (*Lamentations Rabbah* 1:5:31). A physician who heals for nothing is worth nothing (*Baba Kamma* 85a).

Yet, during talmudic times and even earlier, physicians, judges, teachers, and other public officials were prohibited from accepting fees for their services because they were to emulate God, who heals, judges, and teaches free of charge. If a judge took payment, his judgments were void (*Bechorot* 29a). The legal codes of Jacob ben Asher *(Tur, Yoreh Deah* 336) and Joseph Karo *(Shulchan Aruch, Yoreh Deah* 336:2) rule that a physician may only receive compensation for his trouble and loss of time during which he could earn a living by other means. This limitation on physician's fees in antiquity and the Middle Ages is discussed at length by Nachmanides (*Torat Ha Adam,* thirteenth century), Judah the Pious *(Sefer Chasidim #810,* thirteenth century), and Eshtori Haparchi *(Kaftor Vaferach,* ch. 44, fourteenth century).

In modern times, however, the concept of lost time has been reexamined by the rabbinic authorities since physicians no longer derive their income from other endeavors as they did in ancient times.[1] A physician nowadays is entitled to reasonable fees and compensation for his services. In talmudic times when physicians, rabbis, teachers, and judges served the community on a part-time basis only and had other occupations and trades, their compensation was limited to lost time and effort. Nowadays, however, when physicians have no other occupation, they can charge for their expert medical knowledge and receive full compensation.[2] Excessive fees are discouraged but are not prohibited if the patient agrees to the fee in advance. Indigent patients should be treated for reduced or no fees at all. These principles are applicable to both a salaried physician and a physician in private practice who charges fee-for-service.

---

1. F. Rosner and J. Widroff, "Physicians' Fees in Jewish Law," *Jewish Law Annual*, vol. 12 (1997), pp. 115–126.

2. F. Rosner (trans.), *Julius Preuss' Biblical and Talmudic Medicine* (Northvale, NJ: Jason Aronson, 1993), pp. 31–33.

PHYSICIANS' LIABILITY—A physician who unintentionally harms a patient during his caring for the patient is held blameless "because of the public good" (*Tosefta Gittin* 4:6). If physicians were held liable for every error, no one would practice medicine. This exceptional position of a physician not being held liable for honest mistakes does not preclude heavenly judgment, however (*Tosefta Baba Kamma* 6:17). Blamelessness in case of error only applies to well-trained and licensed physicians (*Shulchan Aruch, Yoreh Deah* 336). If a physician is negligent in the care of a patient he is liable (*Tosefta Baba Kamma* 9:11). Such a physician or medical practitioner who is a negligent bloodletter or circumcisor should be

dismissed from his position (*Baba Batra* 21b; *Shabbat* 133b).

If a patient dies of an oversight, inadvertently, while being treated, the physician, like any other person who kills accidentally, should be exiled to one of the cities of refuge (*Tosefta Makkot* 2:5) where he must stay until the death of the High Priest. The biblical admonition about "slaying with guile" (Exodus 21:14) specifically excludes a physician who accidentally causes the death of a patient, and a father, teacher, or court-appointed bailiff who deliberately inflicts corporal damage as discipline or punishment with a fatal outcome (*Yalkut*, Exodus 21:14) because they had no evil intentions (*Mechilta*, Exodus 21:14). The father who inadvertently slays his son, the teacher who beats his pupil, and the bailiff who flogs a sinner are all exempt from going into exile because they acted while performing their duty (Maimonides, *Rotzeach* 5:5–6). The same applies to a physician (*Shulchan Aruch, Yoreh Deah* 336:1). A physician is obviously not liable if the patient fails to follow instructions and is noncompliant with therapeutic recommendations (*Pesikta de Rav Kahana* 14).

In summary, Jewish law requires a physician to be well trained and licensed by the local authorities. An unlicensed physician is liable to pay compensation to the patient for unintentional errors or side effects. A negligent physician is obviously culpable even if he is licensed. However he is not liable for misjudgments or side effects or a bad outcome if he acted responsibly. Judaism protects the physician from undeserved liability but stresses that the physician recognize the limits of his or her abilities and demands that physicians consult with more experienced colleagues in situations of doubt.[1]

1. F. Rosner (trans.), *Julius Preuss' Biblical and Talmudic Medicine* (Northvale, NJ: Jason Aronson, 1993), pp. 27–31.

PHYSICIANS' LICENSE TO HEAL—In Jewish tradition, God is considered to be the Healer of the sick (Exodus 15:26). Nevertheless a physician is given specific Divine license to practice medicine[1] based on a biblical passage (Exodus 21:19) that the talmudic sages interpret as Divine authorization for a physician to heal the sick (*Baba Kamma* 85a). The biblical precept of restoring a lost object (Deuteronomy 22:2) includes the restoration of one's lost health. Thus, Maimonides considers healing to be a biblical mandate (*Mishnah Commentary, Nedarim* 4:4). A physician who refuses to care for a patient with resultant adverse consequences is guilty of transgressing the biblical prohibition against "standing idly by the blood of one's neighbor" (Leviticus 19:16). The saving of human life requires all biblical and rabbinic laws and rules

(except murder, idolatry, and forbidden sexual relations) to be waived for the overriding consideration of saving a human life. He who saves one life is as if he saved a whole world (*Sanhedrin* 37a). Jewish law also requires a physician to be well trained and licensed by the local authorities (*Shulchan Aruch, Yoreh Deah* 336). [*See also* PHYSICIANS' LIABILITY and PHYSICIANS' FEES]

1. F. Rosner, "Physician and Patient in Jewish Law," in *Medicine in the Bible and the Talmud*, 2nd ed. (Hoboken, NJ: Ktav and Yeshiva University Press, 1995), pp. 165–175.

PHYSICIANS' OATHS—The oldest Hebrew medical manuscript is ascribed to Asaph Judaeus, who lived no earlier than the third century and no later than the seventh. The deontologic sermon, or physicians' oath, that Asaph imposed on his pupils testifies to a high moral standard in the practice of medicine.[1] The physician's prayer attributed to Moses Maimonides was in fact written by Marcus Herz in Germany in 1783.[2] Other famous physicians' oaths or prayers that demonstrate deep piety and gratitude for Divine help are those of Judah Halevy,[3] Abraham Zacutus,[4] and Jacob Zahalon.[5] All recognize God as the ultimate healer of disease but also emphasize the ethical and moral responsibilities of the physician as a Divine agent in the alleviation of human suffering.

Pigeons–Placenta

1. F. Rosner, "The Oath of Asaph," in *Medicine in the Bible and the Talmud*, 2nd ed. (Hoboken, NJ: Ktav and Yeshiva University Press, 1995), pp. 182–187.
2. F. Rosner, "The physician's prayer attributed to Moses Maimonides," *Bulletin of the History of Medicine*, 41 (1967), pp. 440–454.
3. H. Freidenwald, *The Jews and Medicine*, vol. 1 (Baltimore; Johns Hopkins Press, 1944), pp. 27–30.
4. Ibid., pp. 295–321.
5. H. Savitz, "Jacob Zahalon and His Book *The Treasure of Life*," *New England Journal of Medicine*, 213 (1935), pp. 167–176.

PIGEONS—A paste of dough over a roast pigeon enhances its flavor (*Pesachim* 74b). Mushrooms and pigeons were eaten as dessert after meals (*Pesachim* 119b). Pigeon dung was used as an ingredient in certain medical therapies (*Gittin* 69b). After childbirth a woman brought young pigeons or turtledoves as offerings in the Temple (Leviticus 12:8). So, too, a Nazarite (*Numbers Rabbah* 10:25). Pigeons are qualified for sacrifice when small but not when fully grown. The reverse is true of turtledoves (*Chullin* 22a). Young turtledoves are subject to the law of sacrilege but not old pigeons (*Meilah* 12a). The Talmud describes pigeon holes (*Eruvin* 3a), pigeons with broken legs (*Chullin* 76b), and flying pigeons (*Niddah* 50b). People who train and race pigeons for wagers are considered gamblers (*Eruvin* 82a; *Rosh Hashanah* 22a) and are ineligible to be witnesses (*Eduyot* 2:7) or judges (*Sanhedrin* 24b).

Ladders are used to retrieve young pigeons from dovecotes (*Taanit* 28a). Young pigeons found within fifty feet of a cote belong to the owner of the cote (*Baba Batra* 23b). [*See also* DOVES; BIRDS, CHICKENS, and GEESE]

PLACENTA—The biblical term for placenta or afterbirth is *shilyah* (Deuteronomy 28:57). One talmudic sage compares the placenta to the stomach of a hen out of which the small bowel (i.e., the umbilical cord) issues (*Niddah* 26a). Other sages say that the placenta first resembles a thread of the woof and later resembles a lupine. It is hollow like a trumpet (ibid.). There is no placenta without an accompanying fetus. Therefore, if a woman discharges a placenta, there must have been an embryo that probably became mashed (*Bechorot* 46a). Part of a placenta can emerge without a fetus (*Baba Kamma* 11b). A placenta can emerge from a woman partly on one day and partly on the next day (*Baba Kamma* 11a). Rarely, the placenta can be expelled up to twenty-three days after the birth of a child (*Niddah* 27a). Normally, however, for the first three days after childbirth, the placenta is attributed to the child; after that the possibility of a second child must be considered (*Niddah* 26b). A newborn infant who does not cry or breathe should be rubbed with its afterbirth to stimulate breathing (*Shabbat* 134a).

The token of a valid birth is the discharge of a placenta, both in women (*Niddah* 25a) and in animals (*Chullin* 68a). A woman who aborts a placenta must observe the rules of ritual impurity relating to childbirth (*Niddah* 24b). A placenta in a house renders the house unclean because of the dead fetus that must be in it (*Niddah* 18a and 26a; *Bechorot* 22a). A placenta is not susceptible to the defilement of food unless one intends to boil it *(Eruvin* 28b). The placenta of a consecrated animal must be buried (*Temurah* 33b). The placenta found in a slaughtered animal may be eaten (*Chullin* 77a).

According to homiletical literature (*Numbers Rabbah* 4:3) the placenta was brought out (*Niddah* 27a) and preserved in a bowl (*Niddah* 9:2) for the purpose of warming the child. Princesses used to hide their placentas in bowls with oil, wealthy women in wool fleeces, and poor women in oakum (*Shabbat* 129b). Alternatively, placentas were placed in straw baskets (*Tosefta Shabbat* 15:3), in straw, or on sand, and later preserved in earth (i.e., buried) to pledge that the person once attached to the placenta will eventually be buried (*Jerushalmi Shabbat* 18:16). It was forbidden to bury the placenta at a crossroads or hang it from a tree because such was consid-

ered a heathen practice (*Chullin* 77a). The placenta of a black cat was once used for demonic exorcism (*Berachot* 6a). [*See also* PREGNANCY, CHILDBIRTH, and MIDWIFE]

PLAGUE—The biblical terms for plague or pestilence include *dever* (Leviticus 26:25; 1 Kings 8:37; Ezekiel 7:15; Amos 5:10), *magefa* (Numbers 17:13 and 25:9; 2 Samuel 24:21), *negef* (Exodus 30:12; Numbers 17:11), and *nega* (Leviticus 13:2). The scouts died of *magefa* (Numbers 14:36), which some writers interpret to mean *askara* or epidemic diphtheritic croup (*Sotah* 35a). The pestilence that afflicted Korach and his followers (Numbers 17:46) killed 14,700 people. Another plague killed 24,000 people (Numbers 25:8). The epidemic that afflicted the Philistines (1 Samuel 5:6ff.) was probably bubonic plague.[1] The Israelites who lusted for meat in the desert and were Divinely provided with quail[2] died of a plague (Numbers 11:33) that Ibn Ezra explains as "pestilence" and the Septuagint translates as "cholera." The ten plagues with which God afflicted the Egyptians are well known (Exodus 7:14–12:36; *Avot* 5:4). The *schechin* plague in Egypt (Exodus 9:8–11) was a skin disease characterized by boils, perhaps pustular eczema or furunculosis.[3] The entire body may be covered (*Taanit* 21a) and it may affect garments (*Yebamot* 4b) and houses

(*Yoma* 11b; *Baba Batra* 164b; *Yeba-mot* 103b). Poor skin hygiene may also lead to *schechin* (*Nedarim* 81a). Various folk remedies are suggested to treat this disease (*Gittin* 86a).

Plague is an illness that kills many people in a short time (*Taanit* 21b). Three deaths on three consecutive days in one town is defined as the beginning of a plague (ibid.). Epidemics of plague occur where large numbers of people aggregate (Leviticus 26:25). Plague or pestilence spreads from town to town through active people who traffic between them (*Taanit* 21b). Even rivers cannot prevent its spread because of ferryboats (ibid.). Swine or other animals can be affected and spread the disease (ibid.). Some plagues (Haggai 2:17) affect grains and crops rather than humans (*Ketubot* 8b). Plagues or epidemics may last up to seventy years (*Sanhedrin* 29a). Death from plague usually occurs quickly, sometimes even the same night (Ezekiel 24:18).

Some plagues and famines are Divine punishments for delay, perversion, or erroneous judgments (*Shabbat* 33a), and for other sins (*Avot* 5:8). Prayer and fasting may reverse them (*Taanit* 8b). Hence, fasts were decreed when an epidemic broke out, to atone for the sins that caused it (*Avot* 5:12). The *shofar* or ram's horn was blown (*Taanit* 3:4), either as a supplication to God (Numbers 10:9) or to warn the people (Ezekiel 33:6). The incense brought by the High Priest that stopped the plague afflicting Korach and his followers was not a disinfectant but a Divine signal (Numbers 17:10–13). The best remedy for plague is to flee (Jeremiah 21:9; *Baba Kamma* 60b). One should also close one's windows (*Baba Kamma* 60b) because death comes in through the windows (Jeremiah 9:20). When dogs howl, the angel of death has come to town (*Baba Kamma* 60b). [*See also* ISOLATION, SYPHILIS, SKIN and FAMINE]

1. F. Rosner, (trans.), *Julius Preuss' Biblical and Talmudic Medicine* (Northvale, NJ: Jason Aronson, 1993), pp. 154–157.
2. F. Rosner, *Medicine in the Bible and the Talmud*, 2nd ed. (Hoboken, NJ: Ktav and Yeshiva University Press, 1995), pp. 293–294.
3. F. Rosner (trans.), *Julius Preuss'*, pp. 342–347.

PLASTERS AND POULTICES— Among the popular remedies in antiquity and the Middle Ages were plasters and poultices (salves or ointments) for whose bases tallow and wax were used (*Shabbat* 133b). Three types of plaster are mentioned in classic Jewish sources: *retiya, ispelanit,* and *melugma* (*Tosefta Kelim* 6:9; *Tosefta Kilayim* 5:25). *Retiya* is applied to a wound (*Mechilta*, Exodus 14:24), even on a healed wound for protection (*Jerushalmi Shabbat* 6:8). A person whose whole body is injured from a fall from the roof is completely covered with plaster (*Exodus Rabbah* 24:9). It must be applied evenly (*Shabbat* 75b) or it will fall off (*Tosefta Shabbat* 5:5). Its ingredients are unknown except for wheat flour (*Tosefta Pesachim* 2:3; *Tosefta Demai* 1:25). A plaster can be applied on a wound on the Sabbath (*Shabbat* 18a). A plaster detached from a wound may be replaced on the Sabbath (*Eruvin* 102b; *Betzah* 11b).

Ispelanit may represent a pasty cloth used to cleanse a wound (*Tosefta Shabbat* 5:6) or plastered onto the wound. If it hurts, the plaster must be removed (*Jerushalmi Abodah Zarah* 2:40). The plaster was made of leather or material (*Kelim* 28:3), or linen or wool rags (*Jerushalmi Kilayim* 32). A wise woman once recommended a poultice for pain, consisting of seven parts of fat and one part of wax (*Shabbat* 133b).

Melugma refers to cataplasms. It is like mixing dough on a wound (*Jerushalmi Shabbat* 7:10). Some cataplasms are made of plants or fruits such as wheat or figs (*Sheviit* 8:1). King Hezekiah placed a fig cake (cataplasm?) on his boils (2 Kings 20:7). If a *melugma* stands for a long time, it becomes foul-smelling (*Tosefta Pesachim* 2:3). [*See also* COLLYRIA and BANDAGE]

PLETHORA—The expression "I, blood, [i.e., an excess of blood] am the cause of all illness" (*Baba Batra* 58b) might recall the Galenic teaching concerning plethora and its detrimental consequences. Plethora (polycythemia?), however, plays a major role in the pathology of antiquity as well as in the Talmud and other classic Hebrew sources. The homiletic commentary known as Midrash considers plethora to be the cause of leprosy: The body of a normal person has equal quantities of blood and water; if the water gains over the blood, the person becomes hydropic; if the blood gains over the water, the person becomes leprous (*Leviticus Rabbah* 15:2). The talmudic sage Resh Lakish also said that "much blood produces much leprosy" (*Bechorot* 44b).

Elsewhere, the Talmud asserts that human beings and animals "overcome by blood," i.e., who suffer from blood congestion or plethora, are placed in cold water to cool off (*Shabbat* 53b). An animal "overtaken by blood" should be phlebotomized, although one thereby creates a body blemish that renders it unfit to be offered as a sacrifice (*Tosefta Bechorot* 3:17). If an animal is very hot because of an excess of blood but later becomes cooled off, its flesh is not harmful to man (*Tosefta Chullin* 3:19). A special part of general plethora is "the blood of the head," for which several folk remedies are discussed in detail in the Talmud (*Gittin* 68b). This condition more likely represents the heterocrania or hemicrania of the ancients from which the French derived the term "migraine."

The only modern disease for which the initial treatment of choice is phlebotomy is polycythemia vera. Such patients are plethoric, suffer from headaches, have beefy red tongues, conjunctival suffusion, and occasionally intense itching of the skin. It is likely that those patients in ancient and medieval times who benefitted from bloodletting were afflicted with this disease. Plethora and headache are two of the signs and symptoms for which phlebotomy was recommended in talmudic times. [*See also* BLOOD-LETTING]

POISONS—Snake poison is usually lethal (*Jerushalmi Terumot* 8:45). Someone pierced with a poisoned spear should be given strong stimulants such as undiluted wine and fat meat roasted on coals (*Gittin* 70a). Poisoning is a method of murdering one's enemies (*Megillah* 13b). Wet nurses who want to kill the baby rub poison on their breasts and have the baby suckle (*Abodah Zarah* 26a). Human respiration was thought to be poisonous (*Jerushalmi Terumot* 8:45), as was black cumin (*Berachot* 40a). Some people consider onion roots to be poisonous (*Eruvin* 56a). Shredded gourd stew was said to be poisonous (2 Kings 4: 39–40), perhaps because gourds are intensely bitter and difficult to digest (*Nedarim* 49b).

Uncovered liquids left overnight are prohibited lest a snake drank and injected some of its poison (*Sanhedrin* 70a; *Baba Batra* 97b). A snake's poison is lodged in its fangs (*Sanhedrin*

78a). The venom of young snakes sinks to the bottom whereas that of an old snake floats on top (*Abodah Zarah* 30b). Animals can accidentally eat poison (*Chullin* 58b) or be intentionally poisoned (*Baba Kamma* 47b). [*See also* SNAKES AND SERPENTS]

POLYGAMY—In biblical times when polygamy was permitted, a man could marry other wives in addition to his first wife provided he was able to support them (*Yebamot* 65a). A man with two wives, one old and one young, became bald because one plucked out his gray hairs and one plucked out his black hairs (*Baba Kamma* 60b). A king could take many wives provided they not turn his heart away (*Baba Metzia* 115a; *Sanhedrin* 21a) as King Solomon's wives did to him when he was old (1 Kings 11:4). A High Priest, however, could marry only one woman (*Yoma* 2a). Even in talmudic times, some rabbis prohibited polygamy (*Yebamot* 65b).

Rabbi Gersham ben Judah (960–1028 C.E.) instituted a ban against polygamy that has been nearly universally accepted ever since the eleventh century. [*See also* MARRIAGE]

POMEGRANATES—The pomegranate is one of the fruits with which the land of Israel is blessed (Deuteronomy 8:8). Pomegranates are scraped and peeled before being consumed (*Shabbat* 115a). The peel is discarded (*Chag-*

igah 15b). The pomegranate cannot be preserved without its peel (*Ketubot* 108b). The blossom does not protect the pomegranate after it is plucked (*Berachot* 36b) but the point is included with the fruit (*Chullin* 118b; *Uktzin* 2:3). The fruit is split open and then eaten (*Ketubot* 61b). It can also spontaneously rupture (*Orlah* 3:8). The red pomegranate is especially beautiful (*Baba Metzia* 84a). Pomegranates can be wormy (*Sanhedrin* 108b) or not (*Uktzin* 2:3). They are not usually squeezed for juice (*Shabbat* 143b) although some people did so (ibid., 144b). They are stored suspended in bags (*Shabbat* 139b), in receptacles (*Shabbat* 84a), or in storerooms (*Baba Batra* 20b) and are served to guests (*Baba Metzia* 22a), usually as a separate course at a meal (*Berachot* 41b), or sent to one's beloved (*Song of Songs Rabbah* 4:12:2). After eating pomegranates, one says Grace of three blessings (*Berachot* 44a).

The pomegranate is one of the trees from which one must leave some fruits for the poor (*Peah* 1:5). The laws of the Sabbatical year apply to the husks and blossoms of pomegranates (*Sheviit* 7:3). One can decorate a Festival booth (*sukkah*) with pomegranates (*Betzah* 30b). The pomegranate is an accepted measure of size for certain legal matters (*Berachot* 41b; *Shabbat* 112b; *Sukkah* 6a; *Eruvin* 4b, 24a, and 29a; *Chullin* 138a; *Kelim* 17:1). The pomegranates of Baden (*Betzah* 3b; *Yebamot* 81b; *Zevachim* 72b) are usually numbered and counted when sold (*Abodah Zarah* 74a). Children hollowed out pomegranates to measure sand or they fashioned them into scales (*Chullin* 12b). In the absence of dice, pomegranate peels were used for gambling (*Sanhedrin* 25b).

Homiletically, the phrase "Thy temples are like a pomegranate" (Song of Songs 6:7) is interpreted to mean that the merits of the most unworthy Jews are as plentiful as the seeds of a pomegranate (*Eruvin* 19a; *Chagigah* 27a; *Megillah* 6a; *Sanhedrin* 37a; *Genesis Rabbah* 32:10).

PRAYER—Are prayers efficacious in the healing of human illnesses?[1] The patriarch Abraham prayed for the recovery of Abimelech (Genesis 20:17) and God healed him. David prayed for the recovery of his son (2 Samuel 12:16) but his son died. Elisha prayed for the recovery of the Shunammite woman's son (2 Kings 4:33) and the boy recovered. King Hezekiah prayed for his own recovery (2 Chronicles 32:24) and God added fifteen years to his life.

The Bible is replete with descriptive prayers (Psalms 6:3, 30:13, 38:1–10, 102:4–6, and 107:6), figurative prayers (Psalms 13:4, 34:21, and 147:1), philosophic prayers (Psalms 39:5), prayers of youth (Psalms 102:24), and prayers of old age (Psalms 71:9). The shortest prayer on record is the famous prayer uttered by Moses for the recovery of his sister, Miriam, who was afflicted with leprosy. Said Moses: *El na refa na la* ("O God, heal her, I beseech Thee"), and she recovered (Numbers 12:13).

The Talmud describes private prayers (*Shabbat* 30b; *Abodah Zarah* 4b and 7b) and public prayers (*Berachot* 82, *Baba Batra* 91a), morning prayers (*Berachot* 6b) and afternoon prayers (ibid.), prayers to be recited on entering a house of worship (*Berachot* 28b) and on leaving a house of worship (ibid.), on going to the privy (ibid., 60b) and on entering a bathhouse (ibid., 60a), on going to bed (ibid., 60b) and upon arising in the morning (ibid., 28b), and on passing through a city (ibid., 54a and 60a). The Talmud further discusses the prayer shawl (*Chagigah* 14b), the time for prayer (*Shabbat* 118b; Berachot 28b, 29b, and 31a), the language of prayer (*Shabbat* 12b), the place for prayer (*Berachot* 8a, 10b, 28b, and 39a), preparation for prayer (ibid., 32b; *Shabbat* 10a), washing before praying (*Berachot* 15a and 22a), and sacrifices that accompany prayers (*Pesachim* 82a; *Taanit* 27b; *Megillah* 3a).

The rapidity with which prayers can be answered is described by the Midrash Rabbah in its interpretation of the biblical phrase "whensoever we call upon Him" (Deuteronomy 4:7). The Talmud also discusses the efficacy of prayer (*Berachot* 32b) and concludes that the claim that God *must* answer a prayer is presumptuous and represents a transgression in Judaism (*Baba Batra* 164b).

Another circumstance in which prayers are said to be efficacious is the need of the community for the sick person (*Eruvin* 29b). The distinction and righteousness of the person who utters the prayers is also of importance (*Yebamot* 64b; *Berachot* 34b; *Chagigah* 3a).

Judaism seems to sanction certain alternative therapies, such as prayers, faith healing, amulets, incantations, and the like, when used as a supplement to traditional medical therapy. However, the substitution of prayer for rational healing is condemned. Quackery, superstition, sorcery, and witchcraft are abhorrent practices in Judaism, but confidence in the healing powers of God through prayer and contrition is encouraged and has its place of honor alongside traditional scientific medicine.[2]

1. F. Rosner, "Therapeutic Efficacy of Prayer," in *Medicine in the Bible and the Talmud,* 2nd ed. (Hoboken, NJ: Ktav and Yeshiva University Press, 1995), pp. 204–210.

2. F. Rosner, "Unconventional Therapies," in *Modern Medicine and Jewish Ethics,* 2nd ed. (Hoboken, NJ: Ktav and Yeshiva University Press, 1991), pp. 419–432.

PREGNANCY—There exists an extensive homiletical literature relating to pregnancy and birth. If a bottle of water is turned upside down, all the water therein is spilled out (*Niddah* 31a)—yet an embryo lies in the mother's womb and does not fall out (*Leviticus Rabbah* 14:14; Midrash Psalms 103:6). God built a woman like a storehouse: narrow at the top and broad on the bottom to hold its contents (*Berachot* 61a). Eve was cursed in Paradise with discomfort of pregnancies (*Genesis Rabbah* 20:6). Only pious women are exempt from this curse (*Sotah* 12a). During the generation of the Flood, women became pregnant and gave birth in three days (*Leviticus Rabbah* 5:1), yet righteous women such as Sarah found pregnancy more difficult to obtain than rubies (*Genesis Rabbah* 45:1). Tamar's pregnancy ended in the birth of twins delivered by midwives (Genesis 38:27–30).

Menses cease with the beginning of pregnancy and menstrual blood is converted to milk (*Niddah* 9a). Occasionally, menses occur during pregnancy (*Niddah* 10b). Pregnancy may occur at a very young age, even before menarche (*Niddah* 45a). Bathsheba, wife of King David, gave birth at six years of age (*Sanhedrin* 69b). Pregnancy and childbirth at such a young age are considered dangerous. Hence, the rabbis allow a married young girl to use a contraceptive absorbent tampon during marital relations (*Yebamot* 12b).

Pregnancy after menopause is a rarity. At ninety years of age, Sarah gave birth to Isaac by Divine intervention (Genesis 17:17). Rabbi Chisda said that a woman less than twenty years old who marries begets children until age sixty; if she marries at age twenty she begets until age forty; if she marries at age forty, she begets no more (*Baba Batra* 119b).

A pregnant woman is said to be repulsive and loathsome (*Song of Songs Rabbah* 2:14:8). Her head and limbs become heavy (*Niddah* 10b) and she has fancies of the mind (*Sirach* 34:5). Pregnant women may have bizarre cravings or pica. If such a craving for food occurs on the day of Atonement and she becomes faint, she should be fed until she feels restored (*Yoma* 8:5). Ordinarily, however, pregnant women must fast on the Ninth of Av and on the Day of Atonement (*Pesachim* 54b). A pregnant woman is allowed to eat a quantity of unclean food smaller than the standard size, because of her serious condition (*Keritot* 13a). If she craves for prohibited food such as pork, she is first offered permitted food dipped in the juice of the prohibited meat. If that does not suffice, she is fed the meat itself because all biblical and rabbinic laws are waived in the face of danger to the life of the mother or the fetus. These cravings were thought to represent a bad omen as fetal indiscretions (*Yoma* 82a–b). Esau struggled to get out of his mother's womb when he smelled the aroma of idolatrous Temple worship (*Genesis Rabbah* 6 3:6). When Esau and Jacob struggled in her womb and caused her pain (Genesis 26:22), Rebecca suggested she might have been better off not becoming pregnant (*Genesis Rabbah* 63:6).

Pregnancy can be externally recognized at three months (*Niddah* 8b). The twin pregnancy of Tamar was also first recognized at three months (Genesis 38:24). The pregnancy of a young primigravida such as Zilpah is the most difficult to recognize (*Genesis Rabbah* 71:9). Following divorce or the death of her husband, a woman may not remarry for three months so that if she is pregnant, one can distinguish between the seed of the first and that of the second husband (*Yebamot* 33b and 42a). A woman whose abdomen is "between her teeth" is certainly pregnant (*Tosefta Ketubot* 1:6). This became a proverbial expression (*Rosh Hashanah* 25a).

The normal duration of human pregnancy is nine months or 271 to 273 days (*Niddah* 38a), or 274 days in the opinion of the Jerusalem Talmud (*Niddah* 1:49b). Exceptionally, pregnancy can last even up to twelve months (*Yebamot* 80b). Preuss points out[1] that both Hippocrates and Aristotle speak of an eleven-month pregnancy. The shortest pregnancy duration is 212 days (*Jerushalmi Niddah* 1:49b). Varying lengths of pregnancy for a variety of animals are also cited in the Talmud (*Bechorot* 8a).

During the first three months of pregnancy, cohabitation is harmful to both mother and fetus; during the next three months, it is harmful to the mother but beneficial to the fetus; during the final months, it is beneficial for both because the child becomes well formed and of strong vitality (*Niddah* 31a). Pregnant women should eat light foods. When God told Moses to lead the Jews out of Egypt, he asked Him: Have you prepared soft food for the pregnant women? (*Exodus Rabbah* 3:4). Pregnant women ate *zard* together with barley groats (*Yoma* 47a). Egyptian *zithom,* a potent laxative made from barley, safflower, and salt, is dangerous for pregnant women (*Pesachim* 42b). Samson's mother drank no wine when she was pregnant with him because Samson was to be a Nazarite, to whom wine is forbidden (Judges 13:4).

Preserving stones were worn by pregnant women to prevent miscarriages. They were also worn by women trying to become pregnant (*Shabbat* 66b). The nature of this preserving stone is discussed by Preuss. Pregnant women were expected to breast-feed their babies after birth (*Yebamot* 42a). A pregnant woman may use an absorbent tampon during marital intercourse to prevent her from becoming pregnant again (superfetation), which might cause the second fetus to be crushed and aborted as a flat, fish-shaped abortus called a *sandal (Yebamot* 12b and 42a). The Talmud also alludes to the possibility of a woman being pregnant at one time from two men (superfecundity) (*Yebamot* 42a–b). Elsewhere, the Talmud rejects this possibility (*Niddah* 27a). The Jerusalem Talmud says that it is only possible during the first forty days of pregnancy (*Jerushalmi Yebamot* 5c). [*See also* FETUS, CHILDBIRTH, PLACENTA, and MIDWIFE]

1. F. Rosner (trans.), *Julius Preuss' Biblical and Talmudic Medicine* (Northvale, NJ: Jason Aronson, 1993), pp. 381–387.

PREGNANCY REDUCTION—The use of "fertility" pills and the introduction of assisted reproduction to help previously barren couples have children frequently results in multiple pregnancies. Is it permissible for a woman carrying five or six or more embryos to undergo pregnancy reduction or selective abortion of some of the embryos to give the other fetuses a chance to survive? Does the Judaic axiom that one may not sacrifice one human life to save another human life extend even to the unborn fetus?

Most rabbis permit pregnancy reduction, in part because of the increased danger of maternal complications in multiple pregnancy. The number of fetuses to be destroyed is a medical question to be decided by physicians to insure a good prognosis for both mother and remaining fetuses.[1,2,3] [*See also* ABORTION]

1. R.V. Grazi, *Be Fruitful and Multiply* (Jerusalem: Genesis Press, 1994), pp. 175–208.
2. F. Rosner, *Modern Medicine and Jewish Ethics*, 2nd ed. (Hoboken, NJ, and New York: Ktav and Yeshiva University Press, 1991), pp. 155–162.
3. F. Rosner, *Pioneers in Jewish Medical Ethics* (Northvale, NJ: Jason Aronson, 1997), pp. 104 and 180.

PROCREATION—The commandment "Be fruitful and multiply" was articulated by God to Adam and Eve (Genesis 1:28) and later to Noah and his sons (Genesis 9:1 and 9:7) and Jacob (Genesis 35:11). The world was created for procreation (*Pesachim* 88b). Both man and woman are subject to the precept of procreation (*Genesis Rabbah* 5:12), which is derived and discussed in the Talmud (*Yebamot* 65b). The definition of procreation is a minimum of two children (*Yebamot* 61b). If one fails to procreate, it is as if one sheds blood and diminishes the Divine Image (*Genesis Rabbah* 34:14; *Yebamot* 63b). Even if one foresees, as did King Hezekiah, that one's children will be wicked, one is not allowed to refrain from procreation (*Berachot* 10a). A Torah scholar should never be without a wife (*Yoma* 10a), even in old age (*Genesis Rabbah* 61:3). Even a High Priest had to be married (*Yoma* 1:1). Examples of prophets who were married and had children are Samuel (1 Samuel 8:2), Isaiah (Isaiah 8:18), Ezekiel (Ezekiel 24:18), and Hosea (Hosea 1:2). When man is led to judgment in the next world, he will be asked: "Did you engage in procreation?" (*Shabbat* 31a)

One should not marry a woman who has never menstruated because she is incapable of bearing children (*Niddah* 12b). Eunuchs are incapable of procreation as are men with hypospadias (*Yebamot* 76a). The younger one marries, the longer one can procreate (*Baba Batra* 119b). In Egypt, the Israelite women each bore six children at one birth (*Exodus Rabbah* 1:8). One may, but is not obligated to, use modern assisted reproductive techniques to overcome infertility and to thus fulfill the precept of procreation.[1] [See also CELIBACY, CHILDLESSNESS, and MARRIAGE]

1. F. Rosner, *Modern Medicine and Jewish Ethics*, 2nd ed. (Hoboken, NJ, and New York: Ktav and Yeshiva University Press, 1991), pp. 85–121.

PROSTHESES—Amputees were fitted with artificial legs, some of which were padded (*Shabbat* 6:8; *Yoma* 78b). For additional support, stilts were tied to the thighs and hand crutches were used (Rashi, *Yebamot* 102b). Some amputees wrapped the stumps of their arms and legs with thick, soft rags (*Baba Batra* 20a). Knee stilts were also used. For people who could not use their knees for locomotion, a low stool was specially built and attached to the body. When the amputee wished to move, he supported himself on his hands with small benches, lifted his body from the ground, and propelled himself forward (*Shabbat* 6:8; *Yoma* 78b; *Chagigah* 3a; *Yebamot* 102b and 103a). The preparation of prostheses for leg amputees was done by skilled professionals (Shabbat 11b). A prosthesis for an animal is also described in the Talmud: Rabbi Simeon ben Chalafta once fashioned a reed tube as support for a chicken whose hip was dislodged or torn out, and it recovered (*Chullin* 57b). For dental prostheses, see ARTIFICIAL TEETH. An artificial eye of gold is cited in the Jerusalem Talmud (*Nedarim* 9:41). [*See also* AMPUTEE]

PROSTITUTION—The term *zonah*, for prostitute (*Yebamot* 61b), or a variant thereof, is found more than sixty times in the Bible.[1] Another biblical term for a Jewish prostitute is *kedeshah* (Deuteronomy 23:18). Harlots in biblical times (Isaiah 23:15) placed myrrh and balsam vials in their shoes. When they saw handsome young men, they stepped on the vials, splashing the fragrant spices on them and thereby arousing them to immorality (*Yoma* 9b; *Shabbat* 62b). Jewish women were secluded from the outside world to protect them from immorality. Dinah, daughter of Jacob, was raped because "she went out" (Genesis 34:1). Even her mother Leah was reproached for "going out to meet her husband" (Genesis 30:16). Protection from prostitution was by early marriage (*Pesachim* 113a) and by work because "idleness leads to lewdness" (*Ketubot* 5:5). A special biblical admonition against prostitution is addressed to a priest's daughter (Leviticus 21:29) and is discussed at length in the Talmud (*Sanhedrin* 50b–52a). A priest is not allowed to marry a harlot (Leviticus 21:7). Harlots are executed by stoning or strangulation (*Ketubot* 45a and 48b). A harlot's hire cannot be devoted to the Temple (Deuteronomy 23:19) except under certain circumstances (*Abodah Zarah* 62b). In biblical times, immorality was rampant in Arabia (*Kiddushin* 49b) and Egypt (*Exodus Rabbah* 1:18; *Esther Rabbah* 1:17).

The Talmud states that whoever has intercourse with a harlot will later become impoverished (*Sotah* 4b). He who yields to prostitution suffers premature aging (*Shabbat* 152a). Men seek out female harlots more often than the reverse (*Ketubot* 64b). It takes a strong-willed person to live and work on a street of prostitutes and not be enticed (*Pesachim* 113a–b). Harlots paint each other to conceal blemishes (*Shabbat* 34a). They may also hate each other (*Pesachim* 113b). A harlot who hires herself out will at the end be despised by all (*Abodah Zarah* 17a). Harlots may cover their faces (*Megillah* 10b), as did Tamar when Judah first met her (Genesis 38:15). Some harlots use absorbent tampons to prevent conception (*Ketubot* 37a; *Yebamot* 35a). Other harlots make twisting movements after coitus to expel sperm and thereby avoid pregnancy (ibid.). One harlot asked for four hundred gold dinars for her hire (*Menachot* 44a).

One of the descendants of the famous Rahab the harlot was Chulda the prophetess (*Megillah* 14b). Elijah the prophet once appeared as a harlot (*Abodah Zarah* 18b). Jezebel painted pictures of harlots on King Ahab's chariot to sexually arouse him from his frigid nature (*Sanhedrin* 39b). The disciples of Rabbi Ishmael performed a postmortem examination on an executed prostitute to ascertain the number of bones and limbs in a human being (*Bechorot* 45a).

---

1. A. Even-Shoshan, *Concordantzia Chadashah* (Jerusalem: Kiryat Sefer, 1981), pp. 334–335.

PUBERTY—In Judaism, puberty is defined not only by signs of sexual maturity (i.e., two pubic hairs) but also the attainment of a certain age—twelve or thirteen full years for girls and boys, respectively (*Niddah* 45b and 52a). Physical signs of puberty in a girl are the appearance of a wrinkle beneath the breast, the hanging down of the breasts, the darkening of the ring around the nipple, or the sinking in of the nipple when one presses on it (*Niddah* 47a). Pubic hair may precede breast development but not usually the reverse (ibid., 48a). Breast development is called the "upper sign" and pubic hair is called the "lower sign" (*Kiddushin* 16b). These are biblically portrayed as "Thy breasts are fashioned and thine hair is grown" (Ezekiel 16:7). The beauty of the breasts is also portrayed in the Bible (Song of Songs 4:5). [*See* BREASTS]

Among townswomen, the pubic hairs develop earlier because they take frequent baths; among village women, the breasts develop earlier because they grind with millstones and thereby constantly exercise their arms (*Niddah* 48b). The right breast develops earlier in rich girls because it rubs against their scarves, which are worn on the right side close to the body (*Leviticus Rabbah* 2:4). In poor girls, the left breast develops earlier because they carry water jugs and their siblings on the left side (*Niddah* 48b). A woman matures earlier than a man (*Yebamot* 80a; *Niddah* 47b). In men, there is no upper sign of puberty.

Not all children develop signs of puberty at the same time. If a boy aged seven to nine years grows two pubic hairs it is considered to be a mole, but at thirteen years it is a sign of puberty (*Kiddushin* 16b; *Niddah* 46a). The two pubic hairs proving puberty must have their own hair follicles (*Niddah* 52a). When girls grow pubic hair before the proper age, they apply depilatory plasters to remove the hair (*Shabbat* 80b). If a minor girl gives birth to a baby, she has proven her puberty and requires no physical signs (*Yebamot* 12b). Such childhood pregnancies are dangerous to both mother and child (*Jerushalmi Pesachim* 8:35).

Before puberty, girls are automatically considered to be ritually clean (*Niddah* 10b). Daughters are married off shortly after attaining puberty to avoid their becoming unchaste (*Sanhedrin* 76b). An adolescent girl may not make herself unsightly even when she is in mourning for a parent (*Taanit* 13b).

Although acts of minors usually have no validity, children six or seven years old may purchase or sell movable property (*Ketubot* 70a) and girls at age eleven have valid vows (*Yebamot* 105b; *Niddah* 45b). A boy nine years old has a certain status (*Yebamot* 96b). A priestly boy is qualified to serve in the Temple as soon as he grows two pubic hairs (*Chullin* 24a). A congenital eunuch has no pubic hair (*Tosefta Yebamot* 10:6). So too for a barren woman (*Yebamot* 80b).

Jewish women were renowned for their beauty (Ezekiel 16:14) because they had neither pubic nor axillary hair (*Sanhedrin* 21a). It was considered lewd for women to "make their opening like a forest" *(Shabbat* 62b). Men were prohibited, however, from using depilatories. [*See also* DEPILATORIES and HAIR]

PUERPERAL ILLNESS—Puerperal bleeding is considered part of normal birthing (*Niddah* 21b) and renders the parturient woman ritually unclean. Such a woman's limbs are disjointed and her natural strength does not return for two years (*Niddah* 9a). The puerperal illness known as *kuda* (*Abodah Zarah* 29a) is, according to the commentaries, a cold that the woman caught on the birth stool. A herbal potion is prescribed for its treatment (ibid.). Death during childbirth is frequently mentioned in the Talmud, sometimes as punishment for not fulfilling religious precepts (*Shabbat* 2:6). Preuss interprets the death of a woman in confinement (*Eruvin* 41b) to be due to puerperal sepsis.[1] Rachel (Genesis 35:18); the wife of Phinehas (1 Samuel 4:20); Michal, wife of King David (2 Samuel 6:23; *Sanhedrin* 21a); and Queen Esther (*Megillah* 13a) all died during childbirth. [*See also* PREGNANCY and CHILDBIRTH]

1. F. Rosner (trans.), *Julius Preuss' Biblical and Talmudic Medicine* (Northvale, NJ: Jason Aronson, 1993), p. 428.

PURGATIVES—Water from the spring of palm trees is a powerful purgative (*Nazir* 51b; *Shabbat* 110a). Bread, fish brine, and beer have strong purgative effects (*Shabbat* 108a). Egyptian *zythom* is dangerous for pregnant women and ill people (*Pesachim* 42b) because of its powerful purgative effect. Cucumbers have a laxative effect (*Abodah Zarah* 11a). Dates are wholesome, act as a laxative, and strengthen the body (*Ketubot* 10b). Severe fright or fear can also act as a laxative (*Megillah* 15a; *Song of Songs Rabbah* 3:4). [*See also* DIARRHEA, INTESTINES, and DEFECATION]

PURITY AND IMPURITY—Ritual purity and impurity *(tumah* and *taharah)* are not hygienic terms indicating physical cleanness or uncleanness. Rather, these words connote a religious concept whereby an impure person cannot have contact with the Temple or its services. The state of ritual impurity is contracted through contact with a corpse (Numbers 19:11) or unclean dead animal; through leprosy (Leviticus 14:8), menstruation (ibid., 5:19), or male genital emissions (ibid., 15:13); from eating forbidden food (ibid., 17:15); from the waters of sprinkling (Numbers 19:21) and from the scapegoat (Leviticus 16:26). The terms "pure" and "impure" are also used in regard to the uncircumcised (Isaiah 52:1), countries other than Israel (Joshua 22:19; Hosea 9:3), idols (Genesis 35:2; Isaiah 30:22), and to serious biblical transgressions such as sexual immorality (Leviticus 18:27–28). The state of ritual impurity can be corrected by the performance of specified rituals, mainly including ablution or immersion in a ritual bath.[1,2]

Twelve entire tractates of Talmud are devoted to the laws of ritual purity and impurity, the categories of impurity, the methods of contracting impurity, food and utensil impurity, hands and body impurity, the consequences of impurity, and the methods of purification. Purity and impurity are understood in the correlative sense of "holiness" (*Abodah Zarah* 20b). With the destruction of the Temple, many of the laws of purity and impurity have lost their practical signifi-cance. The main laws still in force to-day relate to the consumption of forbidden foods and the ritual impurity of the menstruating woman. Purity is a religious ideal. Repentance and good deeds are conducive to purity and holiness (*Berachot* 17a). More detailed discussions are available elsewhere. [*See also* MENSTRUATION, GONORRHEA, and RITUAL BATH]

1. C. Roth (ed.), *Encyclopedia Judaica*, vol. 13 (Jerusalem: Keter, 1971), pp. 1405–1414.

2. F. Rosner (trans.), *Julius Preuss' Biblical and Talmudic Medicine* (Northvale, NJ: Jason Aronson, 1993), pp. 506–511 .

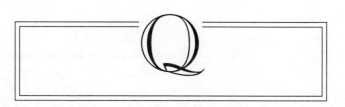

QUACKS—Judaism has always held the physician in high esteem. Ancient and medieval Jewish writings are replete with expressions of admiration and praise for the "faithful physician." Therefore, the derogatory talmudic statement "The best of physicians is destined for Gehenna" (*Kiddushin* 4:14) generated extensive discussion and commentary throughout the centuries.[1] "To hell with the best of physicians" was never understood as a denunciation of the conscientious practitioner. Physicians are among a group of communal servants who have heavy public responsibilities and are warned against the danger of negligence or error. The talmudic epigram with its curse is thus limited to physicians who are overly confident in their craft, are guilty of commercializing their profession, lie and deceive as do quacks, fail to acknowledge God as the true Healer of the sick, fail to consult with colleagues or medical texts when appropriate, perform surgery without heeding proper advice from diagnosticians, fail to heal the poor and thus indirectly cause their death, fail to try

hard enough to heal their patients, consider themselves to be the best in their field, or who otherwise fail to conduct themselves in an ethical and professional manner.

Jewish law requires a physician to be skilled and well educated. If he heals without being properly licensed, he is liable for any bad outcome. If he is an expert physician and fully licensed but errs and thereby harms the patient, he is exempt from payment of damages "because of the public good" (*Tosefta Gittin* 4:6). The Divine arrangement of the world requires and presupposes the existence of physicians. If one were to hold the physician liable for every error, very few people would practice medicine. The physician, however, is still liable in the eyes of Heaven (*Shulchan Aruch, Yoreh Deah* 336:1).

If a physician causes an injury deliberately or acts without proper license, he can be sued for damages no matter how competent he is (*Tosefta Gittin* 3:13). A physician who kills a patient and realizes that he was in error is exiled to the cities of refuge just like anyone else who kills another person through error (Numbers 35:11; Deuteronomy 19:3).

Blamelessness in case of error applies only to a *rophe umman*, who is an expert or well-trained physician and who heals "at the request of the authorities"—that is to say, a licensed physician. A nonlicensed physician is subject to the general law and can be sued and must pay for damages he inflicts. Error and ignorance are used as excuses by quacks, whom Judaism looks upon with disdain. [*See also* PHYSICIANS' LIABILITY and PHYSICIANS' LICENSE TO HEAL]

---

1. F. Rosner, "The Best of Physicians Is Destined for Gehenna," in *Modern Medicine and Jewish Ethics,* 2nd ed. (Hoboken, NJ: Ktav and Yeshiva University Press, 1991), pp. 21–28.

QUAIL—The biblical story of the consumption of quails by the Israelites in the desert, as described in the sixteenth chapter of Exodus and the eleventh chapter of Numbers, continues to intrigue medical historians as well as biblical scholars. The subsequent sudden death of the Israelites is explained in various ways.[1]

An alternate explanation of the quail affair is that the entire happening was an act of God. Some biblical commentators, in fact, state that many of the people who died had not consumed any quail at all but were stricken as soon as they raised the meat to their mouths. This is the interpretation of the phrase "while the meat was yet between the teeth, before it was consumed" (Numbers 11:33). It is conceivable to attribute the deaths to both Divine intervention as well as organic food poisoning if we interpret that God punished the people by medical means.

Further reference to the quail incident is found in the Psalms (78:26–31 and 106:13–15) and in the Babylonian Talmud (*Yoma* 75b; *Sanhedrin* 17a; *Avot* 5:4; *Chullin* 27b; *Arachin* 15a).

---

1. F. Rosner, "The Biblical Quail Incident," in *Medicine in the Bible and the Talmud,* 2nd ed. (Hoboken, NJ: Ktav and Yeshiva University Press, 1995), pp. 293–294.

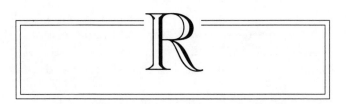

RAATAN—The term *raatan* is usually thought of as a form of leprosy or skin disease associated with trembling and extreme debility of the body. *Raatan* may also refer to a person with an insect in his brain, as described in a lengthy passage in the Talmud (*Ketubot* 77b). One of the elders from among the lepers of Sepphoris (*Tosefta Ketubot* 7:11; *Leviticus Rabbah* 16:1) told Rabbi Jose that there are twenty-four types of skin diseases, and the sages said that coitus is harmful for patients with all types. The greatest harm occurs to those afflicted with *raatan*. According to Preuss,[1] the probable meaning is the premature loss of potency. A homiletical discussion in the Midrash also suggests that the *raatan* sickness is harmful to potency (*Leviticus Rabbah* 16:1). For this reason, the Talmud ascribes the illness of the Egyptian Pharaoh who took Sarah into his harem (Genesis 12:17) as being *raatan*, which hindered him in cohabitation (*Jerushalmi Ketubot* 7:31).

The Talmud states that children with *raatan* are born to parents who cohabited shortly after bloodletting (*Ketubot* 77b). Remedies for this illness are also described (ibid.). Rabbi Yochanan issued the announcement: Beware of the flies of the man afflicted with *raatan* (because they are infectious). Rabbi Zera never sat with such a sufferer in the same draught. Rabbi Eleazar never entered his tent. Rabbi Ammi and Rabbi Assi never ate any of the eggs coming from the alley in which he lived. Rabbi Joshua ben Levi, however, attached himself to these sufferers and studied the Torah with them, confident that the Torah serves as a shield and protects those who study and observe it (ibid.). Rabbi Chaninah said: Why are there no sufferers from *raatan* in Babylon? Because they eat mangold (or beet or tomatoes) and drink beer made from cuscuta of the *hizmi* shrub.

According to Preuss, there is no illness in modern times that conforms to the clinical appearances and anatomical substrates described in the Talmud. He was unable to find a parallel thereto in antiquity. He suggests that the symptoms probably refer to leprosy. The assumption that transmission of this disease can be effected by flies is probably justified since nowadays, says Preuss, it is recognized that sleeping sickness and malaria are transmitted by mosquitoes.

There is no dearth of other explanations of this talmudic passage. Preuss quotes authorities who consider the illness *raatan* to be syphilis, glanders, or even ulcerating lupus. He also presents various contradictory opinions about the sexual instincts of lepers in an attempt to explain the talmudic assertion that *raatan* results from sexual intercourse. He struggles to explain the recommended therapy for sufferers from *raatan*. The softening of the skull by complicated boiled concoctions, instead of the usual trepanning, points to folk medicine. Perhaps no artificial opening of the skull was made, and the talmudic case refers to a brain tumor that bored through the skull. Although the main talmudic commentator, Rashi, clearly states that *raatan* refers to "a person with an insect in his brain," the text can be equally well understood to refer to a tumor whose outgrowths resemble "the feet" of a reptile, and whose removal must be accomplished with extreme caution.

Another famous talmudic passage dealing with an insect in the brain concerns the final illness of Titus (*Gittin* 56b). When Titus landed on dry land after the destruction of the Temple in Jerusalem, a gnat flew into his nose, ascended into his head, and knocked against his brain for seven years. One day, as he was passing a blacksmith, the gnat heard the noise of the hammer and stopped. He said: I see there is a remedy. So every day they brought a blacksmith who hammered before him. This went on for thirty days, but then the gnat got used to it and again began to knock. After Titus died, they opened his skull and found there something like a sparrow (or swallow), two *selas* in weight. One talmudic sage said: like a young dove two pounds in weight. Legend records that its beak was of brass and its claws of iron.

A homiletical source states that the pain-plagued Titus requested that his skull be opened and something like a dove was drawn forth. When it flew away, his soul also flew away (*Genesis Rabbah* 10:7). The entire story may only represent a moral lesson to illustrate the teaching that the Lord can destroy even the mightiest ruler with one of His smallest creatures.

The medical analysis of the case is that of a man plagued by severe headaches for many years, who was temporarily deafened by the noises of the world around him, and in whom, on postmortem examination, a brain tumor was found. According to the other version, through trepanning of the skull the patient lost his life and the tumor was discovered. Both versions are plausible. Trepanning was well-recognized in antiquity. The Talmud refers to a skull borer (*Oholot* 2:3) and reports the case of a trepanation on a person for a condition called *en bul*

(*Tosefta Oholot* 2:4). The skull defect was later covered with the dried shell of a pumpkin.[2] [*See also* SKIN]

---

1. F. Rosner (trans.), *Julius Preuss' Biblical and Talmudic Medicine* (Northvale, NJ: Jason Aronson, 1993), pp. 341–342.
2. F. Rosner, "The Illness *Raatan* (Insect in the Brain?)," in *Medicine in the Bible and the Talmud*, 2nd ed. (Hoboken, NJ: Ktav and Yeshiva University Press, 1995), pp. 74–78.

RABIES—Rabies (hydrophobia) is a disease of great antiquity, having been described in the pre-Mosaic Eshnuna Code of ancient Mesopotamia about four thousand years ago.[1] Bites of a rabid dog are discussed in the Babylonian Talmud as follows: "If one was bitten by a mad dog, he may not be given the lobe of its liver to eat, but Rabbi Matia ben Cheresh permits it" (*Mishnah Yoma* 8:6).

The therapeutic use of parts of the rabid animal, particularly the liver, for individuals bitten by such an animal, was recommended by many ancient physicians. In the Talmud, only Rabbi Matia ben Cheresh, who lived in Rome, advocates this type of therapy, since he believed in its curative values (perhaps a forerunner of modern homeopathics), and hence permitted the consumption of the liver of the rabid animal by the patient. The other Sages of the Mishnah consider it useless, deny its curative value, and hence prohibit its use since it is derived from a nonkosher animal.

The Talmud describes the behavior of a mad dog and cautions against even rubbing against it lest one develop symptoms of hydrophobia. One talmudic sage recommends that one kill the rabid dog and avoid any direct contact with it (*Yoma* 83b). From these talmudic statements, it is obvious that the etiology of rabies was not understood, although the symptomatology was correctly recognized. Folk remedies for the treatment of someone bitten by a mad dog are presented in some detail (*Yoma* 84a).

The Jerusalem Talmud (*Yoma* 8:5) relates that Rebbe (Rabbi Judah the Prince) gave "liver" to his Germanic servant, who had been bitten by a mad dog, but in vain: The effort was futile and the patient died, from which the Talmud concludes: "Let no man tell you that he was bitten by a mad dog and lived." This statement is also found elsewhere in the Jerusalem Talmud (*Berachot* 8:5).

A final statement dealing with the bite of a mad dog is found in the Babylonian Talmud: Rabbi Joshua ben Levi said: "All animals that cause injury [i.e., kill] may be killed [even] on the Sabbath." Rabbi Joseph objected. "Five may be killed on the Sabbath, and these are they: the Egyptian fly, the hornet of Nineveh, the scorpion of Adiabene, the snake in the land of Israel, and a mad dog anywhere" (*Shabbat* 121b).

This ruling is codified by Maimonides *(Mishneh Torah, Shabbat* 11:4*)* and Karo *(Shulchan Aruch, Orach Chayim* 316:10). Other animal bites are mentioned in the Talmud (*Yoma* 49a; *Chullin* 7b; *Baba Kamma* 84a), but the wound inflicted was probably not associated with rabies. Furthermore, snakebites are frequently discussed in the Talmud, but the poisons injected by venomous snakes do not produce the clinical picture of what is today known as rabies. [*See also* DOGS and SNAKES AND SERPENTS]

1. F. Rosner, "Rabies," in *Medicine in the Bible and the Talmud,* 2nd ed. (Hoboken, NJ: Ktav and Yeshiva University Press, 1995), pp. 50–53.

RADISHES—Radishes have large and fibrous roots (*Uktzin* 1:2). Young radishes are soft; they eventually become hard (*Eruvin* 28b). Radishes are a pungent vegetable (*Chullin* 112a) and give off a distinctive aroma (*Baba Batra* 146a). Radishes are constipating (*Shabbat* 108b). They help the dissolution of food and, hence, digestion (*Abodah Zarah* 11a). They are good for fever (ibid., 28b). Radishes are healthy but their leaves are not (*Eruvin* 56a). The juice of sharp radish is healthy. It should not be salted after it is cut into slices (*Shabbat* 108b). Radishes were never lacking on the table of Rabbi Judah the Prince (*Abodah Zarah* 11a; *Berachot* 57b).

RAPE—For raping a virgin maiden, a man must pay a fine and marry her (Exodus 22:15; Deuteronomy 22:29), even if she is lame, blind, or a leper (*Ketubot* 3:5). For seducing a maiden, the punishment is the same but here the man has the right to divorce her (*Ketubot* 39b). The man, in either rape or seduction, must also pay for the disgrace, pain, medical bills, and bodily harm he inflicted (ibid.). For raping a married woman or a prohibited relative, the perpetrator is put to death. Rape applies only to a woman (*Yebamot* 53a), although some rabbis disagree. One may save a betrothed maiden from a rapist even at the cost of the latter's life (*Yoma* 82a). Cases of rape are adjudicated by a court of three judges (*Sanhedrin* 2a). If a girl less than three years of age is raped, her tokens of virginity grow back (*Niddah* 45a).

The story of the Benjaminites in Gibeah raping and abusing a woman all night is well known (Judges 19:1ff.). Through a concocted plan, Amnon raped his sister Tamar (2 Samuel 13:14). Preuss describes in detail the practice of some Roman emperors to have their officers cohabit first with all newly married women, a form of rape known as Hegemonian coitus.[1] [*See also* HOMOSEXUALITY, LESBIANISM, and BESTIALITY]

1. F. Rosner (trans.), *Julius Preuss' Biblical and Talmudic Medicine* (North-

vale, NJ: Jason Aronson, 1993), pp. 468–488.

RAVEN—The raven is not a kosher (i.e., edible) bird (Leviticus 11:15; *Chullin* 61b). Noah sent forth a raven from the Ark (Genesis 8:7). Ravens brought food to Elijah the prophet (1 Kings 17:6; *Chullin* 5a; *Leviticus Rabbah* 19:1). Ravens love each other (*Pesachim* 113b) and care for their young (*Ketubot* 49b). Ravens expectorate their seed into their mate's mouth (*Sanhedrin* 108b). They retire to roost at night and are only seen during the day (*Shabbat* 35b).

Ravens can do considerable damage to date trees (*Baba Batra* 23a). Ravens can also pick someone's eyes out (Proverbs 30:17). They carry flesh or meat in their beaks (*Baba Batra* 91b; *Chullin* 95b). They carry pieces of a corpse (*Niddah* 61a), and they may impart ritual impurity (*Tohorot* 4:4). There are many types of ravens including the starling (*Baba Kamma* 92b), the black raven, the white spotted raven, and the valley raven (*Chullin* 63a). Raven's eggs resemble those of a dove (*Chullin* 64a). [*See also* DOVES, PIGEONS, and BIRDS]

RAZOR—Scissors and razors are used to cut hair (*Nazir* 39a). The latter are also used to shave (Isaiah 7:20; *Sanhedrin* 95b), although shaving the beard and sideburns is frowned upon in Judaism (Leviticus 19:27; *Makkot* 20a). Women sometimes shave their privy parts with a razor (*Moed Katan* 9b). A Nazarite may not use a razor to cut his hair or shave (Numbers 6:5). At the end of his Nazariteship he shaves his head with a razor (*Nazir* 40a). A life-long Nazarite may thin his hair with a razor when it becomes burdensome (*Nazir* 4a). A healed leper also shaves his entire body with a razor, including the head, beard, and eyebrows (Leviticus 14:9; *Negaim* 14:2). At their first consecration for Temple service, the Levites shaved all the hair of their flesh with razors (Numbers 8:7).

REMEDIES, ANIMAL—Numerous animal remedies are discussed throughout this encyclopedia, such as bees' honey for a variety of ailments [*see* HONEY], including honey applied on a scab to heal it (*Shabbat* 77b). A patient with a heart problem was told to drink goat's milk directly from the udder (*Tosefta Baba Kamma* 8:12). The liver of a mad dog was suggested for someone bitten by that dog (*Yoma* 8:6). The gall of a white stork is a therapy for a scorpion bite (*Ketubot* 50a). Goat kidney juice is said to cure earaches (*Abodah Zarah* 28b). Squashed gnats are applied to snake bites (*Shabbat* 77b) and crushed spiders to scorpion bites (ibid.). Dog excrement was used to treat *barsam* (pleuritis) and pigeon dung for *rushata* (*Gittin* 69b). For heart weakness, meat from the right flank of a male beast is suggested (*Eruvin* 29b). [*See also* FOLK MEDICINE]

REMEDIES, NONMEDICINAL—Nonmedicinal remedies are recommended in the Talmud for a variety of ailments. Warm compresses are recommended for abdominal pain (*Shabbat* 40b), perhaps using a hot water bottle called *adasha* (*Tosefta Shabbat* 3:7). Alternatively, a hot cup can be placed on the navel (*Shabbat* 66b). A kettle (ibid., 40b) or a bowl of hot water (*Jerushalmi Shabbat* 9:12) may be dangerous. Gourds are placed on the forehead to cool patients with fever (*Yoma* 78a). Trickling water is used to help sick people fall asleep (*Tosefta Shabbat* 2:8). A light may be turned off on the Sabbath to allow a patient to sleep (*Shabbat* 2:5). An abscess is incised and drained (*Abodah Zarah* 28a). A nail from the gallows of an executed criminal is applied on a site of inflammation (*Shabbat* 67a).

The sun has healing powers (*Nedarim* 8b) and carries healing in its wings (Malachi 3:20). The sun healed Jacob (*Genesis Rabbah* 78:5). Water also has healing effects. Lepers are relieved by rain (ibid., 13:16). Patients and animals overcome by blood are put in cold water to cool off (*Shabbat* 53b). Cold water is used in eye compresses (ibid., 78a). Bathing in mineral or salt water heals (*Tosefta Shabbat* 12:13). River waters have healing powers (Ezekiel 47:9; *Exodus Rabbah* 15:21) and may prevent leprosy in Babylon (*Ketubot* 77b). Children were bathed in wine for healing purposes (*Tosefta Shabbat* 12:13). [*See also* BATHING]

REMEDIES, PLANT—Plant remedies are cited in the Bible, including treebarks, roots, and leaves (Ezekiel 47:12). Plant oils are also used (*Berachot* 36a). Plant remedies are most efficacious in the spring (*Shabbat* 147b) and are usually consumed for several days on an empty stomach (*Gittin* 70a). Sometimes, herbs are pulverized and used as a dry powder or are suspended in water and imbibed as a potion as in the case of an abortifacient (*Niddah* 30b). For a mouth abscess, the remedy is blown into the mouth with a blade of straw (*Gittin* 69a; *Yoma* 8:6).

Plant extracts are used as emetics (*Shabbat* 147b). The herb *samtar* heals injuries to a leg nerve (*Baba Batra* 74b) and wounds from spear or arrow punctures (*Yebamot* 114b). Various ophthalmic salves and collyria are made from plants (*Shabbat* 133b) [*see* PLASTERS AND POULTICES]. Green leaves are applied to inflamed eyes (*Shabbat* 109a). Cress in vinegar is a remedy for an open wound (*Abodah Zarah* 28a). Ashes from burned alkali are applied to rectal fissures (ibid., 28b). Radishes are good for fever and beets for cold shivers (ibid.). Peppercorn counteracts bad mouth odor (*Shabbat* 65a) and salt globules relieve toothache or gum disease (ibid). [*See also* VEGETABLES and specific vegetables and plants]

RIBS—The Hebrew word for rib is *tzela* (Daniel 7:5; *Nazir* 52a). God took one of Adam's ribs to create Eve (Genesis 2:21–22); thus, the phrase "my rib" means "my wife" (*Kiddushin* 6a). The Talmud counts eleven ribs on each side (*Oholot* 1:8), perhaps because the twelfth is not attached to the rib cage (Karo's *Shulchan Aruch, Yoreh Deah* 54:1). Only large ribs are said to contain marrow (*Chullin* 52a). The breast of an animal, together with two pairs of ribs, is one of the priestly gifts (Leviticus 7:31). The liver and the gallbladder are said by one sage to be attached to the fifth rib (*Sanhedrin* 49a). This is where Abner pierced Asahel (2 Samuel 2:23) and Joab stabbed Abner (ibid., 3:27) with their spears. Rib fractures in animals are discussed in some detail *(Chullin* 52a).

RUMINANTS—Ruminants have four sections of their stomach: the *keres hapenimit* (rumen or paunch), the *bet hakosot* (reticulum), *hemses* (omasum), and *kevah* (abomasum) (Deuteronomy 18:3; *Chullin* 3:1 and 134b). The inner *keres* refers to the entrance to the rumen (*Chullin* 50b). *Bet hakosot*

literally means "house of goblets" (*Kelim* 16:2). If the rumen of a ruminant is pierced or if the greater portion of the outer covering (serosa) is torn, the animal is not viable (*Chullin* 52b). Perforations or needles can also occur in the other parts of the stomach (ibid., 50b). The four stomachs of ruminants are among the ten or twelve that rule over digestion (*Ecclesiates Rabbah* 7:3). Ruminants also have a "rose lobe" in the right lung—possibly the median lobe or an extra lobe (*Leviticus Rabbah* 18:1).

RUNNING—In biblical times, runners were cultivated mainly for their military value, and there are numerous biblical references to runners as guards (1 Samuel 22:17; 2 Chronicles 12:11; 2 Kings 11:13; 2 Kings 10:25; 1 Kings 14:27). Swift runners were valued as important military assets; men of the tribe of Gad were said to be "mighty men of valor . . . and as swift as the roes upon the mountain" (1 Chronicles 12:8). They were used as a means of military communication. A man from the tribe of Benjamin ran from Aphek to Shiloh, a considerable distance, arriving the same day to notify the High Priest that the Ark of the Covenant was taken (1 Samuel 1:12). According to rabbinic tradition, the man was Saul, later to become king of Israel. Later, Saul and his son Jonathan were eulogized and said to be "swifter than eagles and stronger than lions" (2 Samuel 7:23). Asahel, one of King David's warriors, was "as light of foot [i.e., swift] as one of the roes in the field" (2 Samuel 2:18).

When Absalom, the rebellious son of King David, was slain by David's general Joab (ibid., 1:14), Achimaaz, son of Zadok, volunteered to run to inform David that "the Lord hath avenged him of his enemies" (ibid., 18:19). Apparently Achimaaz was an experienced long-distance runner and was able to overtake and pass a Cushite runner dispatched by Joab. His running style was recognized in that the watchman was able to identify him at a distance. Perhaps King David is praising swift runners such as Asahel and Achimaaz when he compared the sun to a "bridegroom coming out of his chamber and rejoicing like a strong man to run his course" (Psalms 19:6).

Other biblical runners include the fifty runners who ran before the chariots and horses of Absalom and Adonijah, the sons of David (1 Kings 1:5), and the runners employed by King Solomon as his palace guards. Golden shields were made for them by Solomon; in a later generation, Rehoboam prepared brass shields so that his runner-guards would not be defenseless (1 Kings 14:27) and housed them in a chamber of the runners (ibid., 14:28).

In talmudic times, running was recognized as a form of exercise as well as for mundane purposes. Running as a form of exercise on the Sabbath is ordinarily not permitted (*Tosefta Shabbat* 17:16) but runners may run on the Sabbath (*Shabbat* 147a) for other purposes such as to deliver an important message. The Talmud (*Sanhedrin* 96a) interprets the biblical phrase "If thou hast run with the footmen and they have wearied thee, how canst thou contend with horses?" (Jeremiah 12:5) with a parable. Elsewhere (*Niddah* 24b), the Talmud speaks of a man running three parasangs while pursuing a deer but not reaching it. [*See also* EXERCISE]

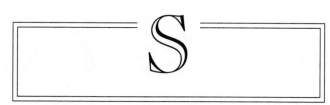

SAFFLOWER—Gallbladder disease is treated with Egyptian *zythom*, which is composed of barley, safflower, and salt (*Shabbat* 110a; *Pesachim* 42b). Safflower, cumin, and fenugreek boiled in wine is a therapy for abnormal vaginal bleeding (*Shabbat* 110ab). Safflower seeds, crushed and boiled in wine, is a remedy for impotence.

SALIVA—The oral cavity is kept moist by spittle or saliva, which is constantly swallowed (Job 7:19). Spittle spurts forth from the mouth when one speaks (*Tohorot* 10:6). Saliva is sweet (*Numbers Rabbah* 18:22) and makes food soft to avoid injury to the intestine (*Exodus Rabbah* 24:1). Kissing on the mouth exposes both people to each other's saliva (*Berachot* 8b). Pomegranates are acrid fruits that stimulate intense salivation (*Ketubot* 61b). Onions also stimulate salivation and expectoration (*Yebamot* 106b). Eating garlic produces unpleasant-tasting spittle (ibid.). Saliva adheres to a spoon that is put in the mouth (*Nedarim* 49b). Saliva flows from a leper's mouth (*Ketubot* 77b).

Spittle from a newborn (*Baba Batra* 126b) and from a fasting person (*Shabbat* 108b) was thought to have healing powers. Such saliva, therefore, could not be used as a routine eye remedy on the Sabbath (ibid.). Tasteless spittle (i.e., from a fasting person) is one of seven substances that, when applied to a red stain, can determine whether it is blood or a dye (*Niddah* 61b–62a; *Sanhedrin* 49b).

Spitting is a mark of ostentation (*Sotah* 47b) and a sign of contempt (*Tosefta Baba Kamma* 9:31). Expectorated saliva should be covered (*Ketubot* 105b). One may not spit before one's teacher unless one has eaten foods very difficult to digest (*Tamid* 27b). Such a pupil suffers dire consequences (*Eruvin* 99a). If a father spits on his daughter's face (Numbers 12:14), he has committed an offense for which a hefty fine may be imposed (*Baba Kamma* 8:6). One may not expectorate on the Temple Mount or in the Temple for it is equivalent to spitting into the Lord's eye (*Berachot* 62b).

Preuss suggests[1] that the view of spitting as being offensive may be related to the tradition that ritual uncleanness is transmitted through spittle (*Shabbat* 14b and 15b; *Pesachim* 19b; *Kelim* 1:3; *Machshirin* 6:6). If a person with a flux (gonorrhea?) spits on a clean person, the latter must wash his clothes (Leviticus 15:8). Saliva from an unclean person cannot be nullified by saliva from a clean person (*Zevachim* 79a). All spittle found anywhere was declared unclean by rabbinic decree (*Tohorot* 4:5), except that found in Jerusalem, where people were scrupulous in matters of purity (*Shekalim* 8:1). Even spittle from Gentiles was declared unclean (*Eduyot* 5:1). Spittle from an Arab (*Yoma* 47a) and a Sadducee (*Niddah* 33b) once flew onto the High Priest's garments, disqualifying him from performing his duties on the Day of Atonement. Spittle defiles when wet or dry (*Eduyot* 5:4; *Niddah* 34a and 35b). Heave offering is burnt if spittle comes in contact with it (*Tohorot* 4:5 and 5:7). The ritual uncleanness of spittle is deduced from the Bible (Leviticus 15:8) by the rabbinic sages (*Niddah* 55b).

Spittle is formed in globules when it is expectorated (*Niddah* 19b). If one spits on the ground and another person is injured, the spitter is liable to pay compensation (*Baba Kamma* 3b). One should not spit on the ground in a bathhouse lest one slip on the stone floor (*Derech Eretz* 10). The ceremony of *chalitzah* (Deuteronomy 25:9), where a man refuses to marry the childless wife of his deceased brother (levirate marriage), requires the woman to

spit before her brother-in-law (*Yebamot* 106b). The judges must see the spittle issuing from the woman's mouth (*Yebamot* 101b and 106b; *Sanhedrin* 49b). [*See also* SPUTUM]

1. F. Rosner (trans.), *Julius Preuss' Biblical and Talmudic Medicine,* (Northvale, NJ: Jason Aronson, 1993), pp. 85–86.

SALT—Although salt does not nourish (*Eruvin* 30a) and becomes neutralized in dough and in cooked food (*Betzah* 39a), people cannot exist without salt (*Jerushalmi Horayot* 3:48). It is regarded as a spice (*Abodah Zarah* 67a) or as produce *(Ketubot* 79b) and is used as a bread seasoning (*Berachot* 2b). A meal without salt is no meal (ibid., 44a). Dry bread and salt is a very meager meal (*Berachot* 2b; *Yebamot* 15b; *Avot* 6:4). Salt is beneficial in small amounts but harmful in large amounts (*Berachot* 34a). Food is stored in salt to preserve it (*Shabbat* 47b).

Salt water or brine is a condiment (*Shabbat* 108b) or preservative for fish (*Abodah Zarah* 35b). Olives are dipped in salt before being eaten (*Betzah* 35a). Salt is collected from a salina or salt deposit (*Shabbat* 73b) and is white or black (*Abodah Zarah* 39b). Salt is pounded in a small cruse or with mortar and pestle (*Betzah* 14a). Salt is used in tanning hides (*Betzah* 11a). Salt placed in a lamp helps the oil burn more clearly (*Shabbat* 67b). Salt must be stored at least three handbreadths distant from a neighbor's wall (*Baba Batra* 2:1)

Medically, salt is an ingredient in remedies for *tzafdina* or gum bleeding (*Yoma* 84a), gallbladder disease (*Shabbat* 110a; *Pesachim* 42b), earache (*Abodah Zarah* 28b), and toothache (*Gittin* 69a). A salt ball is used to clean dentures (*Shabbat* 65a). Using salt on one's food prevents *askara*, which is diphtheritic croup (*Berachot* 40a). Small salted fish can be harmful when washed down with date beer (*Berachot* 44b). Dipping one's finger in salt and licking it helps restore one's memory (*Horayot* 13b). Before bloodletting one should not eat salted meat (*Nedarin* 54b).

Washing the hands after meals is to prevent Sodomite salt on one's fingers from blinding the eyes (*Eruvin* 17b; *Pesachim* 42a; *Chullin* 105a–b). Some sages state that this custom has ceased since no Sodomite salt exists nowadays (*Tosafot, Chullin* 105a, s.v. *mayim*). Salt is used to extract blood from the meat of a slaughtered animal to make it fit for human consumption. Meal offerings in the Temple had to be salted (*Menachot* 20a).

SCAR—When a wound heals, a mound develops (Jeremiah 30:13) and finally a scar, which is paler than the original wound (Nahum 3:19). Scars following dogbites can be quite disfiguring (*Ketubot* 75a). Young people usually do not have venesection scars

(*Sanhedrin* 93b). Flesh and skin do not degenerate; rather, a scar develops there (*Niddah* 55a). Scars are not considered interpositions for ritual immersions (*Niddah* 67a).

SCIATICA—The patriarch Jacob wrestled with the angel of God and was wounded in his sciatic nerve and limped (Genesis 32:26ff.). Since then the consumption of this nerve is prohibited to Jews by divine decree (Genesis 32:33). The Talmud gives instructions about how to remove the sciatic nerve from freshly slaughtered animals (*Chullin* 89b). The removal of this nerve and its tributaries is quite difficult and requires considerable skill.

The talmudic term *shigrona* (*Gittin* 69b) refers to sciatica. A ewe who dragged its hind legs was found at autopsy to be suffering from this malady (*Chullin* 51a and 59a). The treatment for this condition is to rub fish brine sixty times on each hip (*Gittin* 69b). A person with pain in the loins was told to rub his loins with wine and vinegar or with oil, especially rose oil (*Shabbat* 14:4). [*See also* SPINAL CORD]

SCORPIONS—Folk remedies to treat scorpion bites include the gall of a white stork (*Ketubot* 50a), ointment made from black and white lizards (*Shabbat* 77b), old wine (ibid., 109b), warm compresses (*Abodah Zarah* 28b), and crushed spiders (*Shabbat* 77b). A scorpion is more likely to sting than a snake (*Berachot* 33a). The pit into which Joseph was thrown by his brothers (Genesis 37:24) was full of snakes and scorpions (*Shabbat* 22a; *Chagigah* 3a). Modest behavior in the toilet (i.e., outhouse) protects one from a scorpion bite (*Berachot* 62a). Scorpions may be killed even on the Sabbath because of the danger (*Shabbat* 121b). Never did a scorpion bite anyone in Jerusalem (*Yoma* 21a; *Avot* 5:5).

Prayers are recited for afflictions caused by scorpions (*Baba Kamma* 80b). Incantations were recited to ward off scorpions (*Tosefta Shabbat* 7:23). It is forbidden to charm snakes or scorpions (Deuteronomy 18:11; *Keritot* 3b) or to cast a spell over them unless they pose an immediate danger (*Keritot* 3b). Scorpions are said to lay sixty eggs at a time (*Genesis Rabbah* 44:17; *Leviticus Rabbah* 13:5) and to give birth to sixty or seventy at one time (*Exodus Rabbah* 1:8). [*See also* SNAKES AND SERPENTS]

SCROTUM—The scrotum is called *kis*, meaning "sac." Each testicle sits in its own sac (*Tosefta Bechorot* 4:8). A hornet sting to the scrotum can make a man sterile (*Sotah* 36b). An animal with crushed testicles cannot be offered in the Temple (Leviticus 22:24). Testicles crushed while still in the scrotum can retain or regain their vitality; since no air gets into them, they do not putrefy (*Chullin* 93a–b). Normal testicles and scrotum can shrink (i.e., retract inside) and resemble crushed testicles (*Bechorot* 39b). A man once scratched off boils *(chatatim)* from his scrotum and became a castrate (*Jerushalmi Yebamot* 8:9).

SCURVY—A disease called *tzafdina*, in which gum bleeding is the major symptom, is described in the Talmud. *Tzafdina* in most Jewish sources, in both the classic German and English versions of the Talmud, as well as in modern Hebrew dictionaries, is translated as "scurvy." Rabbi Yochanan suffered from *tzafdina* and went to a Roman matron seeking a remedy (*Yoma* 84a). The symptoms of this disease are that the gums bleed if one puts anything between the teeth. The story of Rabbi Yochanan's scurvy and the remedy provided by the Roman matron is found elsewhere in the Talmud (*Abodah Zarah* 28a) with minor variations.

Another talmudic passage states the following: Rabbi Matia ben Cheresh said: "If one has pain in his throat, he may pour medicine into his mouth on the Sabbath because there is a possibility of danger to human life, and every danger to human life suspends the laws of the Sabbath" (*Mishnah Yoma* 8:6). Some talmudic commentators, notably Alfasi and Asheri, interpret this passage literally. Others, however, notably Tur, Bertinoro, and Tosafot

Yom Tov, change the phrase "pain in the throat" to "pain in the teeth so that the gums begin to rot and the palate and throat become secondarily involved." Also supporting the latter viewpoint is Maimonides, who states in his commentary on the Mishnah that "pain in the mouth means the gums, which are rotting, and if nothing is done, the palate will also rot." Whether Rabbi Matia ben Cheresh described scurvy or another malady of the mouth, teeth, gums, and throat cannot be answered with certainty.

Another sage who suffered from presumed scurvy is Rabbi Judah the Prince (*Baba Metzia* 85a). He observed that Rabbi Eleazar, son of Rabbi Simeon, had submitted to much suffering for which he was divinely rewarded in that his body remained intact, defying decomposition and decay, for many years. Thereupon Rabbi Judah the Prince undertook to suffer likewise for thirteen years, six through stones in the kidneys or bladder and seven through scurvy. The talmudic word for scurvy here is *tzipparna*, which is a variation of *tzafdina*. Rabbi Nathan ben Yechiel states that the manuscript versions of the Talmud in fact have the word *tzafdina*. The English translation of the Talmud also renders *tzipparna* as scurvy.

That *tzafdina* is an affliction of the teeth that is a potential hazard to life because it begins in the mouth but spreads to the intestines is also evident from the Jerusalem Talmud (*Abodah*

Zarah 2:2). Whether *tzafdina* represents true scurvy, as appears to be the opinion of most talmudic commentators and translators, or whether it is another ailment, such as pyorrhea, thrush, tooth abscess, or the like, as the medical description in the Talmud would appear to indicate, is a problem that may never be resolved.[1] [*See also* GUMS]

1. F. Rosner, "Scurvy," in *Medicine in the Bible and the Talmud*, 2nd ed. (Hoboken, NJ: Ktav and Yeshiva University Press, 1995), pp. 54–57.

SEX DETERMINATION—The secret of determining one's baby's sex was known to the talmudic sages, who interpret the biblical phrase "if a woman emits seed and bears a male child" (Leviticus 12:2) to mean that if she emits her semen first she will bear a male but if the man emits his semen first, she will bear a female (*Niddah* 31a). Two places in the Talmud raise the question of what happens if both man and woman emit seed simultaneously (*Niddah* 25b and 28a). Several possible answers are given: The offspring may be a hermaphrodite (*androginos*); one whose sex is unknown (*tumtum*); or twins, one male and one female.

Elsewhere the Talmud describes a "village of males" (*Kfar Dikraya*), so called because women used to bear male children first, finally a girl, and then no more (*Gittin* 57a). Another talmudic passage states that if a man's wife is pregnant and he supplicates that God grant that his wife bear a male child, this is a vain prayer (*Berachot* 54a).

Does the phrase "if a woman emits seed" refer to ovulation or to orgasm? The biblical commentaries of Ibn Ezra, Siftei Chachamim, Nachmanides (Ramban), and Seforno on Leviticus 12:2 discuss this issue extensively but do not resolve it. The Talmud emphatically states that if a woman emits her semen first, she will bear a male, and if the man emits his semen first, she will bear a female. We have yet to understand what the Talmud means. The secret of sex predetermination remains hidden.[1]

---

1. F. Rosner, "Sex Determination" in *Medicine in the Bible and the Talmud*, 2nd ed. (Hoboken, NJ: Ktav and Yeshiva University Press, 1995), pp. 248–253.

SHEEP—Sheep are fit for human consumption (i.e., kosher) (Deuteronomy 14:4). Sheep have thick tails that cover their hind parts (*Shabbat* 77b). Sheep have a six-month pregnancy (*Rosh Hashanah* 8a). Sheep with very small kidneys are not viable (*Chullin* 55a–b). Flies are often found in the nasal passages of sheep (*Shabbat* 54b). Sheep in the meadow manure the field (*Moed Katan* 12a). In sheep, one can remove

the brain from the skull without breaking any bones (*Pesachim* 84b).

Moses and David were both tested by God with sheep (*Exodus Rabbah* 2:2). The people of Israel are compared to sheep (*Exodus Rabbah* 24:3 and 34:3). [*See also* LAMBS, CALF, and GOATS]

SHOULDER—In Hebrew, *katef* and *shechem* refer, respectively, to the anterior and posterior parts of the shoulder. When Abraham was commanded to sacrifice his son Isaac, he took wood (Genesis 22:6) and carried it on his shoulder (*Genesis Rabbah* 56:3). Members of the family of Kohot carried the holy vessels on their shoulders (Numbers 7:9). When the Jews eventually return to Jerusalem, they will carry their daughters on their shoulders (Isaiah 49:22). Moses' blessing to Benjamin is that He dwell between his shoulders (Deuteronomy 33:12). A porter carries his load on his shoulders (Genesis 49:15). Women carried water pitchers on their shoulders (Genesis 21:14 and 24:15). Shem and Yafet covered their shoulders with a garment and walked backwards so as not to view their father's nakedness (Genesis 9:23). When Job speaks about his arm falling from his shoulder blade (Job 31:22), he is referring to dislocation of his humerus.

While bathing in the hot springs of Tiberias, a person placed his hand on the shoulder of the person in front of him in order to support himself (*Jerushalmi Shabbat* 1:3). In Babylon, captured Jews had sacks filled with sand placed on their shoulders until they were stooped over (Midrash Psalms 137:3). The shoulder, the cheeks, and the maw are biblically prescribed (Deuteronomy 18:3) priestly gifts (*Leviticus Rabbah* 7:29ff.; *Yebamot* 99b and 100b). There are four bones in the shoulder (*Makkot* 23b; *Oholot* 1:8).

The armpit under the shoulder is referred to as *shechi*. Women used to remove their hair from that location, a practice forbidden for men (*Nazir* 59a). Placing coins under one's armpits is either unappetizing (*Jerushalmi Terumot* 8:45) or unhealthy (Karo's *Shulchan Aruch, Orach Chayim* 170:16). The armpit was examined for signs of leprosy (*Negaim* 2:4).

SKIN—God clothes people with skin and flesh (Job 10:11; Ezekiel 37:6), although the mother contributes that skin to her offspring (*Niddah* 31a). The skin of Jews and other Semites is intermediate in color between that of Germanic people and Ethiopians (*Negaim* 2:1). It becomes dark when exposed to the sun (Song of Songs 1:6) or from anxiety and grief (Job 30:30). Ham, son of Noah, had black skin (*Sanhedrin* 108b). A dark-skinned man should not marry an equally dark skinned woman lest their offspring be pitch black (*Bechorot* 45b). The skin of Moses shined from the glow of divine splendor (Exodus 34:29). Incising the skin as a sign of mourning (Jeremiah 16:6 and 48:37) is prohibited in Judaism (Leviticus 19:28), as is skin cutting for heathen cultic purposes (1 Kings 18:28). Tattooing is also prohibited (Leviticus 19:28). Pallor (anemia) and yellowness of the skin (jaundice) are discussed elsewhere in this encyclopedia.

Fish and meat should not be salted together for this food may lead to skin sickness (*Pesachim* 112a). If a patient's blood is not let periodically, a skin disease may develop (*Bechorot* 42b). If intercourse takes place after both spouses have been bled, they will have children with *raatan* (see below) (*Niddah* 17a). The skin diseases collectively known as *tzaraat* in the Bible (Leviticus 13:1ff.) probably refer to various forms of leprosy including *baheret* (spotty leprosy), *se'et* (nodular leprosy), and *sappachat* (vulgar leprosy or psoriasis). *Nega tzaraat* means "afflicted" by leprosy. The color, depth, location, and character of these skin lesions and their causes, dissemination, diagnosis, and treatment are discussed in detail by Preuss.[1] He also analyzes the skin diseases of Job, Hezekiah, and the Egyptians as well as skin rashes, scars, wounds, burns, and inflammations such as *shechin*, *garab*, *cheres*, *raatan*, *chatatin*, *chaluda*, and others.

Certain snake extracts can cure skin eruptions (*Shabbat* 77b). Oil of olives rubbed on women's skin removes the hair and rejuvenates the skin (*Pesachim* 43a). The skin of a eunuch is smooth and soft (*Yebamot* 80b). Certain skins are thin and tender and legally regarded as flesh. These include the skin of humans, fetuses, and a variety of animals (*Chullin* 122a). Animals were flayed for their skins (*Chullin* 123a). Animals were sold with and without their skins (*Eruvin* 27b). The skin of a stoned ox is forbidden (*Pesachim* 22b; *Sanhedrin* 15b). *Diftera* is a salted animal skin placed in flour but not treated with gallnuts (*Megillah* 19a). Such skins were prepared to serve as parchment for holy writings (*Gittin* 22a). He who sleeps on a tanner's hide may develop leprosy (*Pesachim* 112b). Fish skins were used to polish and smooth the surface of furniture (*Sanhedrin* 20b; *Kelim* 16:1). The Talmud also speaks of skin bags (*Kelim* 20:1) or water skins (*Kelim* 24:11 and 26:4; *Parah* 5:8; *Mikvaot* 6:1), skin bottles (*Abodah Zarah* 33a; *Chagigah* 22a), skin slings (*Eduyot* 3:5), a bed of skins (*Sanhedrin* 20b), and a street of skinners (*Baba Metzia* 24b). [*See also* DEPILATORIES, BALDNESS, and COSMETICS]

1. F. Rosner, (trans.), *Julius Preuss' Biblical and Talmudic Medicine* (Northvale, NJ: Jason Aronson, 1993), pp. 323–353.

SKULL—The temples are at the sides of the skull and that is where Jael smashed Sisera's skull (Judges 4:21). The temples are also the biblical "corners of the head" (Leviticus 19:27), which the Talmud calls "the end of the head" (*Makkot* 20b). The brain is enclosed in the skull (*Chullin* 45a). The anterior fontanelle in a baby is where the skull is soft and pulsates (*Menachot* 37a). An animal's skull is called the *kappa de mocha* (*Chullin* 54a). If the greater part of its skull is shattered, the animal is not viable (ibid., 52b). Skull fractures in birds were carefully examined (ibid., 56ab). In birds, bean-shaped protuberances (cerebral hemispheres?) are seen at the entrance to the cranium (ibid., 45a–b). In sheep, the brain can be removed from the skull through the nose (*Pesachim* 84b) or through the ear (*Jerushalmi Pesachim* 7:35) without breaking a single bone [*see also* EMBALMING].

The Talmud describes people with round-shaped skulls and heads (*Nedarim* 66b) and newborns with "stopped up" skulls (anencephaly?) (*Niddah* 24a). Surgeons' drills were used for trepanning (*Eruvin* 7a; *Oholot* 2:3). The skull can also be split with clubs (*Sanhedrin* 81b). A certain woman broke Abimelech's skull (Judges 9:53). If a man strikes his servant on the brain and water comes out (skull fracture with cerebrospinal fluid leak?), the owner must free his servant (*Tosefta Baba Kamma* 9:27). When Titus died, they opened his skull and found a sparrow-like mass (brain tumor?) (*Gittin* 56b). A procedure is described for softening the base of the skull to extract worms (or tumor?) from the brain (*Ketubot* 77b).

A skull imparts ritual impurity (*Oholot* 2:1). Hillel once saw a skull floating on the water (*Sukkah* 53a; *Avot* 2:6). King Jehoiakim's skull was buried twice and emerged from the ground twice, after which it was burnt in an oven (*Sanhedrin* 82a and 104a). [*See also* BRAIN and HEAD]

SLAUGHTERING—Animals are fit for human consumption only following ritual slaughtering (*Genesis Rabbah* 16:6), which requires the severance by a single sharp cut of the trachea, esophagus, and both carotid arteries (*Chullin* 27a; *Yoma* 75b). The internal organs of slaughtered animals must be carefully examined for defects or blemishes before the meat is declared fit for consumption (*Chullin* 46a–b). Any sharp instrument such as a knife, sickle, flint, or reed is fit for ritual slaughtering (*Chullin* 15b–16a; *Genesis Rabbah* 56:6). To test whether or not a slaughtering knife is completely notch-free, it is examined with the nail of one's finger (*Chullin* 17b).

Cattle are bought and sold for breeding or for slaughtering (*Baba Batra* 92a). One should not live in a city without a ritual slaughterer (*San-*

hedrin* 17b). Liquids in a slaughterhouse are blood and water used to wash the blood away (*Pesachim* 16a). In the Temple slaughterhouse, no fly was ever seen (*Avot* 5:5).

SLEEP—Night was created for sleep (*Eruvin* 65a). The sleep of a laborer is sweet (*Ecclesiastes Rabbah* 5:10:2). He who stays awake at night imperils his life (*Avot* 3:4). If someone swears to not sleep for three days, he is flogged and his oath is invalid (*Nedarim* 15a). On the other hand, excessive sleep is not a good thing either. Lazy people sleep a lot (Proverbs 6:9). Workers sleep more than their masters (*Kiddushin* 49b). The royal servants of Ahasuerus, however, complained they slept little because they worked so hard (*Megillah* 13b). Priests on duty in the Temple could not sleep and were rudely awakened if they did (*Tamid* 28a). During the water-drawing ceremony in the Temple, the Levites did not sleep but dozed on each other's shoulders (*Sukkah* 53a). A man who becomes a surety for another may not sleep until he has paid his debt (Proverbs 6:4). The High Priest was not allowed to sleep on the night prior to Yom Kippur (*Yoma* 19b). He was, therefore, not fed a large meal on Yom Kippur eve (*Yoma* 1:1) and was made to walk to and fro on the cold marble floor (*Yoma* 1:7).

In the hot Middle East, people nap or sleep at midday or early afternoon, as did Abraham (Genesis 18:1) and Ishboshet (2 Samuel 4:5). Shepherds' flocks also rest at noon (Song of Songs 1:7). Work begins early in the morning as did Abraham (Genesis 22:3), Balaam (Numbers 22:21), and others. Morning sleep is decried (Proverbs 26:14; *Avot* 3:10) and early rising is recommended (Psalms 119:62). Sleep at dawn is like a steel edge to iron (*Berachot* 62a). Only royalty sleeps late (*Berachot* 1:2). King David arose at midnight to serve the Lord so that he awakened the dawn (Psalms 57:9; *Berachot* 3b).

Moderation in sleep is praiseworthy (*Avot* 6:5). Torah study day and night is required (Psalms 1:2) and those who sacrifice sleep for it will inherit the future world (*Baba Batra* 10a) as will their wives who allow it (*Ketubot* 62a). One should not sleep in the house of Torah study (*Megillah* 28a). Several talmudic sages slept only on the Sabbath (*Sukkah* 28a). One should only nap and not sleep during the day (*Sukkah* 26b). Sleep is good if it is followed by Torah study (*Genesis Rabbah* 9:5 and 44:17). One can sleep sufficiently after one is dead (*Eruvin* 65a).

Sleep is one-sixtieth part of death (*Berachot* 57b). The incomplete experience of death is sleep which is like a premature fruit and death is the ripe fruit (*Genesis Rabbah* 17:5). Divinely induced sleep is described in relation to Adam (Genesis 2:21). He who

wishes to taste death should sleep in his shoes (*Yoma* 78b). When a person sleeps the soul warms the body to keep it alive (*Genesis Rabbah* 14:9). God restores one's soul every morning (Deuteronomy 5:15). Choni the circle drawer slept for seventy years (*Taanit* 23a).

Medically, sleep is beneficial in moderation but harmful in excess (*Gittin* 70a). Sleep is a favorable sign in a convalescing patient (*Genesis Rabbah* 20:10; *Berachot* 57b). Wine induces fatigue and sleep (*Eruvin* 64b). Sleep overcomes the effects of the wine (*Ecclesiastes Rabbah* 7:26:2). Dozing is not sleep and not wakefulness (*Taanit* 12b). Eating a large meal also induces sleep (*Berachot* 61b). Nocturnal emissions occur during sleep (*Yebamot* 53a). One should not sleep in a house alone (*Shabbat* 151b) nor in the shadow of a palm tree (*Pesachim* 111a). [*See also* INSOMNIA and SOPORIFICS]

SNAKES AND SERPENTS—The Talmud (*Avot de Rabbi Nathan* 29:3) states that in the Bible the snake is designated by six Hebrew words: *nachash* (twenty-nine times), *saraf* (Numbers 21:8; Deuteronomy 8:15, Isaiah 30:6), *tannin* (Genesis 1:32; Exodus 7:10–12; Isaiah 27:1), *zifoni* (Proverbs 23:32; Isaiah 11:8, 14:29, and 59:5; Jeremiah 8:17), *efah* (Job 20:16; Isaiah 30:6 and 59:5), and *achshub*

(Psalms 140:4). The term *shefifon* is also found (Genesis 49:17). *Saraf* may be identical to *peten*, the Egyptian cobra (Deuteronomy 32:33; Job 20:14–16; Psalms 58:5–7).

Nachash is the snake or serpent that transmitted its spiritual venom to the first woman in the Garden of Eden (Genesis 3:1–14). "And God made the beast of the earth" (Genesis 1:25) refers to the serpent (*Genesis Rabbah* 7:5). "And God created the great sea monsters" (Genesis 1:21) refers (*Baba Batra* 74b) to Leviathan the slant (i.e., male) serpent (Job 26:13, Isaiah 27:11) and to Leviathan the tortuous (i.e., female) serpent (Isaiah 27:1). Elsewhere the Bible speaks of a flying serpent (Isaiah 30:6) and a sea serpent (Isaiah 27:1). These seem to represent mythological land, sea, and air dragons.

Moses cast his rod on the ground and it became a snake (Exodus 4:3 and 7:15). When Aaron and the Egyptians cast rods, they turned into *tanninim*, which Rashi interprets as snakes (Exodus 7:10–12). The punishment for evil or slander is to be bitten by a serpent (Amos 5:19 and 9:30; Ecclesiastes 10:8). There is no advantage in being a slanderer or master of the evil tongue (Ecclesiastes 10:11), for "The vipers' tongue shall slay him" (Job 20:16). Such Jews will lick the dust like a serpent (Micah 7:17). The serpent eats dust as its food (Genesis 3:14; Isaiah 65:25). Impenitence will bring retribution in the form of serpents and

basilisks, which cannot be charmed but will bite (Jeremiah 8:17). The biblical brazen serpents are discussed in detail elsewhere.[1]

In the Midrash, a serpent is called *aviya* (*Genesis Rabbah* 26:7). A serpent is said to bear offspring after seven years (ibid., 20:4). Some snakes are harmless and can be domesticated. When they live in a house, they are fond of garlic (ibid., 54:1). Some snakes may even be afraid of man (ibid., 34:12). A serpent's eyelid quivers after death (ibid., 98:14). A serpent can be rendered harmless by snake charmers. (ibid., 19:10; *Deuteronomy Rabbah* 6:11 and 7:10; *Song of Songs Rabbah* 7:8:1).

The snake as the symbol of evil and of slander is found throughout the Midrash. Even Moses spoke slanderously of the Children of Israel (Exodus 4:1) and followed the example of the serpent that spoke slanderously of its Creator (Exodus Rabbah 3:12). The conversion of Moses' staff into a serpent as he threw it on the ground (Exodus 4:3) may have been a sign of God's displeasure, as if to say: "You, Moses, did what this serpent did" (ibid.). Alternatively, the rod was converted into a serpent to symbolize Pharaoh (ibid; *Exodus Rabbah* 9:4), who is called a serpent (Ezekiel 23:3; Isaiah 27:1). Numerous additional references to snakes and serpents are found in the Midrash.[2]

The Talmud describes the anatomy and physiology of snakes (*Niddah* 23a;

Bechorot 8a; *Chullin* 64a and 127a; *Shabbat* 77b; *Berachot* 33a), habits of snakes (*Pesachim* 8a and 112b; *Abodah Zarah* 30b; *Betzah* 7b; *Yoma* 75a), snake charmers (*Pesachim* 10b; *Baba Metzia* 84b; *Sanhedrin* 65a and 101a; *Keritot* 3b), giant snakes (*Baba Batra* 73b; *Shevuot* 29a; *Nedarim* 24b), snake bites and snake venom (*Berachot* 33a and 62a; *Abodah Zarah* 30b; *Sanhedrin* 78a; *Yebamot* 116b; *Eduyot* 1:12; *Chullin* 94a; *Terumot* 8:6), remedies for snakebites and venom (*Shabbat* 109b and 156b), and the prevention of snakebites (*Pesachim* 111a; *Shabbat* 110a). Many other references to snakes and serpents are found in the Talmud.[3]

Many of the statements in the Bible and Talmud concerning snakes and serpents have primarily homiletical connotations. Perhaps because of this, only a few of such statements have any scientific validity. The midrashic assertion that a serpent bears offspring every seven years is contrary to scientific fact. Most snakes and serpents have a litter every year. It is possible that the species referred to in the Midrash is now extinct. More likely is the explanation that the seven years is not meant to be taken literally. Rather, the Divine punishment on the snake for all times for enticing Eve in the Garden of Eden is to suffer more and for longer during pregnancy and parturition than does a woman. Other interpretations are possible.

That snakes are fond of garlic (*Genesis Rabbah* 54:1) and dust (Genesis 3:14; Isaiah 65:25) and dislike vinegar (*Abodah Zarah* 30b) is also not to be understood literally. Since snakes are exclusively carnivorous, their diet consists entirely of meat and meat products. For a snake to copulate with a toad or a lizard (*Chullin* 127a) seems impossible from a scientific viewpoint. The venom of young snakes is identical to that of old snakes; hence, the talmudic assertion that the venom of a young snake sinks to the bottom of a container of fluid whereas that of an old one floats on top (*Abodah Zarah* 30b) is unexplained. The incident of the biblical brazen serpent (Numbers 21:5–9) seems inexplicable from a purely scientific viewpoint. The danger of drinking from uncovered water or wine is extremely remote and essentially nonexistent. Snakes do not discharge venom into fluid from which they drink. They inject their victims with poison to kill them in order to eat them or fight off an enemy, such as man. Only if a snake has recently discharged venom and still has a few drops of fresh, moist venom on its fangs could it possibly exude poison into fluid from which it drinks. Even then there is no danger to a human being who imbibes such fluid since snake poison is not absorbed through the intestinal tract of man if taken in orally.

The use of snake poison to prepare an antidote for a person bitten by a snake (*Shabbat* 3a and 107a; *Eduyot* 2:5) does have scientific merit. Such antidotes were already prepared in the twelfth century and earlier, as described by Maimonides.[4] The prevention of snakebites by a variety of means (vide supra) is also a modern concept. To confuse a snake with an unusual scent or object to force the snake away from oneself (*Shabbat* 110a) finds its analogy in present-day use of shark repellents.

---

1. F. Rosner, "Snakes and Serpents in Bible and Talmud," in *Medicine in the Bible and the Talmud*, 2nd ed. (Hoboken, NJ: Ktav and Yeshiva University Press, 1995), pp. 254–268.
2. Ibid.
3. Ibid.
4. F. Rosner, *Moses Maimonides' Treatise on Poisons, Hemorrhoids, and Cohabitation* (Haifa: Maimonides Research Institute, 1984), pp. 21–115.

SNEEZING—According to legend, originally there was no illness in the world at all; rather, whenever a healthy person's time to die arrived, he sneezed and his soul left him through his nose. Thus, when Jacob went to bless his sons, he began to sneeze, and in anticipation of his imminent death prayed, "I have waited for Thy salvation, O Lord" (Genesis 49:18). He said, "Give me enough time to bless my sons." Thus when a person sneezes, he is obligated to thank God that he remains alive.

Sneezing at the table was considered by the ancients to be a bad omen (Pliny 28:5). Even those who did not

ordinarily offer the traditional "Bless you" after a sneeze might here be inclined to do so. The Jerusalem Talmud states (*Berachot* 6:10) that it was necessary specifically to forbid the exclamation "Bless you" during meals because of the feared danger of choking. Many historians and some clerics report that the origin of the thesis that sneezing is a sign of great danger is the bubonic plague, in which people died suddenly while sneezing or yawning.[1] The Babylonian Talmud (*Niddah* 9:8) points out that yawning and sneezing in a woman may be signs of impending menstruation.

Although the legend of the ill patriarch Jacob (Genesis 48:1) considers sneezing to be a bad and feared omen, the teaching of the Talmud states that the same phenomenon is prognostically a good sign in a patient (*Berachot* 57b) and indicates healing: "His sneezing signifies the light of healing" (Job 41:10). The Talmud (*Berachot* 24b) also considers it to be a favorable omen if someone sneezes while he is praying. It indicates that just as God looks favorably toward him here on earth, so too the angels look favorably toward him in heaven.

The son of the Shunammite woman, who seemed to have died of sunstroke, sneezed seven times and opened his eyes (2 Kings 4:35). Sneezing occurs forcibly and involuntarily (*Berachot* 24b). A concealed eavesdropper once revealed his presence thereby (*Jerushalmi Yoma* 3:40). A strong external stimulus such as frankincense can induce sneezing (*Jerushalmi Sukkah* 5:55). After a suspected adulteress drinks the "bitter tasting waters," she sneezes until her body becomes unsettled (spasmodic sneezing) (*Niddah* 9:8). [*See also* NOSE]

---

1. F. Rosner (trans.), *Julius Preuss' Biblical and Talmudic Medicine* (Northvale, NJ: Jason Aronson, 1993), pp. 74–76.

SOAP—Biblical soaps include *neter* (Jeremiah 2:22) neutralized with vinegar (Proverbs 25:20); *nitron*, a mineral alkaline salt; and *borit* (Jeremiah 2:22), the alkaline plant salt prepared from burned plants that are rich in potash and used by washerwomen (Malachi 3:2). The Talmud describes *ashleg* (*Shabbat* 9:5 and 90a; *Niddah* 9:6 and 62a; *Sanhedrin* 49b), a kind of alkali or mineral used as a soap or detergent to determine whether a red stain on a garment is blood or dye. Also used for this purpose are *borit* (sometimes translated as "lye" or "sulfur") and *ahala* (soapwort), another alkaline plant used as a soap [*see* FORENSIC MEDICINE]. The *ashleg* plant is found between the cracks of pearls, from which it is extracted with an iron nail (*Niddah* 62a).

Preuss[1] postulates that when Job washed himself with *mei sheleg* and *bor* (Job 9:30–31), these terms refer to *ashleg* (soapwort) and *borit* (potash).

Perfumed soap powder contained soapwort, myrtle, or violet as a base. Also used were frankincense powder soaked with jasmine roses. Pepper powder is also mentioned as a soap-like material. These powders are wild and do not loosen the hair (*Shabbat* 9:5 and 90a; *Niddah* 9:6 and 62a), as does *nitron* (*Shabbat* 50a).

Soapwort was also recommended for the healing of a pus blister or abscess (*Gittin* 69b). Hair cleansing was accomplished with *nitron* (soda), *ahala* (soapwort), and *adama* (earth). Soda and earth tear the hair loose (*Niddah* 66b) whereas soapwort causes the hair to stick together (*Shabbat* 50a). Newborn babies were washed in water and "salted" (Ezekiel 16:4–5; *Shabbat* 129b). Sometimes they were washed in wine (*Tosefta Shabbat* 12:13). [*See also* WASHING and BATHING]

---

1. F. Rosner (trans.), *Julius Preuss' Biblical and Talmudic Medicine* (Northvale, NJ: Jason Aronson, 1993), pp. 371–372.

SOPORIFICS—Tiredness after a full meal is well known (*Yoma* 18a). A full stomach induces a person to sleep (*Berachot* 61b; *Taanit* 23a). That is why the High Priest was not given a large meal on the eve of Yom Kippur (*Yoma* 19b). After a meal, one should go for a walk and not to bed (*Moed Katan* 11a). The best soporific is physical activity. A laborer has sweet sleep no matter how little or much he eats (Ecclesiastes 5:11). Wine is also a powerful sleep inducer (*Eruvin* 64b). The sleep of the wicked benefits the world because it is spared of their wickedness while they sleep (*Sanhedrin* 72a).

A sleeping potion was given to a very obese patient before he underwent an extensive operation to remove much of his fat (*Baba Metzia* 83b). A person being led to his execution is given a potion of frankincense and wine to "benumb his senses" (*Sanhedrin* 43a). Sick patients can be helped to sleep by the sound of flowing water (*Tosefta Shabbat* 2:8; *Eruvin* 104a) or by turning off the lights (*Shabbat* 2:5). Wearing a fox's tooth is a folk remedy to help one fall asleep (*Shabbat* 67a). Putting one's hand on one's forehead is a step to sleep (*Pesachim* 112a). [*See also* SLEEP and ANESTHESIA]

SORCERY—Judaism categorically prohibits sorcery as the first and foremost abhorrent practice of the nations. These practices also include augury, soothsaying, divining, casting spells, consulting ghosts or familiar spirits, and inquiring of the dead. "Anyone who does such things is abhorrent to the Lord" (Deuteronomy 18:9–14). Witchcraft in general is also outlawed: "Thou shalt not suffer a witch to live" (Exodus 22:17). Crimes of sorcery are considered tantamount to the idola-

trous crime of human sacrifice (Deuteronomy 18:10). The various forms of sorcery are defined in detail in the Talmud (*Sanhedrin* 65a). Balaam conducted some type of sorcery (*Sanhedrin* 105a). A sorcerer (*Sanhedrin* 53a) or sorceress should be stoned (*Berachot* 21b) but not if he only creates illusions (*Sanhedrin* 67a). Necromancers and charmers are included among the sorcerers (*Yebamot* 4a). Judges in the Sanhedrin had to have a knowledge of sorcery to be able to convict those who seduce and pervert by means of witchcraft (*Sanhedrin* 17a; *Menachot* 65a). Noahides are also prohibited from practicing sorcery (ibid., 60a). Sorcery is forbidden because it overrules the laws of nature (*Chullin* 7b).

Whether the use of sorcery for medical or healing purposes was exempted from the prohibition was a much-debated question in the writings of medieval Jewish authorities.[1] One view is that the practices prevalent in the Middle Ages were not of the idolatrous type prohibited in the Bible as sorcery (S. Habir, Responsa *Nachalat Shiva* #76). Another view is that the prohibition of sorcery can be waived in cases of grave danger to life (J. Ettlinger, Responsa *Binyan Zion* #67). Yet another view is that sorcery or witchcraft may be resorted to only for conditions thought to have been caused or induced by sorcery or witchcraft (S. Luria, Responsa *Maharshal*

#3). [*See also* MAGIC, INCANTA-TIONS, and AMULETS]

---

1. H. J. Zimmels, *Magicians, Theologians, and Doctors* (London, Goldston & Son, 1952), pp. 179–180.

SOTAH—Adultery is biblically prohibited (Exodus 20:13; Deuteronomy 5:17) and both partners are put to death (Leviticus 20:10) by strangulation (*Sanhedrin* 11:1), if premeditation is proven and the act itself is verified by the testimony of two or more eyewitnesses. If both conditions are not fulfilled, the death penalty cannot be carried out.

At the time of the Temple, if a man seriously suspected his wife of infidelity, he could subject her to the biblically described "ordeal of jealousy" (Numbers 5:11–31) for a *sotah* (suspected adulteress). Following the destruction of the Temple, this procedure was abolished by Rabbi Yochanan ben Zakkai. The ordeal, including the drinking of the water of bitterness by a wayward woman or suspected adulteress, is the subject of lengthy discussion by the biblical commentators and talmudic sages.[1] An entire tractate of Talmud is devoted thereto *(Sotah)*. The "falling away" of the thigh and the swelling of the abdomen (Numbers 5:22) followed by the woman's death if she is, in fact, guilty of infidelity, require exposition and explanation.

Rashi (Numbers 5:12) states that the Hebrew word *sotah* has the same derivation as *shoteh*, or "fool." Adulterers never sin unless a spirit of madness or folly enters them *(Sotah* 3a). Rashi further explains that even though the *sotah*'s entire body suffers (vide infra) when she drinks the bitter waters (*Numbers Rabbah* 9:18), only the thigh and belly are mentioned in Numbers 5:21 and 27 "because the sin began there." This explanation is based on the talmudic assertion *(Sotah* 8b) that she began the transgression (i.e., committed adultery) with the thigh and afterwards with the womb; therefore, she is punished first in the thigh and afterwards in the womb (Numbers 5:21).

The water that the *sotah* is made to drink is called the "water of bitterness that causeth the curse" (Numbers 5:18). Many commentators state that Scripture describes the water in terms of its final effect, for there will be bitterness in it, God will deal bitterly with the *sotah*, and it will effect a curse upon her (Rashi, Ibn Ezra, Sifre Hirsch, and others). What was the result of the curse? Not only did her abdomen swell and her thigh "fall away," but her face turned green, her eyes protruded, and she became filled with veins *(Sotah* 20a). Rashi explains that the veins over her mandible swelled and appeared distended and her skin or flesh became very swollen.

There is no dearth of medical explanations of these signs and symptoms.[2] Suggestions include hydrops of the ovaries, swelling due to pregnancy complicated by dropsy, and abortion with peritonitis. None of these rationalizations is satisfactory. Maimonides opines that the entire "ordeal of jealousy" is to instill fear into the woman to induce her to confess if she is guilty. Nachmanides and others state that the swelling of the belly, the falling away of the thigh, and the ultimate death of the woman occurred solely by Divine intervention and have no medical connotations. [See also ADULTERY]

1. F. Rosner, "The ordeal of the Sotah (Wayward Woman)," in Medicine in the Bible and the Talmud, (Hoboken, NJ: Ktav and Yeshiva University Press, 1995), pp. 239–247.

2. F. Rosner (trans.), Julius Preuss' Biblical and Talmudic Medicine (Northvale, NJ: Jason Aronson, 1993), pp. 473–474.

SOUL—Lengthy discussions of the soul can be found elsewhere.[1,2] The Bible uses the word soul (nefesh) to refer to a person (e.g., Leviticus 2:1). The soul is in God's hand (Job 12:10; Deuteronomy Rabbah 5:4). The soul is heard around the world (Yoma 20a; Genesis Rabbah 6:7; Exodus Rabbah 5:9). The soul departs like rushing waters from a channel (Leviticus Rabbah 4:2 and 6:6:1). The souls of the righteous are placed in the Divine treasure (Ecclesiastes Rabbah 3:21:1).

There are three partners in the creation of a human being: the father, the mother, and God. God provides the spirit of life, the soul, and understanding and discernment (Niddah 31a). The soul is implanted by God (Genesis Rabbah 32:11) in the fetus at the moment of conception, when the embryo is formed (Sanhedrin 91b), or when the baby is born (Genesis Rabbah 34:10). The soul that God gives us is pure (Niddah 30b). The soul sees but is not seen (Berachot 10a). Man is given an additional soul for the Sabbath (Taanit 27b). A person's soul resembles a winged grasshopper chained by one foot. When a person sleeps, his soul roams around the world and these are his dreams (Midrash Psalms 11:6). Were it not for the spittle in the mouth, one's soul would depart (Numbers Rabbah 18:22). In ancient times, when people sneezed their souls departed. Thus, when a person sneezes, he should thank God if he is still alive (Pirke de Rabbi Eliezer 52). That is why we say "Bless you" when someone sneezes. [See also SNEEZING]

1. C. Roth (ed.), Encyclopedia Judaica, vol. 15 (Jerusalem: Keter, 1972), pp. 172–181.

2. F. Rosner, Medical Encyclopedia of Moses Maimonides (Northvale, NJ: Jason Aronson, 1998), pp. 206–207.

SPEECH—The mouth (including the tongue and palate) is the main organ of speech (Berachot 61a). Moses said he had a speech defect (Exodus 4:10) but meant that he was not an eloquent speaker. Legend relates that his tongue was burned when he was a child (*Exodus Rabbah* 1:26). To be someone's mouth (Exodus 4:16) means to be his spokesman (*Exodus Rabbah* 3:16). The mouth of God speaks (Isaiah 1:20). To Moses, He spoke mouth to mouth (Numbers 12:8). The speech of God is equivalent to action (*Genesis Rabbah* 44:22). The voice of Divine speech instills fear and fright in those who hear it (*Leviticus Rabbah* 1:11–12).

The Ephraimites had a lisp (Judges 12:6). Isaiah describes stammerers (Isaiah 32:4). Amos had a "loaded tongue" and spoke with difficulty (*Ecclesiastes Rabbah* 1:2). Stutterers and stammerers are considered to be lame with the tongue (Micah 4:6; Zephaniah 3:19). Talking is harmful to patients with headache or eye pain (*Nedarim* 41a). Speaking excessively may bring one to sin (*Avot* 1:17; Proverbs 10:19). He who engages in profane talk sins (*Yoma* 19b) and violates biblical law (Deuteronomy 6:7; Ecclesiastes 1:8). If the tongue articulates idle speech, the throat becomes dry (*Yoma* 77a). Incense atones for the sin of evil speech (Numbers 17:12; *Yoma* 44a). Even the ordinary talk of scholars needs studying (*Abodah Zarah* 19b). [*See also* TONGUE and MOUTH]

SPERM—Sperm emission is called *shichvat zera* and pollution is called *mikreh* (Deuteronomy 23:11) or *keri*

(*Moed Katan* 25a). Any ejaculation, even involuntary as in nocturnal pollution, renders a man ritually impure (Deuteronomy 23:11; *Abodah Zarah* 68b), requiring purification in a ritual bath (Leviticus 15:16; *Chullin* 24b). Ejaculation normally occurs with great force so that nothing remains (*Mikvaot* 8:2–4). Sperm that impregnates "shoots forth like an arrow" (*Niddah* 43a). According to one sage, ejaculation is always accompanied by admixture of urine (*Jerushalmi Shabbat* 1:3). During the time of the Temple no officiating High Priest ever suffered from nocturnal pollution (*Avot* 5:5) although he was separated from his wife for the week before the Day of Atonement (*Yoma* 2a). Certain foods and beverages increase the likelihood of nocturnal pollution (*Yoma* 18a–b; *Kiddushin* 2b; *Tosefta Zavim* 2:5). Pollution is a good prognostic sign for sick patients (*Berachot* 57b). Gonorrheal flux issues from a flabby penis, whereas sperm flows from an erect penis (*Niddah* 56a). Erections can occur while a person is sleeping (*Yebamot* 53a), especially if one sleeps on one's back (*Berachot* 63b). Fear of danger inhibits erection (*Zevachim* 115b).

Emission of semen for naught is prohibited (Genesis 6:13). Bloodletting decreases the sperm (*Gittin* 70a) whereas garlic (*Baba Kamma* 82a), mandrakes, and milk (*Tosefta Zavim* 2:5) increase it. Sperm is "bound" and resembles the white of nonincubated eggs (ibid., 2:4). The semen of a eunuch is like water (*Yebamot* 80b). Semen becomes faint when near fire (*Gittin* 57a). Fertilized semen in a woman's uterus up to forty days of pregnancy is considered as mere fluid (*Yebamot* 69b). A woman can become pregnant by accidental insemination in a bathhouse where a man previously ejaculated (*Chagigah* 15a). Sperm remains viable and capable of fertilizing an egg for up to three days after ejaculation (*Shabbat* 86a). Harlots practiced violent movements following coitus in an attempt to expel the sperm and avoid conception (*Ketubot* 37a). A man whose testicles were pierced by a thorn issued forth semen like a thread of pus but he still sired children (*Yebamot* 75b). [*See also* ONANISM, MASTURBATION, TESTICLES, and GONORRHEA]

SPIKENARD—Anointing oil was made of spikenard and other fragrant leaves (*Shabbat* 62a). Even in a pile of garbage, the fragrant aroma of spikenard can be detected (*Sanhedrin* 108a). Spikenard oil was kept in flasks (*Shabbat* 65a and 78b; *Kelim* 30:4).

SPINAL COLUMN—According to the Talmud, there are eighteen vertebrae in the spinal column (*Oholot* 1:8). At the bottom is a small bone called *luz* that resembles an almond. (*Ecclesiastes Rabbah* 12:5). This bone is indestructible (*Leviticus Rabbah* 18:1).

The vertebral column and the ribs together form the skeleton (*Niddah* 28a; *Baba Kamma* 31b; *Moed Katan* 25a). Dislocation of the vertebral column with injury to the spinal cord may explain the lameness of Mephiboshet (2 Samuel 4:4). A newborn's spinal column and limbs may be straightened even on the Sabbath (*Shabbat* 147b). A baby may be born with two backs and two spinal columns (*Niddah* 24a). Perhaps this is the crooked back or hunchback referred to in the Bible (Leviticus 21:20).

SPINAL CORD—The spinal cord is known as the "string of the vertebral column" *(chut hashedra)* or poetically as "the silver cord" (Ecclesiastes 12:6). The cauda equina represents "the partings" or nerves at the end of the spinal cord (*Chullin* 45b). Breaking the neck bone of an animal severs the cervical spinal cord, rendering the animal unfit for human consumption (*Chullin* 113a). A widespread belief in antiquity was that, after death, the spinal cord turns into a snake (*Baba Kamma* 16a).

An animal with a severed spinal cord is considered nonviable (*Chullin* 45b). Liquefaction or gelatinous degeneration of the spinal cord is also a lethal condition (ibid.). Mephiboshet was lame because of a spinal cord injury (2 Samuel 4:4). An animal dragging its hind legs was found at autopsy to have spinal cord damage (*Chullin* 51a and 59a).[*See also* SCIATICA]

SPLEEN—The spleen is called *techol* and its convex side is named the splenic breast or *dad*. The capsule is referred to as the skin or *kerum,* and the vessels of the hilum are called strings or *chuttim* (*Chullin* 93a). The consumption of hilar vessels and splenic capsule is forbidden since they are included in the prohibition of eating fat and blood (Leviticus 3:15). Although some blood exudes from the splenic hilum (*Keritot* 21b) and is subject to this prohibition, the substance of the spleen, or *shumna,* is considered to be primarily composed of fatty juice (*Chullin* 11a) and is permitted.

The spleen was thought to produce laughter (*Berachot* 61b). The book of Jewish mysticism known as *Zohar* (3:234) also considers the spleen to be the seat of laughter. In his *Book of Kuzari* (4:25), Judah Halevy describes the laughing function of the spleen "because it cleanses blood and spirit from unclean and obscuring matter." Moses Maimonides also mentions the blood-purifying properties of the spleen.[1] An alternate function of the spleen cited in the Talmud is the crushing action of this organ (*Avot de Rabbi Nathan* 31:3). Spleen is said to be good for the teeth but bad for the bowels (*Berachot* 44b). Thus, one should chew it well and then spit it out. It is also considered beneficial to drink spleen broth on the day one is phlebotomized (*Chullin* 111a) or to eat a dish of pieces of spleen (*Shabbat* 129a).

Numerous prescriptions from folk medicine are cited in the Talmud to shrink an enlarged spleen (*Gittin* 69b). Asparagus brewed in wine, but not in beer, is good for the spleen (*Berachot* 51a). Surgical splenectomy is described in the Talmud (*Sanhedrin* 21b). Piercing or puncturing of the spleen has a fatal outcome, whereas removal of the spleen may not (*Chullin* 55a). Many references to the spleen, its anatomy, functions, and disorders are found in the works of medieval Jewish writers such as Asaph, Donnolo, Maimonides, and others.[2]

---

1. F. Rosner, *The Medical Aphorisms of Moses Maimonides* (Haifa: Maimonides Research Institute, 1989), p. 28.

2. F. Rosner, "The Spleen," in *Medicine in the Bible and the Talmud,* 2nd. ed. (Hoboken, NJ: Ktav and Yeshiva University Press, 1995), pp. 102–106.

SPUTUM—Bleeding from the lung that comes out through the mouth is sticky (*Gittin* 69a). Expectorated blood is mixed with saliva (*Yebamot* 105a). A folk remedy is prescribed for lung bleeding (*Gittin* 69a). Noah is said to have coughed up blood in the Ark because of the cold (*Genesis Rabbah* 32:11). Sputum from a patient with gonorrhea imparts ritual defilement to other people (Leviticus 15:8) whether or not the sputum is bloody. [*See also* SALIVA]

STERILITY—A hornet sting in the testicles (*Sotah* 36a), other serious injury to the testicles (*Yebamot* 75b), or severe brain injury can produce sterility (*Chullin* 45b). An oral potion used to treat jaundice may produce sterility (*Shabbat* 109b–110b; *Yebamot* 65b). A eunuch and an *aylonit* are obviously sterile [*see* EUNUCH and AYLONIT]. Famous barren women in the bible are discussed elsewhere [*see* CHILDLESSNESS]. Men may be the infertile partner in some sterile marriages (*Numbers Rabbah* 10:5). Isaac is said to have been infertile at first (*Yebamot* 64a). Some Torah scholars become impotent because of long talmudic discourses during which they hold back their micturition (*Yebamot* 64b). The sickness *raatan* (leprosy?) may interfere with potency (*Leviticus Rabbah* 16:1). Illness in a man may lead to impotency (ibid.), as may psychic causes (*Jerushalmi Nedarim* 11:42) and severe hunger (*Ketubot* 10b). A man with hypospadias is sterile (*Yebamot* 76a) unless it is surgically corrected. [*See also* CASTRATION and TESTICLES]

STOMACH—The word *kevah* means "stomach." The word *libba* refers to both the stomach and the heart (Psalms 105:15; *Gittin* 70a; *Chullin* 59a). The stomach is the organ that grinds the food (*Leviticus Rabbah* 4:4). Homiletically, to have a broad stomach means to be stout (*Pesachim* 86b) and to have a full stomach means to be haughty or arrogant (*Berachot* 32a). Ruminants have four stomachs (*Chullin* 3:1); the rumen *(keres hapenimit)*, the reticulum *(bet hakosot*, literally "house of goblets") (*Kelim* 16:2), the omasum *(hemses)*, and the obomasum *(kevah* or rennet bag). In birds, the *hemses* corresponds to the *kurkevan* or stomach (gizzard), in front of which, in ritually clean birds, is the *zephek* or anterior stomach (crop). It is lacking in the eagle (*Chullin* 61a) and other unclean birds. It is not clear whether *murah* (Leviticus 1:16) refers to the crop or the gizzard. The Talmud also describes a *kurkevan* in human beings (*Shabbat* 152a; *Avot de Rabbi Nathan* 31:2). In humans, the stomach not only grinds food but, when full, brings on sleep. (*Berachot* 61b). Tiredness after a full meal is a well known phenomenon (*Yoma* 18a). In old age, the sound of the grinding is low (Ecclesiastes 12:4) because the stomach grinding is weak (*Shabbat* 152a). Digestion of food begins in the stomach and lasts until one becomes hungry or thirsty again (*Berachot* 53b).

Cheese was prepared by curdling milk with rennet (*Abodah Zarah* 2:5) or by coagulating the milk directly in a calf's stomach (*Chullin* 8:5). Cheese made from fresh milk is difficult to digest (*Berachot* 57b) and a milk-containing dish called *kutach* blocks digestion in the stomach (*Pesachim* 42a).

A diet limited to barley bread may cause the stomach to swell and burst (*Sanhedrin* 81b). Asafetida ground in water or vinegar is a remedy for weakness of the stomach (*Nedarim* 26b). The daily consumption of mustard weakens the stomach (*Berachot* 40a). Unripe bitter dates are also harmful to the stomach (*Baba Metzia* 113b). Asparagus brewed in wine is good for the stomach (*Berachot* 51a). People with weak stomachs should eat sparingly and not overfill their stomachs (*Sukkah* 27a). [*See also* INTESTINES, ABDOMEN, ESOPHAGUS, etc.]

SUFFOCATION—Murder by suffocation is depicted in the Bible (2 Kings 8:15). In the absence of a Sanhedrin or Jewish Supreme Court, capital punishment cannot be imposed. People who are worthy of strangulation either drown in a river or die of suffocation (*Sanhedrin* 37b). *Tashnuk* (*Jerushalmi Berachot* 4:7) is interpreted to refer to death by suffocation since the Aramaic word *shanek* means "to choke."[1]

Overturning a vat on someone may cause his death by suffocation (*Sanhedrin* 77a). Asphyxia and death from fumes or lack of oxygen can occur if a person is in a sealed chamber with a lit candle (ibid.). Bloodletting was used in medieval times to treat asphyxia (*Yoma* 84a). [*See also* ASKARA]

---

1. F. Rosner (trans.), *Julius Preuss' Biblical and Talmudic Medicine* (Northvale, NJ: Jason Aronson, 1993), p. 188.

SUICIDE—The suicides of Samson (Judges 16:23–31), Achitophel (2 Samuel 17:23), and Zimri (1 Kings 16:18), and the attempted suicide of King Saul (1 Samuel 31:1–7 and 2 Samuel 1:5–10) are recorded in the Bible. Two cases of suicide are described in the Apocrypha (2 Maccabees 10:12 and 14:41–46).

The Talmud is replete with stories concerning suicide and martyrdom. The death of Rabbi Chaninah ben Teradion by burning at the hand of the Romans, and the suicide of his executioner, who jumped into the flames, are well known (*Abodah Zarah* 18a). The suicide of the Roman officer who saved the life of Rabbi Gamliel is portrayed in the Talmud (*Taanit* 29a). King Herod set his eyes on a certain maiden from the Hasmonean house of the Maccabees. Rather than submit to him, she threw herself off the roof and died. Herod preserved her body in honey for seven years (*Baba Batra* 3b). A child was inadvertently killed by his enraged father. Both parents in grief threw themselves down from the roof and died (*Chullin* 94a). A woman whose seven sons were martyred by Emperor Antiochus Epiphanes threw herself down from the roof and was killed (*Gittin* 57b). A rabbinic student took his own life by throwing himself from a roof because he was falsely accused of immorality by a harlot (*Berachot* 23a). A man hanged himself out of shame (ibid.). Rabbi Meir's wife is said to have committed suicide by strangulation (*Abodah Zarah* 18b). A mass suicide of four hundred boys and girls is described (*Gittin* 57b). They were being carried off for immoral purposes and chose, rather, to jump into the sea and drown.

Jewish law rules that a willful suicide is not entitled to funeral rites or eulogies *(Mishneh Torah, Avel* 1:11; *Shulchan Aruch, Yoreh Deah* 315). Judaism views suicide as a criminal act and strictly forbidden. The cases of suicide in the Bible, Apocrypha, Talmud, and Midrash took place under unusual and extenuating conditions.[1] In general a suicide is not accorded full burial honors. The Talmud and the codes of Jewish law decree that rending one's garments, delivering memorial addresses, and other rites of mourning that are an honor for the dead are not to be performed for a suicide victim. The strict definition of a suicide for which these laws apply is one who had previously announced his intentions and then killed himself immediately thereafter by the method he announced. Children are never regarded as deliberate suicides and are afforded all burial rites. Similarly, those who commit suicide under extreme physical or mental strain, or while not in full possession of their faculties, or in order to atone for past sins, are not considered as willful suicides, and none of the burial and mourning rites are withheld.

These considerations may condone the numerous acts of suicide and martyrdom committed by Jews throughout the centuries, from the priests who leaped into the flames of the burning Temple to the martyred Jews in the time of the Crusades, from the Jewish suicides during the medieval persecutions to the martyred Jews in recent pogroms. Only for the sanctification of the Name of the Lord would a Jew intentionally take his own life or allow it to be taken as a symbol of his extreme faith in God. Otherwise intentional suicide would be strictly forbidden because it constitutes a denial of the Divine creation of man, of the immortality of the soul, and of the atonement of death.[2]

---

1. F. Rosner, "Suicide," in *Medicine in the Bible and the Talmud* 2nd ed. (Hoboken, NJ: Ktav and Yeshiva University Press, 1995), pp. 273–287.

2. F. Rosner (trans.), *Julius Preuss' Biblical and Talmudic Medicine* (Northvale, NJ: Jason Aronson, 1993), pp. 513–516.

SUNSTROKE—Elisha the prophet promised the birth of a son to a barren woman from the town of Shunam who gave hospitality to Elisha. The prophecy was fulfilled but was followed by the tragic death of the boy from sunstroke (2 Kings 4:17–20). The child's revival by Elisha is described in the Bible (ibid., 34–35).

Some interpret this incident as of purely miraculous connotation. Radak, however, states that Elisha attempted to breathe on the child in order to provide warmth from the natural body heat that emanated from his mouth and eyes. Radak further states that most miracles are performed with direction and guidance from worldly and natural actions. Metzudat David states that Elisha tried to pour some of the life of his own body into the limbs of the child. Ralbag gives an identical interpretation but adds that "he [Elisha] did this after he prayed." Ralbag and Radak thus seem to consider a combination of natural and miraculous events as having contributed to the child's revival.

The type of illness that afflicted the child is clearly enunciated in the Jerusalem Talmud: "Rabbi Manna stated that at harvesttime accidents happen because the sun only blazes on a person's head at harvest time, as it is written: 'And when the child was grown, it happened on a day that he went out to his father to the reapers'" (*Yebamot* 15:2).

The talmudic commentary *Korban Ha'Edah* explains that at harvesttime a person may faint from the scorching sun, and die thereof. Another talmudic commentary, *Penei Moshe,* states that sickness or even death occurs at harvesttime because of the torrid sun, as in the case of the Shunammite boy. The same two commentaries interpret the phrase "who hast protected my head in the day of battle" (Psalms 140:8) to refer to sunstroke. The "day of battle" is thought to be the "day

when winter kisses the summer"—that is, when summer ends and winter begins, one should cover one's head to avoid sunstroke in accordance with the aphorism "The end of the summer is worse than the summer."

Another incident, nearly identical to that of Elisha and the Shunammite woman's child, is described in chapter 17 of 1 Kings. Here the prophet Elijah, the predecessor of Elisha, warns King Ahab of Israel (reigned ca. 875–853 B.C.E.) of a drought that would last for several years. To escape the drought, Elijah traveled to Zarephath, where he received hospitality from a widow who had an only son who fell sick and died because "there was no breath left in him" (I Kings 17:17–22). This phrase is interpreted by Josephus to mean that he appeared to be dead (*Antiquities* 8, 13, 3). Most biblical commentators, however, including Rashi, Ralbag, Metzudat David, and Radak, believe that the boy actually died.

Whether or not this boy also died of sunstroke is impossible to state, nor do the commentaries shed any light on the question. Although the precise clinical picture of heatstroke is not described in the Bible and Talmud, there seems little doubt that this medical entity was recognized at that time and was the cause of death in the case of the Shunammite boy.[1]

---

1. F. Rosner, "Sunstroke," in *Medicine in the Bible and the Talmud,* 2nd ed.

(Hoboken, NJ: Ktav and Yeshiva University Press, 1995), pp. 65–68.

SUPERFECUNDATION AND SUPERFETATION—Successive fertilization of two or more female eggs from the same ovulation, especially by different sires, is called superfecundation. To conceive again while already pregnant is called superfetation.

The Talmud (*Niddah* 27a) discusses the possibility that one woman can be pregnant at one time from two men (i.e., superfecundation). Since conception occurs within three days of cohabitation, states the Talmud, if the woman copulates with another man during this period, mixing of the sperm may occur, and the child may, in fact, have two fathers.

Also discussed in the Talmud is the possibility that a pregnant woman will become pregnant again from a later cohabitation (i.e., superfetation). The Jerusalem Talmud (*Yebamot* 5c) opines that a pregnant woman can only become pregnant again within the first forty days. Earlier than the Talmud, Aristotle (*De Generationis* 4:87) and Hippocrates assumed that a human uterus has two horns; one horn was thought to become pregnant first, and then the other horn at a later date. In his classic book on biblical and talmudic medicine,[1] Preuss points out that superfetation is possible in the very rare case of a complete duplication of the female genital tract. In a normal uterus, however, superfetation might occur during the first month or two of pregnancy but not later. Such an opinion is already expressed in the Talmud. {*See also* PREGNANCY]

1. F. Rosner (trans.), *Julius Preuss' Biblical and Talmudic Medicine* (Northvale, NJ: Jason Aronson, 1993), pp. 386ff. and 417ff.

SUPERSTITION—In general, Judaism is opposed to superstitious practices (*Sanhedrin* 65b–66a) since they are considered as heathen customs (Exodus 23:24). It is a superstitious practice to believe in a "lucky hand" (*Tosefta Shabbat* 6:12), to wear one's shirt reversed, to sit on a broom in order to dream (ibid., 6:7), or to apply fat from an executed ox on a wound as a therapeutic measure (*Pesachim* 24b). Also prohibited as a superstitious or heathen custom is to bury a placenta at the crossroads or to hang it from a tree (*Chullin* 77a). When Rav died, people took dirt from his grave as a remedy for quotidian fever (*Sanhedrin* 47b). Some people are superstitious and do not lend their bags or purses (*Yebamot* 120b; *Baba Metzia* 27b). [*See also* DEMONS, ASTROLOGY, AMULETS, and MAGIC]

SURGEON—Surgical and orthopedic practices, including the instrumentation therefor, are described in the

Talmud as follows: A surgeon wears an apron to protect himself from spurting blood (*Kelim* 26:5), straps the patient tightly to the table (*Tosefta Shekalim* 1:6), and uses a special box to keep his instruments (*Kelim* 16:8). Drugs are kept in a different receptacle (ibid., 12:3) and may be dispensed with the physician's ladle (ibid., 17:12). The surgeon opens abscesses skillfully (*Tosefta Eduyot* 1:8) and opens the skull with the physician's small drill or trepan (*Oholot* 2:3; *Bechorot* 38a). A physician was once called to cut into an abscess of Joseph ben Pisces (*Semachot* 4:2). The surgeon cuts away gangrenous parts (*Chullin* 77a) and amputates limbs for leprosy (*Keritot* 15b). He also heals fractures (*Moed Katan* 21b). For a fall from the roof, the surgeon applies plaster to the head, hands, and feet (*Exodus Rabbah* 27:9). Physicians "knowledgeable with the knife" (*Avot de Rabbi Nathan* 23:4) obviously refers to surgeons. The prophet may be referring to surgeons when he speaks of "binding up that which was broken" (Ezekiel 34:4 and 34:16). [*See also* PHYSICIAN and OPHTHALMOLOGIST]

SURGERY—In talmudic times, the surgeon wore a leather apron (*Kelim* 26:5), strapped the patient to the table (*Tosefta Shekalim* 1:6), and used his knife (*Exodus Rabbah* 26:2) or other instruments that he kept in a special box (*Kelim* 16:8). Rabbi Eleazar was given a sleeping potion (anesthetic?), taken into a marble chamber (operating room?), had his abdomen opened (laparotomy), and a lot of fat was removed (adiposectomy) (*Baba Metzia* 83b–84a). An operation to "smooth" a fissured penis (hypospadias repair?) is described (*Yebamot* 75b). Operations to undo circumcision were performed in ancient times for social and personal reasons [*see* EPISPASM]. Surgical removal of the spleen was carried out without fatal results (*Sanhedrin* 21b). Needles were used for extracting thorns (ibid., 84b). A surgeon who operates to save a person's life is not liable for the "wound" he inflicts (ibid.). [*See also* AMPUTEE, CESAREAN SECTION, CIRCUMCISION, and WOUNDS]

SURROGATE MOTHERHOOD—The fertilization of a human egg with human sperm in a test tube or Petri dish and its reimplantation into the womb produces, if successful, what is known as a test-tube baby. The fertilized egg may be implanted into the egg donor's womb or into another woman's womb. In the latter case, the woman serves as a host or surrogate incubator for the baby for the duration of the pregnancy. These and other methods of assisted reproduction are associated with many legal, moral, and religious issues, some of which are identical to those in artificial insemination. The use of surrogate mothers to carry and give birth to children requires rabbinic guidance as to its permissibility; the status of the child; who is the mother (the egg donor or the birth mother or both or neither); the sperm donor's status regarding paternity, custody, support, and inheritance; the application of rules of the firstborn son; levirate marriage; and a variety of other questions. Similar questions arise following testicular or ovarian transplants. Who is the father of a child sired by a sterile man who received a testicular transplant from his fertile identical twin brother? Who is the mother of a child born to a barren woman who received an ovarian transplant, the birth mother or the donor of the ovary?

These and other questions are discussed at length by several writers, based on biblical, talmudic, and other sources.[1,2,3,4,5] [*See also* ARTIFICIAL INSEMINATION and ORGAN TRANSPLANTS]

---

1. F. Rosner, *Modern Medicine and Jewish Ethics*, 2nd ed. (Hoboken, NJ and New York: Ktav and Yeshiva University Press, 1991), pp. 101–121.

2. R. V. Grazi, *Be Fruitful and Multiply* (Jerusalem, Genesis, 1994), pp. 175–208.

3. E. Feldman, J. B. Wolowelsky, *Jewish Law and the New Reproductive Technologies* (Hoboken, NJ: Ktav, 1997).

4. J. D. Bleich, *Contemporary Halakhic Problems*, vol. 4 (New York: Ktav and Yeshiva University Press, 1995), pp. 237–272.

5. I. Jakobovits, *Jewish Medical Ethics* (New York: Bloch, 1975), pp. 264–265.

SWIMMING—Swimming across a river is described in the Bible (Ezekiel 47:5), as is the spreading of one's hands to swim (Isaiah 25:11). The Apocrypha states that Jonathan and his men jumped into the Jordan and swam to the other side (1 Maccabees 9:48). According to the Talmud (*Kiddushin* 29a) a father is obligated, among other things, to teach his son a craft and to teach him how to swim, the latter because his life may depend on it (ibid., 30b). [*See also* EXERCISE]

SWINE—The skin of a pig is soft and tender like flesh (*Chullin* 122a). A pig gets stronger as it grows older (*Shabbat* 77b; *Abodah Zarah* 30b). Its intestines resemble those of humans (*Taanit* 21b). A swine's pregnancy is sixty days (*Bechorot* 8a; *Genesis Rabbah* 20:4). Pestilence was thought to be spread by swine (*Taanit* 21b). Pigs take everything to the dungheap (*Berachot* 43b). Their snouts are compared to wandering toilets (*Jerushalmi Berachot* 1:4). Ten measures of *nega* (skin illness) descended on the world, nine of which were taken by swine (*Kiddushin* 49b).

The pig is forbidden for human consumption (Leviticus 11:7; Deuteronomy 14:8). For everything forbidden, the Torah provides a permitted substitute. The *turbot* fish (mullet) tastes like swine flesh (*Chullin* 109b; *Leviticus Rabbah* 22:10). One should not breed swine (*Baba Kamma* 79b). He who does so is cursed (ibid., 83a; *Sotah* 49b). Every sow exported from Alexandria had its womb removed to prevent its propagation abroad (*Bechorot* 28b; *Sanhedrin* 33a and 93a).

SYPHILIS—The plague that killed twenty-four thousand people following the Peor cult (Numbers 25:9 and 31:16), the plague that afflicted the Philistines (1 Samuel 5:6ff), and the illnesses of Job and King Hezekiah are all said by some writers to have been syphilis. The illness *tzaraat* (Leviticus 13:1ff.) and several of its skin lesions is interpreted to mean syphilis, as is the term *tachtoniyot*, which usually refers to hemorrhoids. All these suggestions are rejected by the author of the classic work on biblical and talmudic medicine.[1] [*See also* PLAGUE]

1. F. Rosner (trans.), *Julius Preuss' Biblical and Talmudic Medicine* (Northvale, NJ: Jason Aronson, 1993), pp. 154–5 and 185–6.

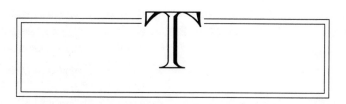

TAMPON—Three categories of women may (or must) use an absorbent tampon in their marital intercourse to prevent conception: a minor, a pregnant woman, and a nursing woman—the minor because otherwise she might become pregnant and possibly, as a result, die; a pregnant woman because otherwise she might cause her fetus to degenerate into a *sandal*; and a nursing woman because otherwise she might have to wean her child prematurely, which would result in its death (*Yebamot* 12b and 100b; *Ketubot* 39a; *Niddah* 45a). Harlots use absorbent tampons to avoid conception (*Ketubot* 37a; *Yebamot* 35a). Absorbent materials were used to examine for vaginal bleeding (*Niddah* 66a).

TASTE—The Hebrew word for "taste" is *taam* and is used to indicate that Jews taste not only food but also cohabitation (*Sanhedrin* 19b), sin (*Pesachim* 87a), sleep (*Jerushalmi Sukkah* 5:55), and death (*Yoma* 78b). "To make one's words tasty" (*Sotah* 21b)

means to offer plausible arguments, and "to taste the goodness of God" (Psalms 34:9) means to trust Him. Taste sensation diminishes in old age (2 Samuel 19:36), although a very old cook may still taste dishes (*Shabbat* 152a). The palate is sweet (Song of Songs 2:3), perhaps because it is an organ of taste (Job 12:11). Blind people develop more their other senses. A blind child knows its mother's breast by the smell and the taste (*Ketubot* 60a). A Nazarite is prohibited from tasting wine or grape products (*Numbers Rabbah* 10:8; *Pesachim* 44b) since the taste is equivalent to the substance itself (*Nazir* 37a; *Chullin* 98b). If something forbidden is mixed with something permitted and imparts its taste thereto, the whole mixture is prohibited (*Nazir* 37a; *Pesachim* 29b and 41a) unless it imparts a deteriorating flavor (*Pesachim* 44b). The sciatic nerve cooked with the thigh imparts a taste into the thigh, making the meat forbidden for consumption (*Chullin* 89b). Tastes of food are neutralized, however, if diluted in a ratio of one to sixty or one to one hundred (*Chullin* 89b; *Numbers Rabbah* 10: 22). [*See also* TONGUE and MOUTH]

TATTOOING—Tattooing is strictly prohibited in Judaism (Leviticus 19: 28). It consists of pricking ink or eye paint into the skin with a needle or a knife (*Makkot* 21a). This is a general prohibition for which one is liable (*Gittin* 86a). Writing on the skin is permissible.[1] In fact, documents were written on the skin and "delivered" by the bearer (*Gittin* 2:3). If one has the Divine Name written on one's skin, one may not bathe or anoint oneself or stand in an unclean place (*Shabbat* 120b). Sprinkling ashes on a wound is prohibited lest the blackness be mistaken for a tattoo (*Makkot* 21 a). A man who tattooed a magic text on his skin was called a fool (*Shabbat* 104b). [*See also* SKIN]

---

1. M. Weiss, "Tattoos: Halacha and Society," *Journal of Halacha and Contemporary Society*, 36 (Fall 1998), pp. 110–123.

TEARS—There are six types of tears (*Shabbat* 151b; *Lamentations Rabbah* 2:15). Those caused by smoke, weeping, or in the privy (from diarrhea or straining at defecation) are harmful, and tears over the loss of a grown-up child are the worst of all. Beneficial tears are those caused by medication,

mustard, or eye salves, and tears of joy are the best of all. The harm of smoke to the eyes is cited in the Bible (Proverbs 10:26). Vision depends on little or no crying since excessive tears can lead to loss of vision (Lamentations 2:11). Clouding of vision results from constant crying (*Shabbat* 151a). The weeping of old age impairs or destroys one's eyesight (*Shabbat* 151b). Putting one's finger in the eyes causes tearing (*Niddah* 13a and 45a). Tears are salty; if they fall on open skin lesions they cause pain (*Shabbat* 33b). Tears on open cheeks can also produce pain (*Lamentations Rabbah* 1:25).

Teleologically, a reason was sought and found for the saltiness of tears. The Midrash is of the opinion that if tears were not salty, a person would continually cry for a deceased individual and he would soon become blind. The saltiness, however, burns his eyes and reminds him to cease (*Numbers Rabbah* 18:22). Salty tears are a microcosm of the salty ocean water (*Avot de Rabbi Nathan* 31:3). Homiletically, a calf is said to have cried (*Baba Metzia* 85a) and the columns of Caesarea cried when Rabbi Abahu died (*Moed Katan* 25b). The altar sheds tears for a man who divorces his first wife (*Sanhedrin* 22a). The angels wept over the destruction of the Temple (Isaiah 33:7). Some Rabbis wept over biblical texts (*Chagigah* 15b). Even God weeps over those who fail to study Torah (*Chagigah* 5b). Tears of supplication to God are efficacious since the gates of tears are never closed.

The secretion of the lacrimal glands accumulates overnight in the corner of the eye and dries out there. This sticky mass is called *lifluf* (*Mikvaot* 9:2 and 9:4; *Niddah* 67a). Water in the eye can be transient if the eye tears normally. The cessation of tear secretion indicates a serious affliction (*Tosefta Bechorot* 4:4), perhaps an allusion to what is today known as Sjogren's syndrome. The signs of the *raatan* illness include tearing eyes, dripping nostrils, and profuse salivation (*Ketubot* 77b). Chronic blepharitis following excessive weeping may cause the eyelashes to fall out. The weeping of Leah (Genesis 29:17) because of her fear of marriage to Esau resulted in her eyelashes falling out (*Baba Batra* 123a). Rabban Gamliel wept in sympathy with a woman whose son had just died, and his eyelashes fell off (*Sanhedrin* 104b). Another woman who wept for her deceased son also suffered from loss of her eyelashes (*Lamentations Rabbah* 1:24). A woman once cried from pain because of an inflamed eye; her eye burst (*Abodah Zarah* 28b). Job complained to his friends of a red face because of his weeping (Job 16:16). Weeping may cause a decrease in one's sperm (*Gittin* 70a). [*See also* EYES, VISION, BLINDNESS]

TESTICLES—The biblical and talmudic terms for testicle are respectively, *ashech* (Leviticus 21:20) and *betzah*

(literally: "egg") (*Chullin* 45a) and less often *kubasin* (*Baba Metzia* 101 b; *Shevuot* 41a). Hair growth around the testicle is a sign of adulthood (*Sanhedrin* 68b). The skin of the testicles is rich in blood vessels (*Chullin* 93a). A priest with *meroach ashech* cannot serve in the Temple (Leviticus 21:20). This term means either absent testicles, softened testicles, crushed testicles, air in the testicles (pneumatocele), or water on the testicles (varicocele).[1] An animal with crushed testicles, hanging testicles (*Bechorot* 39b), or other testicular abnormalities may not be offered in the Temple (Leviticus 22:24). Testicles crushed in the scrotum may retain some vitality (*Chullin* 93a–b). Cutting or crushing the strands of the testicles (spermatic cords) makes a man unfit to marry (*Yebamot* 75b). Falling from a tree can injure the testicles (*Tosefta Yebamot* 10:3).

The Talmud describes a man with only one testicle who can still procreate (*Yebamot* 75a). Congenital absence of both testicles (anorchidism) is associated with sterility (*Jeushalmi Yebamot* 8:9). A newborn of indeterminate or uncertain sex (*tumtum*) may have hidden testicles (cryptorchidism) (*Chagigah* 4a; *Yebamot* 72a and 83b). This condition is also known in animals (*Bechorot* 6:6). [*See also* CASTRATION, ENUCHS and STERILITY]

---

1. F. Rosner (trans.), *Julius Preuss' Biblical and Talmudic Medicine* (Northvale, NJ: Jason Aronson, 1993), p. 220.

THEODUS—Theodus or Theodorus the physician was an expert anatomist and discussed bones, vertebrae, and the skull with the Rabbis (*Nazir* 52a; *Tosefta Oholot* 4:2; *Jerushalmi Berachot* 1:3). He said that every cow or sow in Alexandria was castrated before it was exported to prevent its propagation abroad (*Bechorot* 28b; *Sanhedrin* 33a and 93a).

Theodus should not be confused with Theodosius or Thaddeus, a man of Rome, who is mentioned in the Talmud several times (*Berachot* 19a; *Pesachim* 53b; *Betzah* 23a). [*See also* MAR SAMUEL, AMMI, and BENJAMIN]

THERIAC—Theriac is a mixture of many drugs and ingredients prepared by physicians (*Song of Songs Rabbah* 4:5) in antiquity and the Middle Ages as an antidote for animal bites.[1] The Talmud prescribes it for a person who drinks water left uncovered overnight that was suspected of containing snake poison or leeches (*Shabbat* 109b; *Pesachim* 112a). A legend describes the preparation of theriac for snakebites from ingredients provided by two families of priests (*Song of Songs Rabbah* 4:5). Excised fat was once used to make theriac (*Baba Metzia* 83b). One talmudic sage said, "I do not want fever nor the theriac to treat it" (*Nedarim* 41a-b).

---

1. F. Rosner, *Moses Maimonides' Treatise on Poisons, Hemorrhoids, and Cohabi-*

tation (Haifa: Maimonides Research Institute, 1984), pp. 1–115.

THIGH—The thigh or *yarech* (Psalms 45:4) is where a soldier carries his sword or dagger (Judges 3:16). Smiting one's thigh is a sign of repentance (Jeremiah 31:19) and of mourning (Ezekiel 21:17). The thigh is also a euphemistic expression for the male sex organ. Those who "issue from the thigh" (Genesis 46:26; Judges 8:30) refers to offspring. Thigh is also used figuratively to denote a woman's womb (*Megillah* 13a). In biblical times, an oath was taken by placing the hands "under the thigh" (Genesis 24:9 and 47:29).

The thighbone is called *kulit* in the Talmud. Knife handles were made from this bone (*Tosefta Oholot* 4:3). The marrow of this bone (*Tosefta Uktzin* 2:4), particularly in young lambs, was considered to be a delicacy (*Tosefta Pesachim* 4:10). A thighbone once washed up on the seashore (*Genesis Rabbah* 10:7). It was debated whether or not the flesh outside the bone can be restored by the marrow within (*Chullin* 125a). The thighbone of a dead human or animal conveys ritual impurity (*Chullin* 125a). *Kaf hayerech* is the socket of the hipbone or the head of the femur, which was dislocated when Jacob wrestled with the angel (Genesis 32:36). The Aramaic term is *buka de atma* (*Chullin* 42b). The prohibition of the sciatic nerve in the thigh (Genesis 32:33) applies to both left and right hip (*Chullin* 89b). The entire nerve with its branches must be removed before a ritually slaughtered animal may be consumed (*Chullin* 56a). Luxation of the thigh sinew in an animal is life-threatening (*Chullin* 54b). An ewe suffered from "sciatica" proven at autopsy (*Chullin* 51a and 59a). A painful hip joint was treated by rubbing fish brine sixty times on the painful area (*Gittin* 69b). A person whose hip "is torn off" (*sarua*) drags his leg behind him (*Bechorot* 7:6). Thigh wounds were treated by applying medication to the wound (*Abodah Zarah* 28a). The punishment for a suspected adulteress who is found guilty is that her thigh will fall away and her abdomen swells (Numbers 5:22). This subject is detailed elsewhere.[1,2] [See also LEG, KNEE, ANKLE, and TOES]

1. F. Rosner, *Medicine in the Bible and the Talmud*, 2nd. ed. (Hoboken, NJ: Ktav and Yeshiva University Press, 1995), pp. 239–247.

2. F. Rosner (trans.), *Julius Preuss' Biblical and Talmudic Medicine* (Northvale, NJ: Jason Aronson, 1993); pp. 473–474.

THIRST—If one drinks water to quench one's thirst, one must first recite a benediction (*Eruvin* 14b). Thirst occurs on account of a meal (*Berachot* 53b). Even if a person is thirsty, he should not drink from rivers or pools at night or during the day directly with his mouth since he cannot inspect the water and might swallow a leech or other harmful substances (*Abodah Zarah* 12b; *Pesachim* 112a). [See also BEVERAGES and WATER]

THROAT—The word *garon* for "throat" is used by prophets to denote stretching the neck in a haughty manner (Isaiah 16:6; Ezekiel 16:11). *Askara* is diphtheritic croup that affects the throat [see ASKARA]. For pain in the throat, one may pour medicine in the mouth even on the Sabbath because of the danger (*Yoma* 83a). Boils in the throat (*chinke*) are treated with pyrethrum and other herbs and vegetables such as bran and lentils (*Gittin* 69a). Some writers[1] postulate that King Hezekiah's illness (2 Kings 20:1ff.; Isaiah 38:1ff.; 2 Chronicles 32:24ff.) was a throat abscess [see KING HEZEKIAH'S ILLNESS]. For throat illness, one gargles with various medications (*Berachot* 36a). A foreign object stuck in the throat is considered a medical emergency (*Shabbat* 67a). If a piece of meat is stuck in the throat, one should try to wash it down with water (*Berachot* 45a).

Before entering an outdoor privy, one clears one's throat to discover whether or not the lavatory is occupied (*Berachot* 62a). Esau had to clear his throat because he was choked up from his anger at Jacob for taking his birthright and his father's blessing (*Genesis Rabbah* 67:4). [See also

HOARSENESS, MOUTH, NECK,
and VOICE]

1. F. Rosner (trans.), *Julius Preuss'
Biblical and Talmudic Medicine* (Northvale, NJ: Jason Aronson, 1993), p. 342.

TOES—The word *etzba*, meaning "finger" also means "toe." Walking on the
tips of one's toes is a sign of haughtiness (*Derech Eretz Rabbah* 2:8). A
priest with a swelling protruding from
his large toe is unfit to serve in the
Temple (*Bechorot* 7:6). Other priestly
blemishes include supernumerary or
extra toes (2 Samuel 21:20), which
are either advantageous or unsightly
(*Bechorot* 45b), absence of toes,
crooked large toe (hallux valgus?)
(*Tosefta Bechorot* 5:9), or webbed toes
(*Niddah* 23b). A priest with such defects should not recite the priestly benediction because people would stare at
his feet (*Megillah* 4:7). Squeezing the
two big toes of a recently deceased person together is one way of causing the
eyes to close (*Shabbat* 151b). [*See also*
LEG, ANKLE, THIGH, and KNEE]

TOILETS—In ancient times, public
baths and lavatories were luxuries (*Ecclesiastes Rabbah* 2:8:1). Superior privies had locks (*Tamid* 26a). Wealthy
people had private privies near their
homes (*Shabbat* 25b). Otherwise one
cleared one's throat or blew one's nose
to discover whether the public privy

was free (*Berachot* 62a). Lavatories or
outhouses are mentioned in the Bible
(2 Kings 10:27). Ordinarily, one urinated or defecated near a wall (2 Kings
18:27; Isaiah 36:12; 1 Samuel 25:22)
or in an open field (*Berachot* 62a). In
Babylon it was forbidden to urinate on
the ground for fear of the urine flowing into the well where the High
Priest bathed on Yom Kippur (*Yoma*
31a). It was similarly forbidden to urinate near a river (*Bechorot* 44b). One
should also not urinate or defecate in
the middle of the road but on the side
in semiprivacy (*Sanhedrin* 104b, *Lamentations Rabbah* 1:12).

In outhouses, stones were put together to form a seat (*Betzah* 32b; *Berachot* 61 b). Persians were modest in the
privy (*Berachot* 8b). In fact, privies were
constructed for modesty and privacy
(*Abodah Zarah* 47b). Persian lavatories
had ditches under or behind the stones
(*Berachot* 26a). A fence around such a
privy made it into a permanent toilet or
bet hakise kevua (ibid., 23a), required
before people take up residence in a city
(*Sanhedrin* 17b). Lavatories for the
poor were constructed (*Exodus Rabbah*
31:11) with public funds obtained from
usurers (Proverbs 28:8). In time of
war, outhouses were created for the
soldiers (Deuteronomy 23:10–15).
Money from harlotry or other immoral
practice cannot be used to build even a
lavatory for the High Priest (*Abodah
Zarah* 17a).

When nature calls, one should immediately go to the privy (*Gittin* 70a).

One Sage with severe diarrhea had no access to the privy (*Shabbat* 108a). Hemorrhoids may develop if one strains much or does not sit properly in the toilet (*Berachot* 55a; *Shabbat* 81a). Modesty in the privy requires that one disrobe not while still standing but when one is seated (*Berachot* 62a). A person who sits naked in an outdoor privy is in danger of being bitten by a snake (*Genesis Rabbah* 10:7). A man who threw a Sage out of the privy was bitten by a snake and died (*Berachot* 62b).

One may not recite the *Shema* or pray or wear phylacteries in a privy (*Berachot* 23a–66a), nor recite blessings (ibid., 53a) or study Torah (*Shabbat* 40b and 150a; *Kiddushin* 33a; *Abodah Zarah* 44b; *Zevachim* 102b). One recites a special prayer after washing one's hands upon emerging from the privy (*Sukkah* 46a; *Berachot* 60a). Incantations were recited against the demons of the privy (*Shabbat* 67a). [*See also* DEFECATION and URINATION]

TONGUE—The tongue, known as *lashon*, is an organ of taste [*see* TASTE]. The word *lashon* also means "language" because the tongue speaks (*Berachot* 61a). An animal missing most of its tongue is unfit to be offered as a sacrifice (*Bechorot* 6:8). A man's tongue is his downfall (*Sirach* 5:13). "Death and life are in the power of the tongue" (Proverbs 18:21) means that good or bad (i.e., slander, gossip)

comes from the tongue (*Leviticus Rabbah* 33:1). One who uses his tongue for slander makes his sin reach heaven (Psalms 73:9). "The evil tongue" is the Hebrew term for slander. "Thou deceitful tongue" (Psalms 120:3) is interpreted as God saying to the tongue: "All limbs of man stand and you lie down; all limbs are outside and you are inside" (*Arachin* 15b). Smooth-tongued people are cursed (*Derech Eretz Rabbah* 2:3). One who bears evil tales almost denies the foundation of Judaism (Psalms 12:5) and may develop leprosy (Psalms 101:5; Leviticus 25:30).

Moses was said to have had a heavy tongue because it was burned in his youth (*Exodus Rabbah* 1:26). Legend relates that when the scouts brought back the evil report (Numbers 14:37) their tongues became extremely long and extended down to the navel (*Sotah* 35a). Antiochus cut out the tongues of Jews who refused to eat swine's meat (2 Maccabees 15:33).

TORTURE—Throughout the centuries, Jews have been tortured for practicing and teaching their religion. Hadrian tortured Jews in a variety of cruel ways (*Song of Songs Rabbah* 2:7). Antiochus inflicted torture upon the Jews including excision of the tongue, tearing of the skin, and chopping of the limbs of those who refused to eat swine's meat (2 Maccabees 7:4). In antiquity, Jewish women were "slit open" by their oppressors (2 Kings 8:12). The Romans used iron combs to tear the flesh from the bodies of Jews and others (*Gittin* 57b). Rabbi Akiba and his companions were tortured to death for disobeying the Roman edict forbidding the practice and teaching of Judaism (*Berachot* 61b; *Pesachim* 50a; *Sanhedrin* 110b; *Lamentations Rabbah* 2:2:4). Rabbi Judah ben Baba had three hundred iron spears driven into his body (*Sanhedrin* 14a). Lulianus and Papus were executed in Lydda in the reign of Hadrian (*Pesachim* 50a; *Taanit* 18b; *Baba Batra* 10b). Rabbi Chaninah ben Teradion was burned to death wrapped in a Torah Scroll because he taught Torah, which was specifically outlawed by Hadrian (*Abodah Zarah* 18a). All these prominent Rabbis were martyred while defending their religion with their lives.

TRANSVESTISM—For a man to use cosmetics or dress as a woman violates the biblical prohibition against wearing women's garments (Deuteronomy 22:5). [*See also* HOMOSEXUALITY, LESBIANISM, BESTIALITY, and RAPE]

TURNIPS—Turnips are usually hard (*Sanhedrin* 19a). They were buried beneath vines to keep them fresh (*Kilayin* 1:9; *Shabbat* 50b) since they otherwise wither within twenty-four hours of being pulled out of the ground (*Eruvin* 40a). Turnips were also pickled for preservation and storage (*Pesachim* 56b). Turnips can grow to be very large, up to sixty pounds—large enough to house a fox nest (*Ketubot* 111b).

A stew of turnips containing flour paste shrinks and improves (*Shabbat* 37a). Meat cooked with turnips imparts its flavor to the turnips (*Chullin* 96b). Turnips were considered both harmful and beneficial. On the one hand, the Talmud says: "Woe to the stomach through which turnips are passing" (*Berachot* 44b). Further, if a man eats beets and turnips and lies awake in the summer moonlight, he may develop *achilu*, or fever and chills (*Gittin* 70a). On the other hand, slices of turnip in vinegar can satisfy extreme hunger (*Ketubot* 61a), and Rabba told his servant to purchase turnips in the market as a relish for consumption with bread (*Berachot* 44b).

Roots of turnips serve as a handle like the stalks of apples (*Uktzin* 1:2). Turnip heads are not susceptible to ritual uncleanness.

TWINS—Twins occur if the sperm divides into two parts (*Yebamot* 98b). The talmudic sages recognized the difference between identical twins (one amnion) and fraternal twins (two amniotic sacs) (*Oholot* 7:5). Twin pregnancy can be recognized at three months (Genesis 38:24). One twin may be born alive, the other dead

(*Oholot* 7:5). Many twins are cited in the Bible, including Cain and Abel (*Genesis Rabbah* 23:3; *Sanhedrin* 38b). Cain had a twin sister and Abel had two twin sisters (ibid.). Jacob and Esau were twins (Genesis 25:24–26) as were Lea and Rachel (*Seder Olam Rabbah* 2). Each head of the twelve tribes was born with a twin (*Genesis Rabbah* 84). A twin sister was born with Dinah and an extra twin sister to Benjamin (*Genesis Rabbah* 89:9; *Baba Batra* 123a). During the twin birth of Peretz and Zorach to Tamar, the midwife tied a red thread to the hand of the child that put its hand out first, to assure it its firstborn rights (Genesis 38:28).

The Talmud describes two sets of twins as offspring of Rabbi Chiya. Judah and Hezekiah were twins. Pazi and Tavi were twin sisters (*Yebamot* 65b). If one twin has a headache, the other twin also feels it (*Song of Songs Rabbah* 5:3). The umbilical cord of twins must be cut quickly; otherwise

they would pull on each other endangering their lives (*Shabbat* 129b). If one of two twins stops suckling, so does the other and the mother's breasts run dry (*Song of Songs Rabbah* 4:5:2).

Multiple pregnancies are also portrayed. In Egypt, Jewish women bore six children with each pregnancy (*Exodus Rabbah* 1:7). The reward for tending to the Ark of the Covenant is sextuplet offspring (*Berachot* 63b). Early Jewish sources also portray Siamese twins. Adam was created with two faces (*Eruvin* 18a). A person with two heads (*Menachot* 37a) and twins attached at the head or at the chest are also described (Responsa *Halachot Ketanot*, #245). Numerous Jewish laws and customs pertaining to twins are detailed elsewhere.[1]

---

1. A Steinberg, *Encyclopedia Talmudit Refuit*, vol. 6 (Jerusalem: Falk Schlesinger Institute of the Shaare Zedek Medical Center, 1998), pp. 527–545.

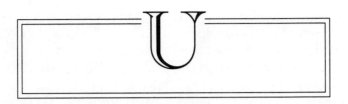

U

URETHRA—Obstruction of the urethra with resultant urinary retention was treated with folk remedies including the insertion of a louse in the urethra (*Gittin* 69b). To force back urine in the urethra produces jaundice (*Bechorot* 44b). Epispadias and hypospadias consist of abnormal urethral openings on the dorsal or ventral surfaces, respectively, of the penis (*Yebamot* 76a). Urethral fluxes and catarrhs are discussed elsewhere [*see* GONORRHEA]. The talmudic sages thought that the sperm and urine are excreted in two adjacent channels; if one of the ducts perforates into the other, the man becomes infertile (*Bechorot* 44b; *Yebamot* 75b–76a). [*See also* BLADDER, KIDNEYS, CIRCUMCISION, PENIS, URINATION, and SPERM]

URINATION—Urination early in the morning is healthy (*Berachot* 62b). One should not defer one's bodily functions (*Makkot* 16b) because that is detestable behavior (Leviticus 11:43). Withholding of micturition causes abdominal swelling (*Bechorot* 44b). It is, therefore, permissible to urinate in public because a delay may endanger health (ibid.). *Yerakon* (jaundice) is said to be caused by the withholding of urination (*Berachot* 62b; *Tamid* 27b; *Bechorot* 49b). One rabbi who withheld urination during a long discourse developed strangury (*Yebamot* 64b). Painful urination may also occur from bladder stones (*Baba Metzia* 85a), for which several folk remedies are recommended (*Gittin* 69b). People urinated in bathhouses (*Abodah Zarah* 3:4). One should not urinate on solid ground or in an earthenware vessel lest the urine contaminate well water (*Yoma* 31a) or river water (*Bechorot* 44b). A man should not urinate against another man's wall (*Baba Batra* 19b), based on a biblical verse (1 Kings 21:21). If the wall is made of boulders, it is permitted (*Tosefta Baba Batra* 1:4).

God despises the act of a man who holds his penis while urinating (*Leviticus Rabbah* 21:8; *Niddah* 12a and 16b). A biblical verse critical of indecent behavior (Amos 6:4) is said to refer to people who urinate naked before their beds (*Shabbat* 62b). One may not pray or recite the *Shema* while urinating (*Berachot* 25a). Urination before idols was an ancient form of pagan worship (*Abodah Zarah* 44b and 53a).

"To cover one's feet" (1 Samuel 24:4) is a euphemistic expression for urination (*Yebamot* 103a). A eunuch's urinary stream does not form an arch (*Yebamot* 80a). Urination cleans out the urethra from sperm after an ejaculation (*Chullin* 24b; *Niddah* 42a). [*See also* URINE, BLADDER, and KIDNEYS]

URINE—Urine is known as "water of the feet" (*Machshirin* 6:5), and "to cover one's feet" (1 Samuel 24:4) means "to urinate" (*Yebamot* 103a). Because urine squirts on the legs, foot washing is required (*Yoma* 29b). Urine is never completely discharged except when sitting (*Berachot* 40a) because a standing person is afraid of drops falling on his legs or clothes. The urine duct (urethra) is separate from the sperm duct (*Yebamot* 75b and 76a). A urine basin or night pot (*Niddah* 9:2), a urine utensil (*Berachot* 25b; *Baba Bathra* 89b), and blood in the urine (hematuria) (*Niddah* 59b) are discussed in the Talmud. A eunuch does not have a strong urinary stream and his urine does not bubble (*Yebamot* 80b). Urine fermented for less than forty days is an effective cleansing agent (*Shabbat* 89b; *Sanhedrin* 49b; *Niddah* 63a). Forty-day-old urine

is said to be efficacious against wasp stings and scorpion bites (*Shabbat* 109b).

Urine can be clear or muddy (bloody?) or white and viscous (semen) (*Mikvaot* 8:2). The urine of a man with gonorrhea is ritually unclean (*Nazir* 66a). The urine of a woman after childbirth defiles only when wet (*Niddah* 34a; *Eduyot* 5:4). Human urine causes ritual uncleanness and also susceptibility to uncleanness (*Machshirin* 6b). A pail of urine immersed in a ritualarium is regarded as though it were water (*Zevachim* 78b; *Mikvaot* 10:6). Urine may not be brought into the Temple Court (*Zevachim* 95a; *Keritot* 6a). Differences in the urine of various animals are depicted in the Talmud (*Bechorot* 7b). Pouring urine before an idol was an ancient form of pagan worship (*Abodah Zarah* 50b). [*See also* URINATION, KIDNEYS, and BLADDER]

UTERUS—God built a woman miraculously in that the baby lies in its mother's womb, whose orifice faces downwards, yet the baby does not fall out (*Berachot* 61a; *Niddah* 31a). God blesses the fruit of the womb (Deuteronomy 7:13), which is derived from both mother and father (Micah 6:7). A child emerges naked from its mother's womb (Job 1:21), its mouth opens, and its navel closes (*Yebamot* 71b). The womb takes in sperm silently and gives forth the baby with a

Uterus

loud cry of the newborn (*Berachot* 15b). A newborn's cry indicates it has come forth from the womb (*Niddah* 42b). A firstborn child is the one who first opens the womb (Numbers 18:15). The pregnant uterus is called *kever* (*Niddah* 21a; *Shabbat* 129a), meaning "heaped up" or "a grave," perhaps because the womb may miscarry (Hosea 9:14). A fetus in utero is said to resemble a nut floating in a bowl of water (*Niddah* 31a). Other portrayals of the fetus in the womb are found in the Talmud (*Niddah* 25a, 25b and 30b). The walls of the womb open wide or are even torn when a baby is born (*Chullin* 70a). Once the womb opens during labor, the mother cannot walk without help (*Oholot* 7:4). A baby endangering its mother's life just before childbirth must be extricated limb by limb from the womb (*Oholot* 7:6).

A barren women is never satisfied (Proverbs 30:15–16). According to legend, Sarah (*Genesis Rabbah* 47:2; *Yebamot* 64b), Rebecca (*Genesis Rabbah* 63:5), and Ruth (*Ruth Rabbah* 8:14) were all born without a uterus. All subsequently had children. Animals born without wombs are also known (*Chullin* 55b). In Alexandria, all cows and pigs for export first had hysterectomies to prevent their breeding outside Egypt (*Bechorot* 28a; *Sanhedrin* 33a). Rebecca carried twins in her womb (Genesis 25:23). The female genital tract including the uterus is detailed in the Talmud (*Niddah* 2:5), which speaks of a woman in a metaphor: She has a chamber (uterus), an antechamber (vagina), and an upper chamber (bladder) (*Niddah* 17b). An embryo born by cesarean section exits the womb from the side (*Niddah* 41a). It is impossible for the uterus to open during parturition without some bleeding (*Niddah* 21b; 38a).

Menses originate from the womb, which is called "the fountain" (*Niddah* 2:5). The womb can also withhold menstrual blood (*Niddah* 3a). A woman who bleeds profusely from the uterus may have a malignant disease there (*Yebamot* 64b). A woman whose uterus is full of blood and who bleeds postcoitally has an incurable disease (*Niddah* 66a). Many folk remedies were recommended to treat vaginal bleeding (*Shabbat* 110a–b). Some sicknesses can be cured by eating uterine meat (*Abodah Zarah* 29a).

[*See also* PREGNANCY and ABORTION]

313

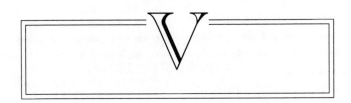

VEGETABLES—Vegetables are usually eaten fresh (*Shabbat* 68a) but are sometimes pickled or preserved (*Sanhedrin* 106b). Fresh and dry vegetables (*Sheviit* 9:6) are consumed by both rich and poor people (*Shabbat* 140b). Even the poor buy vegetables for the Sabbath (*Taanit* 20b) because they are wholesome and cheap (*Eruvin* 55b). The very poor are given three meals for the Sabbath including green vegetables (*Tosefta Peah* 4:8). Vegetables can constitute an entire meal (*Berachot* 44a; *Eruvin* 29a; *Sanhedrin* 94b) or be part of a meal (*Pesachim* 107b). Vegetable seeds and vegetable beds grow in the fields (*Kilayim* 2:10;3:1). Vegetables can shrivel up on the stem during growth (*Chullin* 127b). Flax water can damage a vegetable garden (*Baba Batra* 18a and 25a). Vegetables tied in bundles are due for tithing (*Maaserot* 1:5; *Chullin* 7a) and are stored on the roof to keep them fresh (*Machshirin* 6:2). Vegetables are trimmed before consumption (*Shabbat* 114b) and are grown for personal consumption or sale in the market (*Demai* 5:7; *Sheviit* 7:3) in bundles or by weight (*Sheviit* 8:3; *Eruvin* 37b).

One should not live in a town where vegetables are unobtainable (*Eruvin* 55b). Bitter herbs (*maror*) for Passover use can include lettuce, endives, leeks, coriander, mustard, gourd, and, of course, horseradish (*Pesachim* 39a). The dill plant can be used as seeds, pods, or as a vegetable (*Abodah Zarah* 7b). Animals live simply (i.e., eat grass and vegetables) and are healthy (*Ecclesiastes Rabbah* 1:18). On the other hand, eating raw vegetables can make the complexion pale (*Berachot* 44b), increase bowel movements, bend the stature, and decrease eyesight (*Pesachim* 42a–b). The harm of green vegetables is limited to garlic and leek. A nursing woman may be harmed by green vegetables (*Ketubot* 60b). One should not eat green vegetables on an empty stomach because of the odor one might emit (*Berachot* 44b). Vegetable ashes are spread on wounds to help healing (*Makkot* 21a; *Abodah Zarah* 29a).

Green vegetables were consumed by ancient man before meat became permitted (Genesis 9:3). King David and his entourage were fed vegetables, among other foods (2 Samuel 17: 28–29). Meat is more nourishing than vegetables (*Nedarim* 49b). In the absence of meat, one cooks vegetables in a stew (*Chullin* 84a). Benedictions are recited before and after one eats vegetables (*Berachot* 38b; *Niddah* 51b). [*See also* specific vegetables, e.g., CABBAGE, CUCUMBERS, FENUGREEK, LEEKS, LETTUCE, ONIONS, etc.]

VEGETARIANISM—According to the Talmud (*Sanhedrin* 59b), Adam was originally not permitted to eat meat (Genesis 1:29ff.), but with the advent of Noah, it was permitted (Genesis 9:3). On the other hand, one legend states that the angels roasted meat and cooled wine for Adam in paradise (*Avot de Rabbi Nathan* 1:8). According to Preuss,[1] primitive man did not eat meat because he was not familiar with the killing of animals, not because God prohibited it. When man was banished from the Garden of Eden, he learned to do battle with animals and began consuming their meat. Some people allege that the biblical Daniel was a vegetarian, based on his statement that he ate no meat (Daniel 10:2). Clearly, the reason he ate no meat in the palace of Nebuchadnezzar was because it was not kosher, not because he was a vegetarian.

1. F. Rosner (trans.), *Julius Preuss' Biblical and Talmudic Medicine* (Northvale, NJ: Jason Aronson, 1993), pp. 557–558.

VETERINARIAN—A veterinary house surgeon (*hippiater*) once cauterized a sick she-ass and she bore an offspring with a flame mark (*Numbers Rabbah* 9:5). Veterinarians examined animals to insure the absence of blemishes before they could be offered as sacrifices (*Jerushalmi Shekalim* 6:48). Two famous veterinarians were Ila (*Bechorot* 4:5) and Imla (*Tosefta Bechorot* 4:11). Shepherds help their flock in giving birth (Midrash Psalms 107:4). The Mishnah cites the case of a herdsman who placed his hand into the womb of an animal whose fetus had died (*Chullin* 4:3).

VINEGAR—Vinegar is used for medicinal purposes. It is an ingredient in a remedy for the illness *achilu* (*Gittin* 70a), for leprosy (*Gittin* 86a; *Tosefta Shabbat* 12:11), for worm infestation (*Shabbat* 109a), and for jaundice (ibid., 110b). Eating bread immersed in vinegar prevents intestinal illness (*Gittin* 70a). Cress with vinegar applied to a wound stops the bleeding (*Abodah Zarah* 28a). Hand or foot wounds are fomented with vinegar (*Shabbat* 109a). He who swallows a bee (*Gittin* 70a) or leech (*Abodah Zarah* 12b) should drink strong vinegar. One should not drink vinegar prior to bloodletting, nor after fasting (*Abodah Zarah* 29a). Vinegar may be harmful to the teeth (Proverbs 10:26) but it is good for toothache (*Betzah* 18b; *Abodah Zarah* 28a) and heals the gums (*Shabbat* 111a). For headache, one rubs the head with vinegar, wine, and oil (*Tosefta Shabbat* 12:11; *Tosefta Maaser Sheni* 2:53). For pain in the loins one rubs oneself with a mixture of wine and vinegar (*Shabbat* 14:4). Asafetida soaked in vinegar is useful for medicinal purposes (*Shabbat* 140a) and bread dipped in vinegar is beneficial in hot weather (*Ruth* 2:14; *Leviticus Rabbah* 34:8; *Shabbat* 113b).

Vinegar is also a seasoning (*Ruth* 2:14; *Berachot* 2b) and fruit was steeped in vinegar for that purpose (*Uktzin* 3:4). Although vinegar is not a refreshing drink (*Keritot* 18b), it restores the soul if one feels faint from fasting (*Yoma* 81 b). A drink of lentil flour in vinegar was sent by Barzilai to David (*Abodah Zarah* 38b) when the latter and his entourage were hungry and thirsty (2 Samuel 17:28). Spiced vinegar can be fatal if imbibed (*Abodah Zarah* 38b). Barley soaked in vinegar binds it and prevents fermentation (*Pesachim* 40a). Meat is dipped in vinegar for flavoring (*Eruvin* 29a) and to contract the blood vessels (*Pesachim* 74b; *Chullin* 111a). Mixed wine vinegar and malt vinegar can impart a flavor to each other (*Abodah Zarah* 66a).

Wine can turn sour like vinegar (*Baba Batra* 96a; *Berachot* 5b; Terumot 3:1).

Vinegar is stored in skin bottles (*Baba Batra* 74b), jugs (*Niddah* 2b; *Machshirin* 3:2), casks (*Eruvin* 68a), and cans (*Taanit* 25a). Vinegar deters snakes (*Abodah Zarah* 30b). One may not anoint with wine or vinegar but only with oil (*Sheviit* 8:2). [*See also* OIL and WINE].

VIRGINITY—A virgin is defined as a woman who has never observed a vaginal blood flow (*Niddah* 8b). "A sealed garden" (Song of Songs 4:12) is said to refer to virginity (*Yoma* 75a). The blood of defloration is ritually clean (*Niddah* 11a) and the wound usually heals in four days (*Niddah* 64b). Tokens of virginity return if a girl below age three years has sexual intercourse (*Niddah* 45a). A woman may lose her virginity through an accident (*Ketubot* 36a) or be injured by a piece of wood or other trauma (*Yebamot* 59a; *Ketubot* 13a). Virginity is destroyed by rape or seduction (*Yebamot* 60a). Some women destroy their virginity with their fingers (*Yebamot* 34b). One woman claimed to have lost her virginity because of the high steps of the staircase in her parents' house (*Jerushalmi Ketubot* 1:25). Women in one family in Jerusalem walked with large steps and, as a result, lost their tokens of virginity. They were advised to wear decorative bracelets on their knees, connected by a chain, to force them to take smaller steps (*Shabbat* 63b).

If a husband alleges in court that his newly married wife is not a virgin (*Deuteronomy* 22:14) he may ask for dissolution of the marriage, make a monetary claim, or raise a capital charge (*Sanhedrin* 8b; *Ketubot* 2a, 16b, 36a, and 46a). The parents defend their daughter's honor by presenting proof of her virginity in the form of the bedsheet (Deuteronomy 15:17). If the man's charge is false, he is punished (ibid., 22:18). The rare possibility of a virgin becoming pregnant without losing her virginity (*Chagigah* 14b) is discussed in the Talmud. It may be that the intercourse was only *coitus inter labia* (*Niddah* 64b) or by inclination of the penis (*Ketubot* 6b). An ancient folk practice to verify a maiden's virginity consisted of sitting her on the opening of a wine barrel. If the aroma came through, she was not a virgin (*Ketubot* 10b; *Yebamot* 60b). Famine and starvation can also cause absence of bleeding during the first coitus. When a starved young couple was fed, the blood of defloration appeared (*Ketubot* 10b).

For a virgin, the normal period of engagement is twelve months; for a widow, four weeks (*Ketubot* 57a). A virgin is usually married on a Wednesday, a widow on a Thursday (*Ketubot* 2a). A virgin who marries is entitled to a larger marriage settlement (*ketubah*) than a widow who marries (*Baba Batra* 145a). A High Priest is allowed to marry only a virgin and not a widow or divorcee (Leviticus 21:13). [*See also* CHASTITY, DEFLORATION, and MARRIAGE]

VISION—Vision comes not from the eyes but from higher centers (Isaiah 6:10 and 43:8; *Tosafot, Abodah Zarah* 28b, s.v. *Shuraina*). Visual acuity decreases with advancing age. When Isaac became 123 years old, "his eyes were dim" (Genesis 21:1), a Divine blessing so that he did not have to see the misdeeds of his son Esau (*Genesis Rabbah* 65:10). Eli the priest at age 98 also had dimness of vision (1 Samuel 3:2) and eventually total blindness (ibid., 4:15). Jacob was 147 years old when his eyes became dim "so that he could not see" (Genesis 48:10). Achiya also lost vision in his old age (1 Kings 14:4). Moses was exceptional in that even at 120 years of age, "his eye was not dim" (Deuteronomy 34:7). Eyes that in youth can see at a distance cannot in old age see even near (*Leviticus Rabbah* 18:1).

Clouding of the cornea, or cataract (*dak*), produces diminution of visual acuity (*Bechorot* 6:2 and 38a). Bird droppings that fall into the eyes may produce white spots and loss of vision (*Tobit* 2:10). If the white spots can be dislodged, visual acuity can be restored (*Tobit* 6:2ff., 11:7ff., and 14:2). This occurrence may have represented a corneal erosion. Excessive walking

(*Ketubot* 111 a) or taking big strides (*Taanit* 10b) is said to destroy one-five-hundredth of one's vision (*Ketubot* 111a), which can be restored by religious observances (*Berachot* 43b). Coarse black bread, fresh date wine, and raw vegetables can also decrease one's visual acuity (*Pesachim* 42a–b). Alcohol consumption may alter visual acuity (Proverbs 23:33–35). Smoke is harmful to the eyes and to vision (Proverbs 10:26). Vision is a gift from God to every newborn (*Niddah* 31a). Eyesight is connected to the mental faculties (*Abodah Zarah* 28b). [*See also* BLINDNESS and EYES]

VISITING THE SICK—It is a holy duty (*mitzvah*) incumbent upon everyone to visit the sick. God visits the sick and we must emulate Him as Scriptures state: "Ye shall walk after the Lord your God" (Deuteronomy 12:5). Just as He visited the sick, so too we should visit the sick (*Sotah* 14a). God visited the patriarch Abraham after the latter's circumcision, as it is written: "And the Lord appeared unto him" (Genesis 18:1). God blesses bridegrooms, adorns brides, visits the sick, buries the dead, and recites the blessing for mourners (*Genesis Rabbah* 8:13). "Thou shalt show them the way they must walk" (Exodus 18: 20) is interpreted to refer to the duty of visiting the sick (*Baba Kamma* 100a; *Baba Metzia* 30b). Another example in the Bible of

visiting the sick is when the prophet Isaiah visited King Hezekiah when the latter was ill (Isaiah 38:1). The conversation between the two is vividly described in the Talmud (*Berachot* 10a) and concerns the fact that Hezekiah had never married and was admonished by Isaiah for not having fulfilled the commandment of procreation. The end of the story is a happy one in that Hezekiah did penitence, was cured of his illness, and lived another fifteen years.

Numerous instances of sages visiting their sick colleagues are found in the Talmud. Rabbi Yosei ben Kisma was ill and Rabbi Chaninah ben Teradion went to visit him (*Abodah Zarah* 18a). Rabbi Yannai ben Ishmael was sick and Rabbi Ishmael ben Zirud and others called to inquire about him (ibid., 30a). Comforting mourners, visiting the sick, and the practice of loving-kindness bring welfare into the world (*Avot de Rabbi Nathan* 30:1). Helping to care for the needs of a sick patient may save his life or contribute to the restoration of his health (*Nedarim* 40a).

Another purpose of visiting the sick is for the caller to pray in the patient's behalf (*Shabbat* 12a). When not in the patient's presence, one should pray only in Hebrew since the ministering angels understand only Hebrew. In the patient's presence, one may pray in any language since God Himself ministers to the sick (Psalms 41:4), and the Divine Presence (*shechinah*) rests upon the patient's bed (*Shabbat*

12b). For the same reason, one should not sit on the patient's bed.

There is no limit to the visiting of the sick (*Nedarim* 39b). He who visits the sick takes away one-sixtieth of his illness (ibid., *Leviticus Rabbah* 34:1). One should not be paid for visiting the sick (*Nedarim* 39a). One should not visit patients with illnesses of the bowel (diarrhea), eye diseases, or headaches—the first because of embarrassment and the latter two because speech is harmful to them (ibid., 41a).

Upon recovery from illness, one makes a thanksgiving feast (*Berachot* 46a) and recites the special prayer of thanksgiving (*birchat hagomel*) (*Berachot* 54b). Visiting-the-sick societies are described in the Talmud (*Moed Katan* 27b). Abimi, a member of such a society, used to visit the sick (*Genesis Rabbah* 13:16).

VOICE—The voice emanates from the lungs (*Leviticus Rabbah* 18:1) but the larynx brings it out (*Berachot* 61a). The voice of a eunuch is soft like that of a woman (*Yebamot* 80b) and that of a sterile woman is thick or deep

(ibid.). The voice of a rabid dog is not heard when it barks (*Yoma* 83b). Three things restore a person's good spirits: sounds, sights, and aromas (*Berachot* 57b). In three things people differ from each other: in voice, appearance, and mind (*Sanhedrin* 38a). When man calls to his friend, there is an echo to his voice (*Exodus Rabbah* 29:9). Spoken voices can have good or evil effects (*Leviticus Rabbah* 32:2). A woman's voice can evoke immoral thoughts; therefore, women are silent in the house of God (*Berachot* 24a). A woman's voice should be sweet (Song of Songs 2:14). If it is harsh, it is considered to be a blemish (*Ketubot* 75a).

The voice of the Lord is powerful and full of majesty (*Song of Songs Rabbah* 5:16:3). A heavenly voice, or *Bat Kol,* is described numerous times in the Midrash (*Genesis Rabbah* 35:3; *Exodus Rabbah* 28:6 and 41:7; *Leviticus Rabbah* 6:5; *Numbers Rabbah* 14:1; *Deuteronomy Rabbah* 11:10) and in the Talmud (*Berachot* 3a and 51b–52a; *Taanit* 24b, 25b and 29a; *Baba Metzia* 59b and 85a–86a; *Sanhedrin* 39b; *Horayot* 12a; *Chullin* 44a and 86a–87a). [*See also* SPEECH]

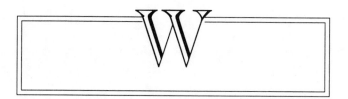

WALKING—Walking as a form of exercise has been practiced by the Jews for centuries. An average man was said to be able to walk ten parasangs (forty *mil*) in a day (*Pesachim* 93b; *Jerushalmi Berachot* 1:1). Walking on the Sabbath is not only permissible but desirable (*Tosefta Peah* 4:10; *Tosefta Shabbat* 16:17), although one should not take long strides when walking because long strides diminish one's eyesight (*Berachot* 43b). Walking was felt to be beneficial to other organ systems: After meals one should perform some exercise; if one eats without walking four cubits after it, the food rots in the intestines and is not digested (*Shabbat* 41a).

Not all scholars were in agreement. Rabbi Judah, perhaps prescient of the risks of exercise, opined that people and beasts die in their prime, or at least age prematurely, in a town built on hills and valleys (*Eruvin* 56a). [*See also* EXERCISE]

WARTS—If one has a wart on one's foot one can cut it away and live in comfort or leave it on and suffer discomfort (*Abodah Zarah* 10b). One removes both moist and dry warts with one's hand or with a knife (*Pesachim* 68b). A wart found on the hide of the paschal offering has legal ramifications (ibid., 88b). An animal with a wart cannot be sacrificed in the Temple (Leviticus 22:22), even if the wart is on the eye or eyelid (*Bechorot* 40b). A woman aborting red hairs was said to have a "wart" (mole?) in her uterus (*Niddah* 22b). A wart (mole?) was seen by a man on his sister's shoulder (*Lamentations Rabbah* 1:46). These may be eczematous or leprous lesions. [*See also* SKIN]

WASHING—Hands are ritually washed every morning upon arising (*Shabbat* 109a). One also washes the hands before and after meals (*Berachot* 43a, 46b, and 51b; *Sotah* 4b; *Chullin* 106a); before prayer and after using the privy (*Berachot* 15a); after bloodletting, a haircut, and nail cutting (*Pesachim* 112a); and after defecation (*Yoma* 3: 12). Soldiers are exempt from washing hands before meals (*Eruvin* 17a). The phrase "Sanctify yourselves" (Leviticus 11:44) refers to washing the hands before the meal, and "Be ye holy" (*ibid.*) refers to washing the hands after the meal (*Berachot* 53b).

One must wash one's face, hands, and feet daily in honor of the Lord (*Shabbat* 50b). On the Sabbath one washes face, hands, and feet, but not the whole body, with water heated on the eve of the Sabbath (*Shabbat* 40a). Travellers are offered water to wash their feet (Genesis 18:4, 19:2, and 24:32; Judges 19:21). After a journey, one washes hands and feet (2 Samuel 18:8; *Menachot* 85b). On retiring at night, one does the same (Song of Songs 5:3).

Medically, washing the hands after meals averts blindness from Sodomite salt (*Eruvin* 17b). Washing the body with mangold water is good for treating skin diseases (*Shabbat* 133b). Washing of the body and one's clothes is part of the ritual cleansing for people with flux (Leviticus 15:13). He who eats cress without first washing his hands will suffer fear for thirty days. He who lets blood without washing his hands will be afraid for seven days. He who trims his hair or pares his nails without washing his hands will be afraid for three days and one day, respectively (*Pesachim* 111b–112a). [See *also* BATHING and BATHHOUSE]

WATER SUPPLY—The world draws its water supply from the waters of the ocean (*Taanit* 9b), which are sweetened by rain water. The world is also watered by rivers and streams (ibid., 10a). In ancient times, water was obtained from wells (*Eruvin* 2:4). Disputes occurred over their use and ownership (Genesis 21:20 and 21:25). Other sources of water included cisterns located in courtyards of large houses (*Avot* 2:8; *Oholot* 11:8; *Baba Batra* 64a; 2 Samuel 17:19), with water channels passing through the courtyards (*Eruvin* 87a; *Chullin* 106a). Large ships carried tanks for sweet water (*Shabbat* 35a). Water reservoirs were repaired before the three pilgrimage festivals (*Shekalim* 1:1). Wells were dug to provide water for the pilgrims (ibid., 5:1; *Baba Kamma* 50a).

Jews in Palestine drank only water from cisterns. When they were exiled to Babylon, they drank water from the Euphrates river and many of them died (Midrash Psalms 137:3). Elisha cast salt into the water supply and "healed" it (2 Kings 2:21). Water fountains and flowing springs have good, cool water (*Abodah Zarah* 12a). Cold, hot, and wholesome water supplies are needed (*Shabbat* 146b). Waters between palm trees are not healthy (ibid., 110a). Cisterns were covered with stones to protect the water (Genesis 29:2). Cities had large public cisterns (*Eruvin* 2:4). Jerusalem's water supply consisted of the well called Gichon (Genesis 29:2), situated outside the city. King Hezekiah (790 B.C.E.) led its water through a canal to the Siloa pool and from there to the city. Another conduit to the Solomonic pools provided water to the southern part of the city. [*See also* DRINKING WATER and BEVERAGES]

WET NURSE—If a woman has twins, she suckles one and hires a wet nurse to suckle the other (*Jerushalmi Ketubot* 5:39). A wet nurse is ordinarily engaged for two years, during which time she may not accept other employment nor nurse another child (*Tosefta Niddah* 2:4), not even her own (*Ketubot* 60b). Heathen wet nurses were suspected of harming babies (*Abodah Zarah* 26a). Both single girls and married women served as wet nurses (ibid.). In the Bible, Deborah was the wet nurse of Rebecca (Genesis 35:8). A wet nurse is held responsible for keeping the baby in good condition (*Genesis Rabbah* 2:2). She must eat more than usual while nursing (*Ketubot* 60b). She must not eat foods that harm the milk or that cause it to decrease flowing (ibid.). [*See also* LACTATION]

WIGS—Women wear wigs made from their own hair, from another woman's hair, or from animal hair (*Shabbat* 64b). Wigs were made from the hair of old women, young women, or mixed (ibid.). Instead of a full wig, women might supplement their own hair with individual strands of hair—

either their own that fell out during combing, or those from another woman or animal. When not in use, wigs were hung on pegs (*Arachin* 7b; *Sanhedrin* 112a). To hold natural hair or a wig in place, women used "needles without perforations" (*Shabbat* 60a; *Jerushalmi Shabbat* 1:3). Women of all ages wore wigs to retain their beauty (*Moed Katan* 9b). Hairnets are also described (*Shabbat* 64b).

A woman is allowed to walk in a public domain on the Sabbath wearing a wig (*Shabbat* 64b). The natural hairs or wigs of women in a condemned city (Deuteronomy 13:13ff.) are forbidden (*Sanhedrin* 112a). A husband has veto power over his wife's Nazarite vow since she would need to shave her head at the end of the Nazariteship and wear a wig, to which the husband can object (*Nazir* 28b).

Wigs for men may also be alluded to in the Talmud where *pekorin* and *cipha* are mentioned (*Tosefta Shabbat* 5:2; *Shabbat* 50a), which Rabbenu Chananel interprets to be wigs that a "bald-headed person puts on his head and it looks as if he has real hair." [*See also* HAIR and BALDNESS]

WINDPIPE—The windpipe consists of cartilaginous rings (*chulyot*) connected by membranous bands (*bar chulya*) (*Chullin* 50a). It extends to the larynx (*pike shel gargeret*) (ibid., 134b). The thyroid cartilage (*kova*) sits on the cricoid cartilage (*tabaat hagedolah*), which ends posteriorly in two round (arytenoid) cartilages (*chitte*) (*Chullin* 18a–b). The cheek is defined as the area from the jaw joint to the prominence of the windpipe (*Chullin* 134b). Slaughtering of animals occurs through the cricoid cartilage or below in the tracheal rings (ibid.). The windpipe and gullet must both be severed during ritual slaughtering (*Chullin* 27a).

Wounds and injuries include the perforation of the windpipe with many holes like a sieve, absence of part of the windpipe, or a lengthwise slit (*Chullin* 45a). The insertion of a tube of reed into a lamb's trachea is one of the earliest descriptions of tracheotomy (ibid., 57b).

One should not eat while reclining because the food may go down the windpipe and endanger the person's life (*Pesachim* 108a). One should not converse during meals for the same reason (*Taanit* 5b). [*See also* LUNGS and VOICE]

WINE—Wine is the most esteemed of alcoholic beverages and is called "the red blood of grapes" (Genesis 49:11). Of the sixty varieties, *tilia* is the worst (*Gittin* 70a). Amoni wine is the most fiery and incites to lewdness (*Jerushalmi Sanhedrin* 10:28). Undiluted Middle Eastern wine was too strong to drink (*Berachot* 7:5). Wine was diluted with three parts of water (*Shabbat* 77a). The word "wine" refers to red wine (*Negaim* 1:2). Boiling improves wine and makes it durable (*Terumot* 11:1). In the desert for forty years, the Israelites drank no wine or date beer (Deuteronomy 29:5). The Rechabites were Jews who never drank wine (Jeremiah 35:6). Wine is permitted to Jews except for priests before and during Temple service (Leviticus 10:9), and for Nazarites (Numbers 6:3). Joseph drank no wine during the twenty-two years that he was separated from his brothers (*Shabbat* 139a). When they were reunited, they drank wine out of joy (Genesis 43:34). Otherwise, abstinence is not a Jewish concept. On the contrary, on every joyous occasion or Festival, wine is imbibed (Ecclesiastes 9:7; Psalms 104:15). Wine delights the soul (*Berachot* 35b).

Wine is nourishing as an accompaniment to bread (Joshua 9:4). Wheat and wine are foods for children (*Nedarim* 8:7). The world can, nevertheless, exist without wine but not without water (*Jerushalmi Horayot* 3:48). Wine is beneficial in small amounts but harmful in large amounts (*Avot de Rabbi Nathan* 37:5, *Gittin* 70a). One glass of wine is becoming to a woman, two are degrading, with three she solicits coitus, and if she has four she solicits even in the street (*Ketubot* 65a). One should drink wine only as part of the meal, otherwise it intoxicates (*Jerushalmi Pesachim* 10:37). Sleep in the morning and wine at midday drive a man from this world (*Avot* 3:10). The bones of people who drink wine are red (*Genesis Rabbah* 98:2). Certain spices are made with wine, honey, and pepper (*Abodah Zarah* 30a). After a bath one drinks a glass of wine (*Genesis Rabbah* 10:7) or a wine-containing beverage (*Shabbat* 140a). In talmudic times, children were bathed in wine for health and other reasons (*Tosefta Shabbat* 12:13).

Wine has a multitude of therapeutic medical uses. Aged wine is good for the intestines, whereas fresh wine is harmful (*Nedarim* 66b). Old wine decreases bowel movements, straightens the stature, and improves vision (*Pesachim* 42a–b). For dysentery, one should drink seventy-year-old apple wine (*Abodah Zarah* 40b) and rub the abdomen with oil and wine (*Shabbat* 134a). For abdominal pain, one should eat pepper kernels soaked in wine (*Gittin* 69b). Drinking wine prevents vomiting if one eats untasty fowl meat (*Shabbat* 145b). For splenic ailments, one should consume water worms (leeches) in wine (*Gittin* 69b). If one swallows poison, quickly drink a cup of strong wine (ibid.). For a heart (or stomach) ailment one should eat certain herbs in wine (*Abodah Zarah* 29a). For heart weakness, lentil flour in wine is recommended (*Eruvin* 29b).

If a fever lasts three days, give the patient red meat and diluted wine (*Gittin* 67b). To treat an abscess, drink a cup of wine in purple-red soapwort (ibid., 69b). Wine or vinegar is applied to traumatic wounds (*Shabbat* 109a). Rubbing painful loins (arthritis) with wine or oil is soothing (*Shabbat* 14:4). Wine-containing ointments can be applied to various skin lesions (*Gittin* 86a). Malodorous perspiration can be neutralized with wine vinegar (*Ketubot* 75a). After bloodletting, one should drink red wine to replenish the blood (*Shabbat* 129a).

Drinking wine as it drips directly from the barrel may lead to poor vision (*Pesachim* 111b). Drinking old wine strengthens vision (ibid., 42a). Eye collyria are sometimes made with wine (*Niddah* 19b). Bread soaked in wine is used for eye compresses (*Shabbat* 108b). Headaches lasting seven weeks can follow the drinking of four cups of wine (*Nedarim* 49b). Blowing into the foam of wine or beer is harmful to the head (*Chullin* 105b). Rubbing the head with wine or oil is soothing for patients with headache (*Tosefta Shabbat* 12:11). Olive oil, wine, and spices restore one's memory (*Horayot* 13b). A woman with heavy vaginal bleeding should drink lots of wine (*Shabbat* 109b–110a). The oral contraceptive potion known as the "cup of roots" is taken with wine (ibid.). [*See also* BEER and DRUNKENNESS]

WORMS—A Sadduccee priest died with worms extruding from his nose (*Yoma* 19b). Antiochus died from a painful abdominal illness with worms growing out of his abdomen (2 Maccabees 9:5ff.). Job complained about his flesh being clothed with worms (Job 7:5), which Preuss suggests were maggots, eczema, or simply poetic exaggeration.[1] Titus's final illness (*Gittin* 56b) may have been maggot infestation known as nasal myiasis.[2] God punished the Israelites who complained about the manna with intestinal worms called *dura* (*Numbers Rabbah* 7:4). Barley flour that is forty days old may be infested with worms (*Berachot* 36a). Hyssop and black dates serve as a remedy (*Shabbat* 109b). In addition to the barley flour worm, worms in cucumbers (*Chullin* 58a and 67b) and in beans left in the ground too long (*Sanhedrin* 65b) are also described. Worms that attack scrolls and silk (*Chullin* 28a and 85a) and infect grapes, figs, and pomegranates are all dangerous if accidentally ingested by human beings (*Shabbat* 90a). Eating worms is forbidden in Judaism (Leviticus 11:41). Worms from a dunghill applied to a wound accelerate healing (*Abodah Zarah* 28a).

One should not drink directly from a waterpipe lest one swallow leeches or other worms and develop abdominal swelling (*Abodah Zarah* 12b). For patients with intestinal worms, various remedies are recommended including a morning snack (*Baba Metzia* 107b), garlic (*Baba Kamma* 82a), macerated hedge mustard (*Gittin* 69b), and wine with laurel leaves (ibid.). A liver fluke (*arketa*) is described in the Talmud (*Shabbat* 109b). It develops in people who eat raw or fat meat or beef or certain cabbage seeds on an empty stomach and then drink water. Various folk remedies are recommended. A liver full of worms is not necessarily a life-threatening situation (*Tosefta Chullin* 3:10). Animals may also suffer from worms entering their nostrils and thence to the lungs or the alimentary tract (*Chullin* 67b). Worms found in the lung of an animal after ritual slaughtering can perforate the lung membrane either during life (*Chullin* 49a) or after death (*Chullin* 47b). Maggots can be found under the skin of animals (*Chullin* 67b). A fish was once seen with a parasite in its nostrils, which killed the fish (*Baba Batra* 73b).

Worm worship is forbidden (*Abodah Zarah* 42b). A man once dreamt that a silk-destroying worm fell into his hand (*Berachot* 56a). Mortal man becomes worm infested in the grave (*Avot* 3:1 and 4:4). Worms are as painful to the dead as a needle in the flesh of the living (*Berachot* 18b; *Shabbat* 13b). [*See also* SNAKES AND SERPENTS and INTESTINES]

---

1. F. Rosner (trans.), *Julius Preuss' Biblical and Talmudic Medicine* (Northvale, NJ: Jason Aronson, 1993), pp. 339–340.

2. F. Rosner, *Medicine in the Bible and the Talmud*, 2nd ed. (Hoboken, NJ: Ktav and Yeshiva University Press, 1995), pp. 740–78.

WOUNDS—Self-wounding (1 Kings 18:28) is biblically prohibited (Leviticus 21:5 and 19:28). Inflicting wounds on one's fellow man (Leviticus 24:19) or a pregnant woman (Exodus 21:22) is a punishable offense (*Shabbat* 106a). A child is forbidden to wound a parent (*Sanhedrin* 84b). Nevertheless, Abner pierced Asahel (2 Samuel 2:23) and Joab pierced Abner (ibid., 3:27). Spear wounds are often fatal (*Yebamot* 114b). Perforation of the aorta is a fatal wound (*Chullin* 45b). A hole in the trachea may not be fatal (*Chullin* 44a). Perforation or cutting of the esophagus is a life-threatening wound (*Chullin* 43a; *Yebamot* 120b). Heart wounds (*Chullin* 45b) are discussed. Severed sinews or arteries usually result in death (*Yebamot* 16:3), although cauterization of the wound may prevent death (ibid., 120b). Defloration is considered to be a wound (*Niddah* 10:1). He who feigns a wound will eventually suffer from one (*Tosefta Peah* 4:14).

Wounds can sprout and granulate (Isaiah 1:6) or be flabby and atonic (Jeremiah 14:17 and 15:18). The wound heals when flesh heaps up (ibid., 30:13) but does so differently in various people (*Baba Kamma* 84a) and more rapidly in children (*Shabbat* 134b). Scraped cynodon root brings on flesh (*Abodah Zarah* 28a). In biblical times, wounds were treated by pressing, bandaging, and oil fomenting (Isaiah 1:6). The balm of Gilead (wound balsam) was a famous wound-healing salve (Jeremiah 8:22; *Sanhedrin* 77b). Cotton or lint cloths and sponges, as well as garlic and onion peels, are bandaged and tied on the wound (*Tosefta Shabbat* 5:3–4). The sponge acts as a wound protector (*Leviticus Rabbah* 15:4). Rushes or reeds were also used and wrapped around an injured finger (*Eruvin* 103b). Flocks of wool were also applied to the wound (*Shabbat* 50a) with or without emollients or plasters (*Yebamot* 114b). The plasters were replaced when necessary (*Eruvin* 102b). Chewed wheat kernels (*Ketubot* 103a) and caraway (*Shabbat* 19:2) are also healing in their effect. Wounds are anointed with oil and hot water even on the Sabbath (*Shabbat* 128a) because they are considered dangerous if not promptly treated.

People also used manure from dung heaps as bandaging material (*Abodah Zarah* 28a). Cauterization of arterial cuts (*Tosefta Yebamot* 14:4), leprous lesions (*Negaim* 7:4), and compound bone fractures (*Tosefta Chullin* 3:6) was also practiced in talmudic times. Cress in vinegar was used as a hemostatic (*Abodah Zarah* 28a). Vinegar also heals wounds on the teeth or gums (*Shabbat* 111a). Medicine was applied to the thigh wound of Rabbi Abbahu (*Abodah Zarah* 28a). Rav Ashi sustained a wound when a donkey trod on his foot. He rubbed it with oil of roses (*Shabbat* 109a).

An animal with a wound from rubbing against a wall or from a heavy saddle is treated with honey (*Shabbat* 8:1; *Baba Metzia* 38b) or squashed snails (*Shabbat* 77b) applied to the wound. It is also given honey to eat (ibid., 154a). In humans, however, ingestion of honey and other sweets is harmful to wounds (*Baba Kamma* 85a). [*See also* INJURIES, BLEMISHES, DEFECTS, FRACTURES, and specific organs]

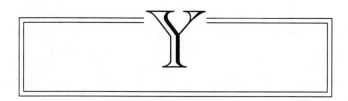

YAWNING—One yawns with the mouth (*Niddah* 9:8). Yawning during prayer recitation is arrogant (*Berachot* 24b). Signs of imminent menstruation include sneezing and yawning (*Niddah* 63a). [*See also* MOUTH]

YERAKON—The term *yerakon* is found six times in the Bible (Deuteronomy 28:22; 1 Kings 8:37; Jeremiah 30:6; Amos 4:9; Haggai 2:17; 3 Chronicles 6:28). With one exception (Jeremiah 30:6), this word always appears in association with the word *shidaphon,* and most English translations render these two words "blasting and mildew." Rashi and others consider *yerakon* to represent diseases that afflict grain in the field, the symptoms of which are that the surface of the grain becomes pale and ultimately turns yellowish green. Other Bible commentators, including Samson Raphael Hirsch, interpret *yerakon* either as jaundice or as chlorosis, illnesses afflicting human beings. The reference in Jeremiah seems to refer to chlorosis or jaundice and not mil-

dew. That the biblical *yerakon* refers to some type of epidemic is clear from talmudic discussions, such as the "alarm is sounded" (*Taanit* 19a) and "prayers are recited" (*Ketubot* 8b) on account of *shidaphon* and *yerakon.* The dual explanation of the word *yerakon* is provided by Bertinoro, when he states: "*Yerakon* is grain whose appearance became pale. And there are some who interpret *yerakon* to be an illness where the facial appearance of a person turns green like the grass of the field" (*Taanit* 3:5).

As no symptoms of this disease are described anywhere in the Bible or Talmud, we are dependent upon the derivation of the word *yerakon* for its proper understanding. There is little doubt that *yerakon is* derived from the word *yerek* or *yarok,* meaning "green." The word *yerek* itself is found many times in the Bible and always refers to a green herb or grass. Also in the Talmud the word *yarok* signifies "green" (*Sukkah* 34b; *Shabbat* 20b; and others). One commentary (*Tosafot Niddah* 19b) states that *yarok* is "yellow," but ordinarily *yarok* or *yerek* means "green." The biblical term *yerakrak* (Leviticus 13:49 and 14:37; Psalms 68:14) is considered to signify "dark green" by some commentators (e.g., Rashi) and "light green" by others (*Tosefta Negaim* 1:5). In the Midrash, dark green vegetables in a vegetable garden (*ginat yerek*) into which a spring flows are said to turn black (*Leviticus Rabbah* 15:3).

A bluish (venous) tinge to the green is implied in the case of a suspected adulteress whose "face turns green, whose eyes protrude, and whose veins stand out" (*Sotah* 3:4). In addition, *Tosafot* (*Chullin* 47b) specifically states that *yarok* is indigo or sky blue. A final interpretation of the word *yerek* or *yerakon* is pallor that may occur due to extreme fear (Jeremiah 30:6). In the Talmud, *yarok* also refers to pallor (as opposed to a healthy ruddy countenance), whether it is due to illness, as in the case of a suspected adulteress (*Numbers Rabbah* 9:21), or to hunger (*Ruth Rabbah* 3:6). If a man is frightened to death, his face may also become greenish, i.e., pale (*Ketubot* 103b; *Abodah Zarah* 20b). If a man is shamed in public, his face blanches (*Avot* 3:11) because the blood is drained from his face (*Baba Metzia* 58b).

Preuss offers the following thought to reconcile the two different interpretations of *yarok*, i.e., anemia (pallor) and jaundice.[1] He cites Rabbi Ishmael, who compares the skin color of Israelites (i.e., Semites) to boxwood (*Negaim* 2:1) and states that the skin color of Semites is in between the dark skin color of Ethiopians and the light skin color of Germanic people. Preuss proposes that pallor in Semitic people thus resembles jaundice.

The human malady of jaundice (*yerakon*) is said by the sages of the Talmud to result from Divine punishment for causeless hatred (*Shabbat* 33a). It is said to be produced by the withholding of urination (*Berachot* 62b; *Tamid* 27b; *Bechorot* 44b).

Numerous therapeutic regimens are recommended in the Talmud for jaundice. Urine from an ass, if imbibed, is good for jaundice (*Bechorot* 7b). According to Rabbi Matia ben Heresh, the flesh of a donkey should be eaten by someone suffering from jaundice (*Yoma* 84a). Water of palm trees and a potion of roots are said to be efficacious for jaundice (*Shabbat* 109b). Water of palm trees was thought to "pierce the gall" (ibid., 110a). A useful potion of roots is cited by Rabbi Yochanan (ibid., 110b). Other remedies are also discussed in the Talmud (ibid.).

The biblical term *yerakon* probably refers to an affliction of grains in the field as Divine retribution for sin. The single exception is the passage of Jeremiah (30:6) where *yerakon* represents a human affliction, either pallor or anemia (chlorosis) or jaundice. The talmudic reference to *yerakon* can, in the final analysis, refer either to jaundice or anemia (chlorosis). As *yerakon* is said to be due to causeless hatred, and hatred and anger were thought to be related to yellow bile or gall, it would seem logical to conclude that *yerakon* is, in fact, jaundice.

1. F. Rosner (trans.), *Julius Preuss' Biblical and Talmudic Medicine* (Northvale, NJ: Jason Aronson, 1993), pp. 164–167.

2. F. Rosner, "*Yerakon*," in *Medicine in the Bible and the Talmud*, 2nd ed. (Hoboken, NJ: Ktav and Yeshiva University Press, 1995), pp. 79–89.

INDEX

Acromegalics, 146
Adam, 107, 127, 140, 194, 214,
    282, 316
  and anesthesia, 18
  created as a hermaphrodite, 165
  rib of, 271
Adam and Eve, 132, 202
  and begetting demons, 96
  and procreation, 257
  sin of, 93
Adasha, 270
Adoni-Bezek, King, 16
Adonijah, 272
Adulteress
  suspected, 11, 154, 187, 221,
    238, 286
Adultery, 14–15, 29, 69, 82, 191,
    204
  suspected, 154, 187
Afsayim, 24
Afterbirth, 248–249
Ahab, 26, 259, 296
Ahasuerus, 106, 161, 175, 191,
    216, 220, 241, 281
Akiba, R., 155, 183, 308
Alcimus, 27, 238
Alcohol
  induced confusion of the mind,
    184
  side effects of, 107
Alfasi, 163, 276
Almonds, 15, 38
Aloes, 15
Alontit, 49
Alopecia areata, 155
Alum, 15–16
  crystals, 15–16
Amenorrhea, 185
Ammi, R., 16, 244, 265

Amnion, 16
Amniotic sac, 16
Amnon, 196, 268
Amos, 290
Amputation
  of arm, 28
  of feet, 189
  of hand, 159
  surgical, 16–17
  of toes, 189
Amputee, 16–17, 28, 189, 258
Amram, 194
Amulets, 17–18, 115, 138, 181
  as remedies, 197, 254
Analgesia, 17
Androginos, 277
Anemia, 55, 107, 279, 330–331
Anesthesia, 17–19
  and alcohol, 19
Angels, 96
  of death, 102, 143, 250
Animal
  antidote for bites from, 304
  births, 21–22
  blemishes, 23–24
  breech delivery of, 131
  cesarean births of, 131
  characteristics of, 20
  copulation, 20
  defects, 23–24
  delivered by cesarean section, 72
  and depilation of, 99
  experimentation, 19–20
  eye disease in, 244
  hybridization of heterogeneous, 21
  internal examination of
    slaughtered, 23
  knee of, 183
  kosher, 23, 278

Flies, 124, 137, 266, 278

Flogging, 137–138
  judicial, 138
  methodology of administering,
    137

Flour, 26, 138
  barley, 138
  paste, 138

Flux. *See* gonorrhea

Foods
  consumption of forbidden, 261–
    262, 299–300
  digestion of, 293

Fontanel, 160

Foot, 189–190
  stools, 190
  washing, 312

Forehead, 139

Fornication, 72

Frankincense, 19, 173, 240, 286–287

Friedenwald, H., 7

Fright, 140

Fruit, 140–141
  juices, 141

Funeral, 81

Furunculosis, 249

Galactorrhea, 186

Galen, 2, 190

Gall, 49–50, 94, 194
  diseases of the, 143
  stones, 143
  of white stork, 269, 275

Gallbladder, 50, 143–144, 271,
    273, 275

Gamiliel, R., 98

Gamliel, R., 155, 223, 294, 303

Gamzu, Nachum, 17, 53, 58

Gangrene, 189, 298

Gargling, 144

Garlic, 26, 144–145, 175, 188, 273,
    283–284, 290, 315, 326, 327

Garon, 305

Gaza, R., 74

Geese, 145

Genitalia, 238
  abnormalities of external, 51
  female, 145–146

Gersham ben Judah, R., 252

Gibeah, 166

Gideon, 120

Gigantism, 146

Ginger, 98, 146, 213

Gintzburger, Wolff, 2–3

Glanders, 266

Gnats, 137, 269

Goats, 146–147, 187
  kidney juice of, 269

God the Healer, 242

Golden Calf, 67, 91, 107, 170

Goliath, 146, 160, 174, 213

Gonorrhea, 84, 147–148, 176, 274,
    290, 292, 311–312

Gordon, M. B., 5

Gourds, 148, 252, 270, 315

Gout, 149, 189, 242

Grapes, 98, 140, 149–150
  medicinal uses, 150

Grasshoppers, 150

Grave, 150–151
  pain in the, 237
  robbers, 151

Graven images, 127

Gullet, 100

Gums, 151, 271, 317

Hackberries, 199

Hadrian, 219, 307–308

Hillel, 155, 189, 281
Hip
  dislocation of, 2, 101
Hippocrates, 190, 256, 297
Hirsch, R. Samson Raphael, 18,
    199, 329
Hisda, R., 56
Histline, 6
Hoarseness, 165
Homosexuality, 69, 165–166, 174
Honey, 38, 40, 47, 65, 125, 138,
    169, 176, 269
  attributes of, 166
  comb, 166–167
  date, 92
  and healing, 167
  from Ziphim, 167
Hormin, 97
Hornets, 47, 276, 293
Horseflies, 21
Horseradish, 315
Horses, 167–168
Hosea, 71, 258
Hospitals, 168
Howard, R. B., 5
Humerus, 278
Huna, R., 45, 97, 191
Hunchback, 168–169, 243, 245,
    291
Hunger, 127–128, 169
  effects of, 169
Hydrakon, 107
Hydrophobia, 267
Hydrops, 100, 107, 251
Hymen, 96
Hypertrichosis, 153
Hypoproteinemia, 107
Hypospadias, 202, 239, 258, 293,
    311

Hyssop, 70, 169–170, 326
  medicinal uses, 169–170
Hysterectomy, 313
Hysteria, 18, 170

Ibn Ezra, 109, 198, 249, 278
Idolatry, 67, 69, 191
Idulatrous customs, 17, 95, 312
Igrat, 97
Illem, 92
Illness, 171–172
  causes of, 171
  exacerbaters of, 171
Imbeciles, 208–209
Impotence, 273, 293
Impurity, 261–262, 269, 281, 290,
    304
Incantation, 117, 172–173, 180,
    254, 275, 307
  for boils, 13
  for epilepsy, 115–116
  against the evil eye, 133, 197
  permissibility of, 172
Incense, 173
  use with corpses, 85
  offered to demons, 96
  for the temple, 38–39
Incest, 29, 69, 173–174, 191,
    203
Indigestion, 112
Infertility, 77–78, 92, 198
  and assisted reproduction, 258,
    298–299
  female, 77–78, 208
  male, 77–78
Inflammation, 174
  corneal, 124
  internal, 48, 199
Insanity, 209

Nose, 63, 191, 223–224
  bleeds, 96, 224
  defects of, 224
  rings, 224
Nutrition, 112
Nuts, 140, 224–225
  gallnut, 225

Obesity, 227
Offerings, 138, 187, 193, 248,
    316
  heave, 274
Og, king of Bashan, 146
Oil, 227–229
  anointing, 228, 230, 291
  embrocations, 229–231
  fragrant, 229
  sources of, 228
  spikenard
  uses for, 227–228
Ointments, 250–251
Old Age, 231, 301
Olives, 52, 232, 274
  oil of, 99, 144, 227, 230, 232,
    280
  wood, 232
Onah, 202
Onanism, 82, 204, 232–233
Onions, 145, 188, 233, 273, 327
  roots, 252
Ophthalmologist, 233–234
Orchiectomy, 69
Organ Transplants, 234
Orpah, 183
Outhouses, 306
Ovarian transplant, 299
Overeating, 234–235
Oxen, 235

Pain, 237
  abdominal, 11, 220, 239, 270
  in animal experimentation, 19–
    20
  bone, 237
  of childbirth, 75–76, 194
  ear, 39, 244, 275
  of edema, 74
  in the eyes, 245
  heart, 88, 237
  in loins, 194
  stomach, 40
  and venesection, 56
Palate, 237
Palga, 96
Pallor, 237–238
Papi, R., 183
Papus, 308
Paralysis, 238
Paraskos, J. A., 6
Paschal lamb, 59, 187, 321
Passover, 7, 40, 62, 83, 99, 143,
    215, 224, 229
  and beets, 48
  bitter herbs for, 315
  Seder, 27, 167, 191
Peaches, 140
Pearlman, Moshe, 4
Peas, 238
Pekiat *ayin*, 124
Penis, 238, 311
  plastic surgery on, 244
Pennyroyal, 175
Pentecost, 62
Pepper, 215, 239
Peppercorn, 271
Peppers, 213
Pepperwort, 26

Worms, 325–326
  eating of, 326
  infestation of, 316
  infestation of in animals, 20–21
  intestinal, 91, 129, 175, 326
  liver, 194
  worship of, 326
Wounds, 52, 326–328
Wunderbar, R. J., 2–3, 7

Yabelet, 122
Yad, 158
Yafet, 278
Yannai ben Ishmael, R., 319
Yarchinai, 33
Yawning, 63, 285, 329
Yerakon, 329–331
Yibbum, 203
Yisrael, Tiferet, 181, 184
Yitzchaki, R. Shlomo *See* Rashi
Yochanan, R., 26, 58, 120, 143,
  169, 172, 183, 184, 243, 244,
  265, 276, 330
Yochanan of Godgada, R., 92
Yochanan ben Zakkai, R., 128–129,
  288

Yom Kippur, 94, 128, 133, 148,
  166, 169, 281, 286, 306
  bathing on, 43
Yonathan, R., 199
Yosei ben Kisma, R., 319
Yotzeh dophen, 71–72

Zabalgan, 124
Zacutus, Abraham, 247
Zaddok, R., 132
Zadok, R., 114
Zagdan, 122
Zahalon, Jacob, 247
Zara'at, 3, 6
Zavir, 122
Zedekiah, King, 53, 86
Zera, R., 265
Zeroa, 28
Zifoni, 282
Zilgah, 256
Zimmels, 173, 181
Zimri, 14, 294
Zipporah, 79, 205
Zonah, 258
Zophar, 143
Zythom, 273

ABOUT THE AUTHOR

Dr. Fred Rosner is Director of the Department of Medicine of the Mount Sinai Services at the Queens Hospital Center and Professor of Medicine at New York's Mount Sinai School of Medicine. Dr. Rosner is an internationally known authority on medical ethics and has lectured widely on Jewish medical ethics. He is the author of six widely acclaimed books on Jewish medical ethics, including *Modern Medicine and Jewish Ethics, Medicine and Jewish Law, Medical Encyclopedia of Moses Maimonides,* and *Pioneers in Jewish Medical Ethics.* These books are up-to-date examinations of the Jewish view on many important bioethical issues in medical practice. Dr. Rosner is also a noted Maimonidean scholar and has translated and published in English most of Maimonides' medical writings.